Springer Series on Evidence-Based Crime Policy

Series Editors
Lawrence W. Sherman
University of Cambridge
Cambridge, UK

Heather Strang
University of Cambridge
Cambridge, UK

Crime prevention and criminal justice policies are domains of great and growing importance around the world. Despite the rigorous research done in this field, policy decisions are often based more on ideology or speculation than on science. One reason for this may be a lack of comprehensive presentations of the key research affecting policy deliberations. While scientific studies of crime prevention and criminal policy have become more numerous in recent years, they remain widely scattered across many different journals and countries. The *Springer Series on Evidence-Based Crime Policy* aims to pull this evidence together while presenting new research results. This combination in each book should provide, between two covers (or in electronic searches), the best evidence on each topic of crime policy.

The series will publish primary research on crime policies and criminal justice practices, raising critical questions or providing guidance to policy change. The series will try to make it easier for research findings to become key components in decisions about crime and justice policy. The editors welcome proposals for both monographs and edited volumes. There will be a special emphasis on studies using rigorous methods (especially field experiments) to assess crime prevention interventions in areas such as policing, corrections, juvenile justice and crime prevention.

More information about this series at http://www.springer.com/series/8396

David Weisburd • David P. Farrington
Charlotte Gill
Editors

What Works in Crime Prevention and Rehabilitation

Lessons from Systematic Reviews

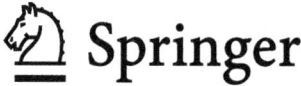

Editors
David Weisburd
George Mason University
Fairfax, Virginia
Hebrew University
Jerusalem, Israel

Charlotte Gill
Department of Criminology, Law & Society
George Mason University
Fairfax
Virginia
USA

David P. Farrington
Institute of Criminology
University of Cambridge
Cambridge
United Kingdom

ISSN 2197-5809	ISSN 2197-5817 (electronic)
Springer Series on Evidence-Based Crime Policy
ISBN 978-1-4939-3475-1	ISBN 978-1-4939-3477-5 (eBook)
DOI 10.1007/978-1-4939-3477-5

Library of Congress Control Number: 2015960898

Springer New York Heidelberg Dordrecht London
© Springer Science+Business Media New York 2016
This work is subject to copyright. All rights are reserved by the Publisher, whether the whole or part of the material is concerned, specifically the rights of translation, reprinting, reuse of illustrations, recitation, broadcasting, reproduction on microfilms or in any other physical way, and transmission or information storage and retrieval, electronic adaptation, computer software, or by similar or dissimilar methodology now known or hereafter developed.
The use of general descriptive names, registered names, trademarks, service marks, etc. in this publication does not imply, even in the absence of a specific statement, that such names are exempt from the relevant protective laws and regulations and therefore free for general use.
The publisher, the authors and the editors are safe to assume that the advice and information in this book are believed to be true and accurate at the date of publication. Neither the publisher nor the authors or the editors give a warranty, express or implied, with respect to the material contained herein or for any errors or omissions that may have been made.

Printed on acid-free paper

Springer Science+Business Media LLC New York is part of Springer Science+Business Media (www.springer.com)

Preface

This volume grew out of a symposium organized in Jerusalem and funded primarily by the Academic Study Group (ASG) of the UK. The ASG brings together UK scholars and Israeli scholars to advance scientific endeavors in a variety of fields. David Farrington was originally approached by the ASG, and he then contacted David Weisburd about the possibility of organizing a meeting focused around what we know about what works in preventing crime. After a series of discussions with John Levy of the ASG, the topic of "what we have learned from systematic reviews" was finalized. Because we wanted to bring together a broader range of scholars, we also solicited and received support from the Center for Evidence-Based Crime Policy at George Mason University, the Jerry Lee Centre of Experimental Criminology at Cambridge University, and the Faculty of Law at the Hebrew University. The Hebrew University also supported the symposium itself, which was held at its Faculty of Law in April 2012. We are very grateful to John Levy for his support of our meeting and his patience in our development of this volume.

The main aim of the symposium was to review what has been learned about the effectiveness of criminological interventions from systematic reviews. Such reviews, pioneered in medicine by the Cochrane Collaboration and in social sciences by the Campbell Collaboration, are relatively recent. Unlike the more traditional narrative reviews, they have explicit objectives, give full details about all sources searched and all searches conducted, try to obtain all potentially relevant evaluation reports (whether published or not), have explicit criteria for including or excluding studies, and focus on studies with the highest methodological quality. There has been no previous effort to summarize what has been learned from systematic reviews in criminology. We were pleased at the outset that Katherine Chabalko, the criminology editor at Springer, was as excited as we were about the possible products of our meeting and offered us early on a contract to publish this work with Springer. Katie was supportive throughout, and we very much appreciate her work on this volume as well as that of Hana Nagdimov, Springer's editorial assistant.

The symposium was extremely useful in allowing all participants to hear and comment on all papers. This was valuable in encouraging uniformity in the style of each paper and in avoiding repetition. It was decided that all chapters should include a systematic search and should include a forest graph of odds ratios from all included systematic reviews. It was also decided that chapters should conclude by addressing the following questions: What works? What is promising? What seems to have no effect? What is harmful? What is uncertain? What is missing?

The conference participants included seven from the UK, five from the USA, and twelve from Israel (supplemented by others from Hebrew University who sat in on sessions). We think that the symposium and subsequently this volume have led to an important contribution to advancing the knowledge base about what works in crime prevention and rehabilitation. Indeed, as readers will see, it provides a remarkable contrast to the negative assumptions regarding these interventions that were prevalent just three decades ago. We also think that this effort has helped to advance cooperation between UK and Israeli scientists, which is a major goal of the ASG, which was the primary funder of our efforts.

Finally, we are extremely grateful to Alese Wooditch, graduate research assistant in the Center for Evidence-Based Crime Policy at George Mason University, who provided substantial analytic and editorial assistance during the preparation of this volume.

George Mason University, Virginia, USA Hebrew University, Jerusalem, Israel	David Weisburd
Cambridge University, UK	David P. Farrington
George Mason University, Virginia, USA	Charlotte Gill

Contents

1. Introduction: What Works in Crime Prevention? 1
   David Weisburd, David P. Farrington and Charlotte Gill

2. Developmental and Social Prevention 15
   David P. Farrington, Maria M. Ttofi and Friedrich A. Lösel

3. Community Interventions 77
   Charlotte Gill

4. Situational Prevention 111
   Kate J. Bowers and Shane D. Johnson

5. Policing 137
   Cody W. Telep and David Weisburd

6. Sentencing and Deterrence 169
   Amanda E. Perry

7. Correctional Programs 193
   David B. Wilson

8. Drug Interventions 219
   Katy R. Holloway and Trevor H. Bennett

9. Qualitative Data in Systematic Reviews 237
   Mimi Ajzenstadt

10. Evidence Mapping to Advance Justice Practice 261
    Michael S. Caudy, Faye S. Taxman, Liansheng Tang and Carolyn Watson

11 Economic Analyses 291
Jacqueline Mallender and Rory Tierney

12 Conclusion: What Works in Crime Prevention Revisited 311
David Weisburd, David P. Farrington and Charlotte Gill

Index 327

About the Editors

David Weisburd is Distinguished Professor of criminology, law and society at George Mason University and executive director of the Center for Evidence-Based Crime Policy. He is also the Walter E. Meyer Professor of Law and Criminal Justice at the Hebrew University in Jerusalem and chief science adviser at the Police Foundation in Washington DC. He is the 2010 recipient of the Stockholm Prize in Criminology and received the Sutherland Award for contributions to criminology from the American Society of Criminology in 2014. In 2014, he also received the Robert Boruch Award for distinctive contributions to research that influences public policy of the Campbell Collaboration.

David P. Farrington is emeritus professor of psychological criminology in the Institute of Criminology, Cambridge University. He received the Stockholm Prize in Criminology in 2013. He is chair of the American Society of Criminology Division of Developmental and Life-Course Criminology. His major research interest is in developmental criminology, and he is director of the Cambridge Study in Delinquent Development, a prospective longitudinal survey of over 400 London males aged from 8 to 56. In addition to over 650 published journal articles and book chapters on criminological and psychological topics, he has published nearly 100 books, monographs, and government reports.

Charlotte Gill is assistant professor of criminology, law and society and deputy director of the Center for Evidence-Based Crime Policy at George Mason University. Her research interests include community-based crime prevention, community policing, place-based criminology, program evaluation, and research synthesis. She has been involved in randomized controlled trials of restorative justice and low-intensity probation and is the coeditor and former managing editor of the Campbell Collaboration Crime and Justice Group. In 2012, she received the Academy of Experimental Criminology's Outstanding Young Scholar award.

Contributors

Mimi Ajzenstadt Hebrew University of Jerusalem, Jerusalem, Israel

Trevor H. Bennett University of South Wales, Pontypridd, UK

Kate J. Bowers Department of Security and Crime Science, University College London, London, UK

Michael S. Caudy The University of Texas at San Antonio, San Antonio, TX, USA

David P. Farrington University of Cambridge, Cambridge, UK

Charlotte Gill George Mason University, Fairfax, VA, USA

Katy R. Holloway University of South Wales, Pontypridd, UK

Shane D. Johnson Department of Security and Crime Science, University College London, London, UK

Friedrich A. Lösel University of Cambridge, Cambridge, UK and University of Erlangen-Nuremberg, Germany

Jacqueline Mallender Optimity Advisors, London, UK

Amanda E. Perry Department of Health Sciences, University of York, Heslington, UK

Liansheng Tang George Mason University, Fairfax, VA, USA

Faye S. Taxman George Mason University, Fairfax, VA, USA

Cody W. Telep Arizona State University, Phoenix, AZ, USA

Rory Tierney Optimity Advisors, London, UK

Maria M. Ttofi University of Cambridge, Cambridge, UK

Carolyn Watson George Mason University, Fairfax, VA, USA

David Weisburd George Mason University, Fairfax, VA, USA
Hebrew University of Jerusalem, Jerusalem, Israel

David B. Wilson George Mason University, Fairfax, VA, USA

Chapter 1
Introduction: What Works in Crime Prevention?

David Weisburd, David P. Farrington and Charlotte Gill

In 1974 Robert Martinson published an article in *The Public Interest* that was to shatter the assumptions of correctional rehabilitation scholars (Martinson 1974). Martinson, who had just completed a review of evidence of the effectiveness of correctional intervention programs with his colleagues Douglas Lipton and Judith Wilks, laid out in simple terms what he viewed as the overall conclusions of this work. The title of the article was composed of a question: "What works? Questions and answers about prison reform." But his answer was clear from the narrative he presented. Although he never actually stated that "nothing works," there could not be much doubt that this was the overarching conclusion of the review.

"Nothing works" was to become the predominant narrative in crime control in corrections, as well as in other areas of criminal justice, such as policing and community supervision (e.g., Bayley, 1994; Cullen & Gendreau, 2001; Sechrest, White, & Brown, 1979; Weisburd & Braga, 2006). Indeed, by the 1990s most criminologists had all but abandoned the idea that programmatic interventions could influence recidivism. The idea that crime prevention or crime control could be effective had literally become a radical idea. Instead most criminologists turned their attentions to broader social and structural impacts on crime (Cullen &

Portions of this chapter are based on Farrington, Weisburd, and Gill (2011).

D. Weisburd (✉)
George Mason University, Fairfax, VA, USA
e-mail: dweisbur@gmu.edu

Hebrew University of Jerusalem, Jerusalem, Israel
e-mail: david.weisburd@mail.huji.ac.il

D. P. Farrington
University of Cambridge, Cambridge, UK
e-mail: dpf1@cam.ac.uk

C. Gill
George Mason University, Fairfax, VA, USA
e-mail: cgill9@gmu.edu

Gendreau, 2001). To argue that specific crime prevention programs could reduce recidivism or deter crime no longer fit within the lexicon of what was known about crime and its control.

Over the past three decades, much has changed. Many pioneering criminologists were unwilling to accept the then accepted wisdom that rehabilitation programs in prison did not affect recidivism, or as David Bayley argued simply in the early 1990s that "(t)he police do not prevent crime" (Bayley, 1994, p. 3). The 1990s was to be a decade of tremendous vitality and innovation in crime prevention and rehabilitation. And it was to produce a host of studies that showed that many strategies *do* work. Many scholars in this period argued that it was time for criminologists and crime prevention scholars to abandon the "nothing works" idea. After reporting on the positive crime prevention outcomes of the Minneapolis Hot Spots Experiment, Sherman and Weisburd (1995, p. 647) argued that "it is time for criminologists to stop saying that 'there is no evidence' that police patrol can affect crime." Frank Cullen (2005), reviewing research in rehabilitation in his 2004 Presidential Address to the American Society of Criminology, noted that "in the space of three decades ... scholars have contributed mightily to transforming the discourse on rehabilitation from the 'nothing works doctrine' to inquiries about 'what works' and 'best practices.'"

Although it is no longer an innovation to argue that many interventions and programs in the criminal justice system work, we know of no collection of essays that review broadly what has been learned about crime prevention and rehabilitation over the past few decades. That is our purpose in this volume, which grew out of a meeting in Jerusalem sponsored by the Academic Study Group, the Jerry Lee Centre of Experimental Criminology at Cambridge University, the Hebrew University, and the Center for Evidence-Based Crime Policy at George Mason University. The meeting was developed to bring together evidence about "what works" in developmental and social prevention, communities, situational crime prevention, policing, corrections, sentencing, and drug prevention. Importantly, it began with a specific approach to answering this question that draws from the methodology used in Martinson's original efforts. Martinson's original work was based on one of the first "systematic reviews" of research evidence in criminology. A systematic review differs from a traditional narrative review in that it has clear and established rules and procedures for identifying the studies that are summarized (e.g., Cooper, 1998; Cooper & Hedges, 2009; Petrosino, Boruch, Soydan, Duggan, & Sanchez-Meca, 2001). Since Martinson's work, methods of systematic review have become more rigorous and have been enhanced by statistical methods that summarize the effect sizes of studies (i.e., meta-analysis). We decided at the outset to capitalize on systematic reviews of research in each of the seven domains listed above, which in turn draw on the results of scores of research studies.

This approach allows us to provide a highly rigorous assessment of what is known about crime prevention and rehabilitation. This is the first comprehensive review of systematic reviews across areas in crime prevention and rehabilitation of which we are aware. As we argue in our conclusions, our findings reinforce strongly the idea that criminal justice programs and interventions can rehabilitate offenders and prevent crime. Not everything works, but overall the portrait of crime prevention and rehabilitation that our work provides is extraordinarily optimistic.

In this introductory chapter, we begin by asking why Martinson's paper had such strong influence on crime prevention and the criminological community. We then turn to a discussion of systematic reviews and how they improve our ability to summarize what works in preventing crime and rehabilitating offenders. After describing systematic reviews, we introduce the work of the Campbell Crime and Justice Group, whose efforts have played a key role in advancing systematic review in the crime and justice arena. Campbell reviews, as we note, are the predominant source for systematic reviews of evidence in our volume. Finally, we briefly describe the focus of each of the chapters in our book.

Martinson and Nothing Works

One question that seems reasonable four decades after Martinson wrote his influential 1974 article is why did it have so much impact on criminologists? It seems unlikely that one article summarizing a specific area of rehabilitation should have such influence on the "tone" of crime prevention and rehabilitation scholarship more generally. One reason for the influence of Martinson's work was that it "debunked" what criminologists and crime prevention specialists seemed to assume at the time—that rehabilitation programs were effective. Debunking conventional knowledge is a very attractive position for scholars. And Martinson developed his paper using a method of presentation focused directly on challenging common assumptions.

Martinson crafted his paper using a rhetorical style that first stated what we had assumed about correctional rehabilitation programs. For example,

> "Isn't it true that a correctional facility running a truly rehabilitative program—one that prepares inmates for a life on the outside through education and vocational training—will turn out more successful individuals than will a prison which merely leaves its inmates to rot?"
> "But when we speak of a rehabilitative prison, aren't we referring to more than education and skill development alone? Isn't what's needed some way of counseling inmates, or helping them with deeper problems that have caused their maladjustment?"
> "All of this seems to suggest that there's not much we know how to do to rehabilitate an offender when he's in an institution. Doesn't this lead to the clear possibility that the way to rehabilitate offenders is to deal with them outside an institutional setting?"

His answer to each of these questions was that we have little evidence that supports such programs, which led him to ask rhetorically:

> Do all of these studies lead us irrevocably to the conclusion that nothing works, that we haven't the faintest clue about how to rehabilitate offenders and reduce recidivism?

While Martinson never actually asserted that "nothing works," his paper led inevitably to that conclusion and set off a storm of controversy and criticism regarding rehabilitation and prevention programs.

A further reason for the paper's influence was the systematic nature of the report by Lipton, Martinson, and Wilks (1975) on which it is based. That report was one of the first truly systematic reviews of evidence in criminology, examining not only the study results but also the nature of the methods used and the specific components of the interventions examined. The report is persuasive, even reading it four decades later. But the influence of Martinson's work was not simply a function of the quality of the report on which it is based. It was also fueled by the reaction of the agency that sponsored it, the New York State Governor's Special Committee on Criminal Offenders. Upon receiving the final report in 1972, they refused to publish it, which led to the report gaining a powerful underground reputation. When it was finally published in 1974 after a court case on prison conditions led to its release, it quickly became one of the most cited publications on crime.

Moreover, Martinson's conclusions were to be reinforced by a National Academy of Sciences panel on correctional interventions in 1979 (Sechrest, White, & Brown, 1979). Importantly, similar conclusions were being developed in other fields, though sometimes the basis of the evidence was cumulative across studies rather than drawn from a single review (Weisburd & Braga, 2006). Evaluations of key police prevention approaches such as generalized preventive patrol and rapid response to citizen calls for service suggested that these programs did little to reduce crime (Kelling, Pate, Dieckman, & Brown, 1974; Spelman & Brown, 1984). Indeed, by the 1990s, David Bayley (1994, p. 3) could argue with confidence (as noted earlier) that:

> The police do not prevent crime. This is one of the best-kept secrets of modern life. Experts know it, the police know it, but the public does not know it. Yet the police pretend that they are society's best defense against crime ... This is a myth.

Although the assumption that nothing works was to gain wide acceptance among criminologists, scholars began almost from the outset to question the broad scope of conclusions that Martinson and others had reached. Palmer (1975), for example, argued that Martinson had overlooked many positive findings in his review in order to come to a strong general statement about the ineffectiveness of crime correctional programs (see Lipton, Martinson, & Wilks, 1975). Sherman and Weisburd (1995) take a similar view of the "nothing works philosophy" in policing, noting that despite studies such as the Kansas City Preventive Patrol Experiment, the 1970s produced examples, albeit isolated, of successful policing initiatives.

It was clear that many crime prevention and rehabilitation efforts did not work. But the conclusion that *nothing* worked was in some ways as naive as the assumptions prevalent before the 1970s, a period in which an unjustified exuberance in crime prevention efforts was common (Visher & Weisburd, 1998). Lipsey (1992) suggests that the debate over the effectiveness of treatment programs was fueled in part by the nature of the distribution of research results. Using the example of juvenile interventions, he illustrates a wide diversity of program effects. Added together, they result in a finding of no difference. But taken study by study, they show that there are programs that have large and significant impacts and others that do not. Similarly, Farrington, Ohlin, and Wilson (1986), while acknowledging the many negative research findings, conclude from a review of randomized experiments that they "do not show that 'nothing works'" (p. 9).

Martinson (1976) himself seemed to have drawn a different conclusion regarding the ability of society to do something about crime in a response to a critique of his 1974 article. He did not conclude that criminologists and policymakers should throw up their hands and close shop. Rather, he argued that we had to pull up our shirtsleeves and get to work to develop smarter crime prevention policies. Martinson wrote:

> The aim of future research will be to create the knowledge needed to reduce crime. It must combine the analytical skills of the economist, the jurisprudence of the lawyer, the sociology of the life span, and the analysis of systems. Traditional evaluation will play a modest but declining role. (1976, p. 181)

Martinson certainly was correct in his expectation that economists would begin to play a more important role in criminology and crime policy (e.g. Bushway, 1998, 2004; Cook, 1980, 1986; Levitt, 1996, 2004). It is also the case that criminologists have taken advantage of basic theory and systems research to understand crime across the life course (Piquero, Farrington, & Blumstein, 2003; Sampson & Laub, 1992). However, Martinson (1976) did not recognize that traditional evaluation, as he defined it, could become a key part of this new knowledge base that would inform crime policy. Martinson (1976) essentially dismissed the potential of focused evaluation research to provide important knowledge about crime control. Our book provides the most comprehensive review of what evaluation evidence tells us about the prevention of crime and rehabilitation of offenders. To do that, we focus on systematic reviews of research evidence.

Summarizing Research Evidence

In 1978, Carol Weiss, one of the early leaders in program evaluation, wrote that evidence should be synthesized to make it more useful to policymakers, rather than expecting them to rely on individual (and potentially conflicting) studies (Weiss 1978). But synthesizing evidence is not only important for policymakers, it is also key to scholars who must reach conclusions regarding what research tells us about prevention and rehabilitation. Deciding what works to reduce crime and delinquency requires us to examine the results of previous evaluation studies whenever they are available. This is better than drawing conclusions about what works from our personal experience, anecdotal evidence, widespread beliefs, or a single study that was well funded or heavily publicized.

Beginning in the 1970s, the traditional methods used in reviews of research evidence began to be seriously criticized (see Petrosino et al., 2001 for a review). One criticism focused on the general lack of explicitness of reviews: Most suffered from a lack of detail about how the reviewer conducted the research. Information was often missing about why certain studies were included while others were excluded from the review. Sometimes this lack of detail was caused by space limitations imposed on reviewers by journal or book editors; however, reports of reviews often did not describe what literature searches were carried out in order to locate relevant evaluation studies. It was often difficult for the serious reader to determine how the reviewers came to their conclusions about what works. Too often, the reader was forced to accept and trust the reviewer's expertise and was not given sufficient information to permit replication of the reviewer's methods. A second criticism focused on the methods used. Most of the reviewers did not attempt to control for problems that could potentially bias their review toward one conclusion rather than another. At its worst, a reviewer advocating a particular conclusion could selectively include only studies favoring that viewpoint in the review. For example, a reviewer in favor of strict gun control laws could ignore evaluations that found little effect of such laws. Such intentional distortion was fortunately rare in academic reviews.

More common than intentional distortion was the failure to deal with potential biases that could compromise the results of a review. For example, some reviewers examining what works relied on easy-to-obtain journal articles as the only source of reports of evaluations. An advantage of journal articles over other documents is that they have usually passed a rigorous peer review process. Unfortunately, research in other fields suggests that relying on journal articles can bias the results toward concluding that interventions are more effective than they really are. This is because researchers in many fields are more likely to submit their papers to journals when they find a positive effect of an intervention and are more likely to bury the manuscript in their file drawer when they do not. Both authors and journal editors are biased against papers reporting no effect, sometimes falsely assuming that such papers do not contribute to knowledge. This is called publication bias (see Rothstein & Hopewell, 2009; Rothstein, Sutton, & Borenstein, 2005).

A third criticism is that inexplicit and unsystematic review methods cannot cope with the incredible increase in research worldwide. For example, the number of journals that now publish materials relevant to crime and justice is enormous compared to that just a few years ago. Relying on journals available in a library or on papers collected in office files will no longer ensure coverage of all available studies. The Internet now makes hundreds—if not thousands—of evaluation reports readily accessible to prospective reviewers. In the same way that it would be difficult to make sense of a large, growing, and scattered collection of police reports or prison files without orderly methods, it is also difficult to make sense of the burgeoning and scattered number of relevant evaluation studies without some systematic method for doing so.

Systematic Reviews

What are systematic reviews? These are reviews that use rigorous methods for locating, appraising, and synthesizing evidence from previous evaluation studies (see Farrington & Petrosino, 2000; Farrington, Weisburd, & Gill, 2011; Littell,

Corcoran, & Pillai, 2008). They contain methods and results sections, and are reported with the same level of detail that characterizes high-quality reports of original research. Other features of systematic reviews include:

1. *Explicit objectives.* The rationale for conducting the review is made clear.
2. *Explicit eligibility criteria.* The reviewers specify in detail why they included certain studies and rejected others. What was the minimum level of methodological quality for inclusion in the review? Did they consider only a particular type of evaluation design such as randomized experiments? Did the studies have to include a certain type of participant, such as children or adults? What types of interventions were included? What kinds of outcome data had to be reported in the studies? All criteria or rules used in selecting eligible studies are explicitly stated in the final report.
3. *The search for studies is designed to reduce potential bias.* There are many potential ways in which bias can compromise the results of a review. The reviewers must explicitly state how they conducted their search of potential studies to reduce such bias. How did they try to locate studies reported outside scientific journals? How did they try to locate studies in foreign languages? All bibliographic databases that were searched should be made explicit so that potential gaps in coverage can be identified (and reviews can be replicated).
4. *Each study is screened according to the eligibility criteria, with exclusions justified.* The searches always locate many citations and abstracts to potentially relevant studies. Each of the reports of these potentially relevant studies must be screened to determine whether it meets the eligibility criteria for the review. A full listing of all excluded studies and the justifications for exclusion should be made available to readers.
5. *Assembly of the most complete data possible.* The systematic reviewer will generally try to obtain all relevant evaluations meeting the eligibility criteria. In addition, all data relevant to the objectives of the review should be carefully extracted from each eligible report and coded and computerized. Sometimes, original study documents lack important information. When possible, the systematic reviewer will attempt to obtain this from the authors of the original report.
6. *Quantitative techniques are used, when appropriate and possible, for analyzing results.* Although there is still some confusion about the meaning of these terms, it is useful to distinguish between a systematic review and a meta-analysis. A meta-analysis involves the statistical or quantitative analysis of the results of previous research studies (see Borenstein, Hedges, Higgins, & Rothstein, 2009; Lipsey & Wilson, 2001). Because it involves the statistical summary of effect sizes and their correlates, it requires a reasonable number of intervention studies that are sufficiently similar to be grouped together. For example, there may be little point in reporting a weighted mean effect size based on a very small number of studies. Nevertheless, quantitative methods can be very important in helping the reviewer determine the average effect size of a particular intervention and under what circumstances it works best.

A systematic review may or may not include a meta-analysis. For example, a reviewer may only find a few studies meeting the eligibility criteria. Although a meta-analysis can in theory be conducted with just two studies, in practice those studies may, for example, differ just enough in the operational definition of the intervention or in the way they were conducted to make formal meta-analysis inappropriate and potentially misleading. It is important not to combine apples and oranges for calculating a weighted mean effect size. Chapters 4 and 5 of this volume include examples of systematic reviews in which meta-analysis was not performed due to a small number of studies and heterogeneity across evaluations.

Qualitative reviews are relatively new in the arena of systematic review, but can provide important information on factors that are ordinarily not easily examined in quantitative systematic reviews. For example, the mechanisms underlying what works have become a key focus of many crime prevention researchers (Laycock & Tilley, 1995). Qualitative studies are particularly well placed to examine such concerns. In Chap. 9 of this volume, Mimi Ajzenstadt discusses the use of qualitative systematic reviews in criminology and also provides examples.

7. *Structured and detailed report.* The final report of a systematic review is structured and detailed so that the reader can understand each phase of the research, the decisions that were made, and the conclusions that were reached. In principle, it should be possible for an independent scholar to replicate both the review and the results.

Campbell Systematic Reviews in Crime and Justice

An important model for the development of systematic reviews has come from the Cochrane Collaboration, which seeks to prepare, maintain, and make accessible systematic reviews of research on the effects of health-care interventions (see http://www.cochrane.org). The Cochrane Library, with more than 1200 completed and maintained reviews on a variety of treatments, is now widely recognized as the single best source of evidence on the effectiveness of health-care and medical treatments, and it has played an important role in the advancement of evidence-based medicine.

In 1999, the founder of the Cochrane Collaboration, Sir Iain Chalmers, made an effort with University of Pennsylvania Professor Robert Boruch to create a similar infrastructure for reviews on what works in areas such as education, social welfare, and criminology (see Petrosino, Boruch, Farrington, Sherman, & Weisburd, 2003a). This resulted in the establishment of the Campbell Collaboration, named after the influential methodologist, psychologist, and evaluation theorist Donald T. Campbell (1917–1996). At a meeting in Philadelphia attended by over 80 persons from 12 different countries, the Campbell Collaboration was inaugurated in February 2000 to prepare, maintain, and make accessible systematic reviews of research on the effects of social, educational, and criminological interventions. At that February 2000 meeting, the Campbell Collaboration established a Crime and Justice Group (C2CJG) and Steering Committee to coordinate the work of this Group (see Farrington & Petrosino, 2001; Petrosino, Farrington, & Sherman, 2003b).

The mission of the C2CJG is to prepare and disseminate systematic reviews of high-quality research on methods to reduce crime and delinquency and improve the quality of justice. Campbell systematic reviews undergo a rigorous editorial process at three stages—the title proposal, protocol (plan for conducting the review), and the final review itself to ensure that the search is comprehensive, the methods are accurate, and the inclusion/exclusion criteria and conclusions are free from bias. Where possible, Campbell reviews also strive to be international in scope (see Farrington et al., 2011; The Campbell Collaboration, 2015).

In the past 15 years since it was founded, the C2CJG has made considerable progress in completing and disseminating systematic reviews. As of June 2015, 38 reviews have been published (some of which have been updated to account for emerging new evidence) and a further 36 reviews are in progress. The topics of the completed reviews range from policing tactics to mentoring at-risk juveniles to corporate crime prevention. Campbell reviews have been downloaded tens of thousands of times, featured at researcher and practitioner conferences around the world, and used in government debates and policymaking (e.g. Woodhouse, 2010).

Reviewing Systematic Reviews

In developing this volume, we did not restrict the authors only to Campbell systematic reviews—we simply asked our authors to analyze systematic reviews in a particular area. However, the Campbell Collaboration remains the most important resource for systematic reviews of what works in crime and justice. Moreover, Campbell reviews provided a baseline for quality that could be used in assessing whether systematic reviews should be included in a comprehensive examination of the research evidence in a field. In the chapters that follow, we review the evidence base from systematic reviews in key areas of crime prevention and rehabilitation across the life course and at each stage of the criminal justice process. We ask: What has been studied? Which programs are most effective? Which programs or interventions appear not to work? How rigorous are research designs in that area? What areas still need to be studied, and how can methods of systematic review be advanced to extend existing knowledge?

In Chap. 2, David Farrington, Maria Ttofi, and Friedrich Lösel examine the evidence base for developmental and social prevention programs on offending outcomes. Developmental and social programs are interventions that are provided in the community to children and adolescents up to age 18. They are designed to alter individual, family, and school risk factors in order to prevent antisocial behavior. Chapter 2 assesses the research on general prevention programs and those aimed at individual children, families, and school students, including early-childhood home visitation, bullying prevention, and interventions for youth with certain conduct disorders.

Chapter 3 focuses on community interventions, broadly defined as civic engagement in crime prevention, supportive interventions for at-risk youth such as mentoring, and community correctional and reentry programs for adjudicated offenders. In this chapter, Charlotte Gill discusses the limited evidence base for community interventions and the challenge of defining "community" and its role in crime prevention, and describes the mechanisms of community prevention most likely to impact crime.

In Chap. 4, Kate Bowers and Shane Johnson discuss what works in situational crime prevention—interventions that seek to prevent crime by reducing opportunities and/or increasing the effort and risk to offenders. In addition to identifying effective situational approaches, Bowers and Johnson assess the contextual factors, such as the time and place of implementation or the type of crime targeted, that explain the variability in effectiveness of these types of approaches.

Cody Telep and David Weisburd examine the effectiveness of policing strategies in Chap. 5. They highlight a substantial growth in the number of systematic reviews in policing over the past decade and assess whether the findings of these reviews counter the "nothing works" claims made about policing as recently as the early 1990s. The review of the evidence concludes with a discussion of the methodological shortcomings the authors identify in many of the primary studies and recommendations for improving future policing research.

In Chap. 6, Amanda Perry reviews the research on deterrence-based sentencing strategies. In the context of increasing prison and jail populations in a number of countries, it has become increasingly important to assess the relative effectiveness of different sentencing practices, the impact of deterrence-based strategies versus individualized treatment, and the choice of custodial versus non-custodial sentences. However, despite a number of systematic reviews and primary studies in this area, there are questions about whether the findings are generalizable to non-US contexts.

In Chap. 7, David B. Wilson assesses what works in correctional programs designed to rehabilitate offenders. In addition to highlighting the most effective rehabilitation programs, this chapter discusses the types of risk factors and focuses on areas that are generally addressed by correctional programming, and the need for further research on which of these factors are most important for successful rehabilitation.

Katy Holloway and Trevor Bennett review what works in drug treatment and prevention interventions in Chap. 8. The impact of drug treatment programs on criminal behavior has not been studied to the same extent as the effect of these programs on more immediate behaviors such as drug use, but there is a growing body of evidence involving crime outcomes. The authors offer directions for future research, including whether drug interventions play a role in crime reduction beyond individual behavior change.

Chapters 9–11 provide insights into how the current use of systematic reviews can be extended to better answer questions about what works. Qualitative research is usually excluded from systematic reviews, which tend to focus highly on assessments of internal validity and quantitative synthesis of findings. In Chap. 9, Mimi Ajzenstadt attempts to bridge the gap between quantitative and qualitative reviews by highlighting the important roles qualitative research can play in understanding the mechanisms of effective programs and generating knowledge for future evaluations.

In Chap. 10, Michael Caudy, Faye Taxman, Lienshang Tang, and Carolyn Watson provide an overview of the Evidence Mapping to Advance Justice Practice project, which focuses on assessing the quality of systematic reviews and meta-analysis. The authors highlight a number of challenges in primary evaluation research and systematic reviews alike, and make recommendations for improving the quality of future research synthesis.

Jacqueline Mallender and Rory Tierney discuss the importance of including economic analyses in systematic reviews in Chap. 11. While an important goal of systematic review is to distill a large amount of information into a manageable summary for policymakers and practitioners, very few reviews or primary studies include the cost–benefit data crucial to policy decision-making. Chapter 11 provides examples of the use of economic analysis in systematic reviews and offers a methodology for combining high-quality research evidence with jurisdiction-specific economic models.

In Chap. 12, we conclude with an overview of what has been learned about the effectiveness of crime prevention and criminal justice interventions based on our review of systematic reviews. As we noted at the outset, we find much evidence for optimism. The "nothing works" conclusion is certainly not consistent with the vast array of studies that show that intervention and prevention programs are effective. Not all programs work, but many do and this provides a basis for guiding crime policies. This concluding chapter also summarizes the additional lessons and areas for improvement highlighted by this exercise, including improving the utility of systematic reviews to policymakers, extending the scope and quality of both primary evaluation research and meta-analytic models, and the need for continuous innovation and improvement in both research and practice.

References

Bayley, D. (1994). *Police for the future*. New York: Oxford University Press.
Borenstein, M., Hedges, L. V., Higgins, J. P. T., & Rothstein, H. R. (2009). *Introduction to meta-analysis*. Chichester: Wiley.
Bushway, S. (1998). The impact of an arrest on the job stability of young white American men. *Journal of Research in Crime and Delinquency, 35*(4), 454–479.
Bushway, S. (2004). Labor market effects of permitting employer access to criminal history records. *Journal of Contemporary Criminal Justice, 20,* 276–291.
Cook, P. J. (1980). Research in criminal deterrence: Laying the groundwork for the second decade. In N. Morris & M. Tonry (Eds.), *Crime and justice: An annual review of research* (Vol. 2, pp. 211–268). Chicago: University of Chicago Press.
Cook, P. J. (1986). The demand and supply of criminal opportunities. In M. Tonry & N. Morris (Eds.), *Crime and justice: An annual review of research* (Vol. 7, pp. 1–28). Chicago: University of Chicago Press.
Cooper, H. (1998). *Synthesizing research* (3rd ed.). Thousand Oaks: Sage.
Cooper, H., & Hedges, L. V. (2009). Research synthesis as a scientific process. In H. Cooper, L. V. Hedges, & J. C. Valentine (Eds.), *The handbook of research synthesis and meta-analysis* (2nd ed., pp. 3–16). New York: Russell Sage Foundation.

Cullen, F. T. (2005). The twelve people who saved rehabilitation: How the science of criminology made a difference—The American Society of Criminology 2004 presidential address. *Criminology, 43*(1), 1–42.

Cullen, F. T., & Gendreau, P. (2001). From nothing works to what works: Changing professional ideology in the 21st century. *The Prison Journal, 81*(3), 313–338.

Farrington, D. P., & Petrosino, A. (2000). Systematic reviews of criminological interventions: The Campbell Collaboration Crime and Justice Group. *International Annals of Criminology, 38*(1/2), 49–66.

Farrington, D. P., & Petrosino, A. (2001). The Campbell Collaboration Crime and Justice Group. *Annals of the American Academy of Political and Social Science, 578*, 35–49.

Farrington, D. P., Ohlin, L. E., & Wilson, J. Q. (1986). *Understanding and controlling crime: Toward a new research strategy*. New York: Springer.

Farrington, D. P., Weisburd, D. L., & Gill, C. E. (2011). The Campbell Collaboration Crime and Justice Group: A decade of progress. In C. J. Smith, S. X. Zhang, & R. Barberet (Eds.), *Routledge handbook of international criminology* (pp. 53–63). Oxford: Routledge.

Kelling, G. L., Pate, A. M., Dieckman, D., & Brown, C. (1974). *The Kansas City preventive patrol experiment: Technical report*. Washington, DC: The Police Foundation.

Laycock, G., & Tilley, N. (1995). Implementing crime prevention. In M. Tonry & D. P. Farrington (Eds.), *Building a safer society: Strategic approaches to crime prevention* (pp. 535–584). Crime and justice, Vol. 19. Chicago: University of Chicago Press.

Levitt, S. D. (1996). The effect of prison population size on crime rates: Evidence from prison overcrowding litigation. *The Quarterly Journal of Economics, 111*(2), 319–351.

Levitt, S. D. (2004). Understanding why crime fell in the 1990s: Four factors that explain the decline and six that do not. *Journal of Economic Perspectives, 18*(1), 163–190.

Lipsey, M. W. (1992). Juvenile delinquency treatment: A meta-analytic inquiry into the variability of effects. In T. D. Cook, H. Cooper, D. S. Cordray, H. Hartmann, L. V. Hedges, R. J. Light, T. A. Louis, & F. Mosteller (Eds.), *Meta-analysis for explanation*. New York: Russell Sage Foundation.

Lipsey, M. W., & Wilson, D. B. (2001). *Practical meta-analysis*. Thousand Oaks: Sage.

Lipton, D. S., Martinson, R., & Wilks, J. (1975). *The effectiveness of correctional treatment*. New York: Praeger.

Littell, J. H., Corcoran, J., & Pillai, V. (2008). *Systematic reviews and meta-analysis*. Oxford: Oxford University Press.

Martinson, R. (1974). What works? Questions and answers about prison reform. *The Public Interest, 35*, 22–54.

Martinson, R. (1976). California research at the crossroads. In R. Martinson, T. Palmer, & S. Adams (Eds.), *Rehabilitation, recidivism, and research*. Hackensack: National Council on Crime and Delinquency.

Palmer, T. (1975). Martinson revisited. *Journal of Research in Crime and Delinquency, 12*(2), 133–152.

Petrosino, A., Boruch, R. F., Soydan, H., Duggan, L., & Sanchez-Meca, J. (2001). Meeting the challenges of evidence-based policy: The Campbell Collaboration. *Annals of the American Academy of Political and Social Science, 578*, 15–34.

Petrosino, A., Boruch, R. F., Farrington, D. P., Sherman, L. W., & Weisburd, D. (2003a). Toward evidence-based criminology and criminal justice: Systematic reviews, the Campbell Collaboration, and the Crime and Justice Group. *International Journal of Comparative Criminology, 3*, 42–61.

Petrosino, A., Farrington, D. P., & Sherman, L. W. (2003b). The Campbell Collaboration Crime and Justice Group: Early development and progress. *Journal of Offender Rehabilitation, 38*(1), 5–18.

Piquero, A. R., Farrington, D. P., & Blumstein, A. (2003). The criminal career paradigm. In M. Tonry (Ed.), *Crime and justice, a review of research* (Vol. 30, pp. 359–506). Chicago: University of Chicago Press.

Rothstein, H. R., & Hopewell, S. (2009). Grey literature. In H. Cooper, L. V. Hedges, & J. C. Valentine (Eds.), *The handbook of research synthesis and meta-analysis* (2nd ed., pp. 103–126). New York: Russell Sage Foundation.

Rothstein, H. R., Sutton, A. J., & Borenstein, M. (Eds.). (2005). *Publication bias in meta-analysis: Prevention, assessment, and adjustments.* Chichester: Wiley.

Sampson, R. J., & Laub, J. H. (1992). Crime and deviance in the life-course. *Annual Review of Sociology, 18,* 63–84.

Sechrest, L., White, S. O., & Brown, E. D. (1979). *The rehabilitation of criminal offenders: Problems and prospects.* Washington, DC: National Academy of Sciences.

Sherman, L. W., & Weisburd, D. (1995). General deterrent effects of police patrol in crime "hot spots": A randomized, controlled trial. *Justice Quarterly, 12*(4), 625–648.

Spelman, W., & Brown, D. K. (1984). *Calling the police: Citizen reporting of serious crime.* Washington, DC: U.S. Government Printing Office.

The Campbell Collaboration. (2015). *Campbell systematic reviews: Policies and guidelines.* Campbell systematic reviews: Supplement 1. http://www.campbellcollaboration.org/artman2/uploads/1/C2_Policies_and_Guidelines_Doc_Version_1_1–3.pdf.

Visher, C. A., & Weisburd, D. (1998). Identifying what works: Recent trends in crime prevention strategies. *Crime, Law and Social Change, 28*(3–4), 223–242.

Weisburd, D., & Braga, A. A. (Eds.). (2006). *Police innovation: Contrasting perspectives.* New York: Cambridge University Press.

Weiss, C. H. (1978). Improving the linkage between social research and public policy. In L. E. Lynn (Ed.), *Knowledge and policy: The uncertain connection.* Washington, DC: National Academy of Sciences.

Woodhouse, J. (2010). *CCTV and its effectiveness in tackling crime.* London: Library of the House of Commons. http://www.parliament.uk/briefing-papers/SN05624.pdf.

Chapter 2
Developmental and Social Prevention

David P. Farrington, Maria M. Ttofi and Friedrich A. Lösel

The main aim of this chapter is to assess systematic reviews of the effects of developmental and social prevention programs (hereafter shortened to developmental prevention programs) on offending outcomes. These programs are defined as community-based programs designed to prevent antisocial behavior, targeted on children and adolescents up to age 18, and aiming to change individual, family, or school risk factors. These programs can be distinguished from situational or physical prevention programs and from criminal justice prevention based on deterrence, rehabilitation, or incapacitation.

Over the past few decades, numerous developmental prevention programs have been implemented in families, kindergartens, schools, family education centers, child guidance clinics, and other contexts to reduce risk factors and strengthen protective factors in child development. *Universal* prevention programs target the whole population, or an age cohort, a neighborhood or a school, irrespective of who is at risk or not. *Selective* prevention includes programs that address specific risk groups such as single parent, lower-class families, or minority families in deprived neighborhoods. *Indicated* prevention programs address families whose children already reveal behavior problems. As with primary, secondary, and tertiary prevention, the categories partially overlap. For example, some "prevention" programs contain treatment for high-risk children and—as in public health care—universal prevention also serves some children or families who are at risk. In principle,

---

D. P. Farrington (✉)
University of Cambridge, Cambridge, UK
e-mail: dpf1@cam.ac.uk

M. M. Ttofi
University of Cambridge, Cambridge, UK
e-mail: mt394@cam.ac.uk

F. A. Lösel
University of Cambridge, Cambridge, UK
e-mail: fal23@cam.ac.uk

universal prevention approaches are more easily implemented because they do not require risk assessment and selection and avoid potential problems of stigmatization. However, for financial reasons, universal programs must be less intensive and thus may not sufficiently meet the needs of high-risk groups.

Many programs focus on individual children or youth by providing training in social competencies, interpersonal problem solving, and other behavioral or cognitive skills. Other programs concentrate on the family by providing training in parenting skills, counseling on child rearing, or coping with family stress. School-oriented programs address issues of school and class climate, the origins of bullying, and authoritative teacher behavior. However, an increasing number of programs are multimodal and contain program components for children, parents, schools, and other social contexts such as peers or neighborhood (e.g. Hawkins, Brown, Oesterle, Arthur, Abbott, & Catalano, 2008; Henggeler, Schoenwald, Borduin, Rowland, & Cunningham, 2009). Developmental prevention programs also vary in numerous other characteristics (see, e.g. Farrington & Welsh, 2007; Lösel & Bender, 2012):

- Breadth of targets, e.g. general promotion of child development, focus on social behavior, or prevention of specific behavior problems such as violence;
- Children's age at intervention, e.g. pregnancy/postnatal, early or late childhood, and adolescence;
- Degree of program structure, e.g. unstructured counseling, semi-structured guidance, or detailed manuals for training in skills;
- Recruitment of participants, e.g. proactive contact with at-risk families, general offers to schools and families, and mandatory intervention for juveniles or families at risk;
- Format of delivery, e.g. individual counseling, group teaching, mixed approaches;
- Intensity and dosage, e.g. a handful of sessions, regular contact over a few months, long-lasting implementation over several years;
- Theoretical foundation, e.g. based on social learning, attachment theory, psychodynamic concepts, or an eclectic integration of different approaches; and
- Evaluation, e.g. no systematic evaluation at all, some methodologically weak process and/or outcome data, controlled evaluation studies, randomized controlled trials, and multiple replications.

Because of these and other issues the field of developmental prevention is extremely varied, and it is difficult to draw consistent conclusions across all areas. Therefore, we had to restrict our inclusion criteria and we excluded reports that may have some criminological relevance (e.g. on child externalizing behavior), but were not directly addressing a criminological topic.

The inclusion criteria for our review were as follows:

1. The report describes a systematic review and/or a meta-analysis. A systematic review has explicit inclusion/exclusion criteria and explicit information about searches that were carried out. A meta-analysis specifies effect sizes and reports a summary effect size. Systematic reviews that yielded no includable studies—so-called "empty" reviews (e.g. the Campbell Collaboration reviews by Fisher, Montgomery, & Gardner, 2008a, b)—were excluded.

2. The report summarizes individual, family, or school programs targeted on children and adolescents up to age 18 and implemented in the community. We classified programs that targeted individual risk factors in schools as school-based programs. In the interests of including more reviews, this criterion was relaxed to include high-quality reviews targeting adolescents aged between 10 and 21 (Wilson & Lipsey, 2000; Wilson, Lipsey, & Soydan, 2003a). Clinic and institutional programs are excluded, but again the criterion was relaxed to include high-quality reviews including a minority of clinic or institutional programs (Sukhodolsky, Kassinove, & Gorman, 2004; Wilson et al., 2003a). Mentoring programs are excluded because they are included in Chap. 3.
3. The report summarizes effects on outcomes of delinquency, offending, violence, aggression, or bullying. Originally we included antisocial behavior, conduct disorder (CD), and conduct problems, but the number of reviews on these topics was too many to include. (Many reviews on these topics are listed in Table 2.1 as excluded reports.) In the interests of including more reviews, we included high-quality reviews that primarily focused on one or more of our outcomes but also included studies of other (disruptive or antisocial behavior) outcomes (Mytton, DiGuiseppi, Gough, Taylor, & Logan, 2002; Park-Higgerson, Perumean-Chaney, Bartolucci, Grimley, & Singh, 2008; Wilson & Lipsey, 2000, 2007). We excluded reports focusing on substance abuse because these are included in Chap. 8.
4. We excluded earlier reviews that were superseded by later reviews (by the same authors), reviews not published in English, and reviews that did not report outcomes separately (e.g. for juveniles vs. adults, or for offending vs. antisocial behavior). We also excluded reviews of juvenile correctional treatment (see e.g. Garrett, 1985; Lipsey, 2009; Walker, McGovern, Poey, & Otis, 2008); reviews of adult correctional treatment are included in Chap. 7.

We searched Google Scholar and PsycINFO up to the end of 2012 using the following keywords: systematic review/meta-analysis, prevention, and delinquen*/offend*/violen*/aggress*/bully*.

Table 2.2 summarizes key features of included reviews, while Table 2.3 summarizes key results of included reviews. Table 2.1 summarizes some reviews that were screened and obtained but excluded, together with reasons for their exclusion. The most common reason was that they did not provide specific information about one of our outcomes of interest. Table 2.4 summarizes weighted mean effect sizes in each review, and their associated confidence intervals (CI). The aim was to convert each effect size into an odds ratio (OR), with OR values greater than 1, indicating an effective program. Where there were two or more effect sizes, a summary effect size was calculated by inversely weighting each effect size by its variance. This is based on the assumption of independence of effect sizes, which may not be true. To the extent that effect sizes are not independent, CI would be wider.

Since 2012, there have been additional systematic reviews of developmental prevention programs. For example, Evans, Fraser, & Cotter (2014) published a review of antibullying programs, and Leen, Sorbring, Mawer, Holdsworth, Helsing, & Bowen (2013) published a review of interventions for adolescent dating violence.

Table 2.1 Excluded reviews

Researchers (Date)	Intervention	Reason for exclusion
Babcock, Green, & Robie (2004)	Cognitive-behavioral therapy for domestic violence	Studies of adults
Baldry and Farrington (2007)	Antibullying programs in schools	Earlier version of Farrington and Ttofi (2009)
Barlow and Parsons (2009)	Parent training	Outcome measures were child problem behaviors
Barlow, Parsons, & Stewart-Brown (2005)	Parent training	Summarizes Barlow and Parsons (2009)
Beelmann, Pfingsten, & Lösel (1994)	Social competence training (SCT)	Outcome measures were social adjustment, social-cognitive skills, social interaction skills, etc.
Bennett and Gibbons (2000)	Cognitive-behavioral interventions	Outcome measures were antisocial behaviors
Brestan and Eyberg (1998)	Psychosocial treatment for conduct disorder	No relevant outcome measures
Cooper, Charlton, Valentine, & Muhlenbruck (2000)	Summer school prevention programs	No program with the stated goal of preventing juvenile delinquency was found. Programs focused on remedial or accelerated learning outcomes or on a positive impact on the knowledge and skills of participants
De Graaf, Speetjens, Smit, De Wolff, & Tavecchio (2008)	Triple P parent training program	Outcome measures were child problem behaviors
DiGiuseppe and Tafrate (2003)	Anger treatment	Studies of adults
Dretzke, Davenport, Frew, Barlow, Stewart-Brown, Bayliss, Taylor, Sandercock, & Hyde (2009)	Parenting programs for conduct disorder	No relevant outcome measures
Durlak, Fuhrman, & Lampman (1991)	Cognitive-behavior therapy	No relevant outcome measures
Durlak, Weissberg, & Pachan (2010)	After-school programs	Outcome measures were child problem behaviors (and other measures such as school performance)
Durlak, Weissberg, Dymnicki, Taylor, & Schellinger (2011)	Social and emotional learning (SEL) programs	Outcomes included improved social and emotional skills, attitude, behavior, and academic performance only

Table 2.1 (continued)

Researchers (Date)	Intervention	Reason for exclusion
Eyberg, Nelson, & Boggs (2008)	Psychosocial treatment for child disruptive behavior	No relevant outcome measures
Fabiano, Pelham, Coles, Gnagy, Chronis-Tuscano, & O'Connor (2009)	Behavioral treatments	Effectiveness of behavior modification for children with attention deficit hyperactivity disorder (ADHD). Mostly clinic studies
Faggiano, Federica Vigna-Taglianti, Burkhart, Bohrn, Cuomo, Gregori, Panella, Scatigna, Siliquini, Varona, van der Kreeft, Vassara, Wiborg, & Galanti, & the EU-Dap Study Group (2010)	School-based prevention of drug use	Outcome measures included drug use and drug knowledge but not offending
Farahmand, Grant, Polo, & Duffy (2011)	School-based mental health and behavioral programs	The meta-analysis did not target any of the desired outcomes
Fisher, Montgomery & Gardner (2008a)	Cognitive-behavioral for gang involvement	No evaluations found
Fisher, Montgomery & Gardner (2008b)	Opportunities provision for gang involvement	No evaluations found
Forness and Kavale (1996)	Social skills training for learning disability	No relevant outcome measures
Furlong, McGilloway, Bywater, Hutchings, Smith, & Donnelly (2012)	Cognitive-behavioral parenting programs	Clinic samples
Gansle (2005)	School-based anger interventions	Outcome measures were child anger and externalizing behaviors
Garrard and Lipsey (2007)	Conflict resolution education in schools	Outcomes were antisocial behaviors
Gilliam and Zigler (2000)	State preschool programs	Outcomes included developmental competence, improving later school attendance and performance, and reducing subsequent grade retention
Gottfredson and Wilson (2003)	Individually focused interventions effective for reducing alcohol and other drug (AOD) use; cognitive-behavioral and behaviorally based interventions	The meta-analysis examined only alcohol or other drug use outcomes
Huey and Polo (2008)	Psychosocial treatments for ethnic minority youth	Outcome measures were not relevant to the current meta-analysis

Table 2.1 (continued)

Researchers (Date)	Intervention	Reason for exclusion
Kaminski, Valle, Filene, & Boyle (2008)	Parent training programs to treat ADHD and conduct problems	The meta-analysis did not examine any of the desired outcomes. It focused on conduct problems, issues of communication, child development, problem solving, etc.
Lauer, Akiba, Wilkerson, Apthorp, Snow, & Martin-Glenn (2006)	Out-of-school time (OST) programs	Outcomes focused on reading and mathematics student achievement and larger positive effect sizes for programs with specific characteristics such as tutoring in reading
Littell, Winswold, Bjorndal, & Hammerstrom (2007)	Certified functional family therapy programs compared with usual services, alternative services, or no treatment	Campbell Collaboration protocol only
Lösel and Beelmann (2003)	Child skills training	Earlier version of Lösel and Beelmann (2006)
Luke and Banerjee (2012)	Studies on emotion recognition and understanding	Outcome measures focus on social understanding (including emotion recognition and understanding, perspective taking, false belief understanding, and attributional biases). The article did not include any of the outcome measures relevant to the current meta-analysis
Lundahl, Risser, & Lovejoy (2006)	Parent training	Outcome measures were disruptive child behaviors and parental behavior and perceptions
McCart, Priester, Davies, & Azen (2006)	Cognitive-behavioral interventions and parent training	Outcome measures were antisocial behaviors
Maggin, Chafouleas, Goddard, & Johnson (2011)	Classroom token economies	No relevant outcome measures
Maggin, Johnson, Chafouleas, Roberto, & Bergren (2012)	School-based group contingency interventions	No relevant outcome measures
Maughan, Christiansen, Jenson, Olympia, & Clark (2005)	Behavioral parent training	Clinic samples
Montgomery, Bjornstad, & Dennis (2007)	Media-based behavioral treatments	No relevant outcome measures
Nowak and Heinrichs (2008)	Triple P parent training program	Outcome measures were child problem behaviors

Table 2.1 (continued)

Researchers (Date)	Intervention	Reason for exclusion
Payton, Weissberg, Durlak, Dymnicki, Taylor, Schellinger, & Pachan (2008)	Social and emotional learning programs (indicated)	Outcomes were conduct problems
Piquero, Farrington, Welsh, Tremblay, & Jennings (2008)	Parent training with children up to age 5	Outcome measures were antisocial behaviors
Prout and Prout (1998)	School-based studies of counseling and psychotherapy	Outcome measures focused on depression, self-esteem/concept, anxiety, social skills/status, attitude, and performance
Reddy, Newman, De Thomas, & Chun (2009)	School-based prevention and intervention programs for children and adolescents with emotional disturbance (ED)	Outcomes were externalizing behaviors and academic skills, internalizing behaviors, etc.
Reyno and McGrath (2005)	Predictors of parent training efficacy for child externalizing behavior problems	This meta-analysis focused on predictors of treatment response and indicators that lead to behavior problems (i.e. low education/occupation, more severe child behavior problems pretreatment, maternal psychopathology). The outcome measures are irrelevant to those in the present review
Serketich and Dumas (1996)	Behavioral parent training (BPT)	Outcome measure was child antisocial behavior which included aggression, temper tantrums, and noncompliance; eventually an overall child outcome was provided which included all the aforementioned. The researchers did not report aggression separately
Shadish and Baldwin (2003)	Marriage and family therapy interventions	Outcomes included drug abuse, marriage and family enrichment, emotional focused therapy, behavioral marital therapy, family therapy for alcoholism, child presenting problems, schizophrenia, and parent effectiveness training

Table 2.1 (continued)

Researchers (Date)	Intervention	Reason for exclusion
Solomon, Klein, Hintze, Cressey, & Peller (2012)	School-wide positive behavior support (SWPBS)	Outcomes focused on school-wide discipline, positive behavior, better class attendance, less expulsions, etc. None of the outcome measures required in our meta-analysis was found
Stanton and Shadish (1997)	Studies on treatment of drug abuse	Outcome examined was prevention of drug abuse based on family and couples treatment. Family therapy appears to be an effective and cost-effective adjunct to methadone maintenance. None of the present outcome measures was found
Stoltz, Londen, Deković, Orobio de Castro, & Prinzie (2012)	School-based interventions for externalizing behavior	No relevant outcome measures
Thomas and Zimmer-Gembeck (2007)	Triple P and parent-child interaction training	Outcome measures were child and parent behavior only
Tong and Farrington (2006, 2008)	Reasoning and rehabilitation	No separate results for adults and juveniles
Weisz, Jensen-Doss, & Hawley (2006)	Psychotherapy	Mostly clinical samples
Welsh and Farrington (2006)	Family-based programs	This article was a somewhat updated but shorter version of Farrington and Welsh (2003)
Wilson, Lipsey, & Derzon (2003b)	School-based programs	Earlier version of Wilson and Lipsey (2007)
Wilson, Rush, Hussey, Puckering, Sim, Allely, Doku, McConnachie, & Gillberg (2012)	Triple P parent training program	This meta-analysis focused on the effects of the Triple P programs on child behaviors. It did not analyze specific outcomes

2 Developmental and Social Prevention

Table 2.2 Characteristics of included reviews

Researchers (Date)	Intervention	Comparison group	Outcome	Design	Searches	Time period
(A) General prevention programs						
Deković, Slagt, Asscher, Boendermaker, Eichelsheim, & Prinzie (2011)	Early prevention programs (p. 535); Nurse-Family Partnership; Infant Health and Development Program; Abecederian program; Chicago Child-Parent Center program; High/Scope Perry Preschool Program; Seattle Social Development Project; The Good Behavior Game; Montreal Longitudinal- Experimental Study; Cambridge-Somerville Youth Study (pp. 537–538)	Control group who did not receive the intervention (p. 535)	Delinquency or criminal offending (p. 535)	Experiments or quasi-experiments (p. 535)	Online databases, Web of Science, PsycINFO, ERIC, PubMed, Sociological Abstracts, Criminal Justice Abstracts, OpenSIGLE, and USA Government Publications; Reviewed bibliographies of several other meta-analyses in the domain of crime prevention; Websites presenting prevention programs were consulted; Emailed the resulting list of eligible studies to leading scholars knowledgeable in the field of crime prevention research to find published and unpublished work. (p. 535)	Up to February 2010 (p. 535)

Table 2.2 (continued)

Researchers (Date)	Intervention	Comparison group	Outcome	Design	Searches	Time period
Manning, Homel, & Smith (2010)	Early developmental prevention (age 0–5)	Control group with no treatment (p. 508)	Relevant outcome measures: juvenile arrest, multiple arrests by 18 years, rates of violent and nonviolent arrest, criminal and antisocial behavior, incorrigible behavior (p. 510)	Randomized or matched groups, quasi-experimental (p. 508)	Key journals (e.g. Monographs of the Society for Research in Child Development, the Future of Children, American Educational Research Journal); Scanning of relevant review articles (p. 508)	1970–2008 (p. 508)
Wilson et al. (2003a)	Interventions designed for White vs. minority delinquent youth (p. 1)	Control receives nothing, minimal contact, school treatment as usual, usual probation services, usual institutional treatment, other treatment as usual, placebo (p. 9)	Juvenile delinquency (p. 3). Others include academic achievement, attitude change, behavior problems, employment status, family functioning, internalizing problems, peer relations, psychological adjustment, school participation, self-esteem (p. 10)	Experimental or quasi-experimental (p. 10)	Not defined	1950–1996 (p. 7)

Table 2.2 (continued)

Researchers (Date)	Intervention	Comparison group	Outcome	Design	Searches	Time period
(B) Individual programs						
(B1) Child training programs						
Fossum, Handega, Martinussen, & Morch (2008)	Behavior therapy (BT), cognitive behavior therapy (CBT), BT and CBT in combination, family therapy (FT), or psychodynamic therapy (p. 440)	Untreated control (waitlist), condition (design 1), or no control (design 2) (p. 442)	Aggression, change in social functioning, and changes in parental distress (p. 438)	Experimental design or randomization procedures, matching, or no control group (p. 442)	PsycINFO; More searches on the authors of these studies; searches in the reference lists of relevant literature reviews; personal request for articles in progress or unpublished material was sent by electronic mail to researchers (p. 440)	January 1987 until January 2008 (p. 439)
Lösel and Beelmann (2006)	Social competence training program (p. 36)	Control group that were compared in an experimental (randomized) design. (p. 35)	Antisocial behavior (p. 36)	Experimental (randomized) design. Stratified modes of randomization were included (e.g. randomized field trial, randomized block design, matching plus randomization) (p. 35)	PsycINFO, MEDLINE, Educational Resources Information Center (ERIC), and Dissertation Abstracts. References from reviews of child skills training and the prevention of antisocial behavior (p. 36)	Up to 2000 (p. 36)

Table 2.2 (continued)

Researchers (Date)	Intervention	Comparison group	Outcome	Design	Searches	Time period
(B2) *Wilderness challenge programs*						
Wilson and Lipsey (2000)	Wilderness challenge programs assessing the impact of delinquent behavior (p. 1)	Control (placebo, wait-list, no treatment or "treatment as usual" group) or comparison group (p. 2)	Delinquency or antisocial behavior (p. 2)	Randomized or non-randomized (p. 2)	First, the bibliographies of previous literature reviews and meta-analyses were reviewed; Second, a research of bibliographic databases, including Psychological Abstracts, Dissertation Abstracts International, ERIC, US Government Printing Office publications, national Criminal Justice Reference Service, and others. Finally, the studies retrieved were examined themselves for additional references (p. 3)	After 1950 (p. 2)
(B3) *Programs targeting odd/cd problems*						
Grove, Evans, Pastor, & Mack (2008)	Psychosocial intervention in programs to prevent oppositional defiant disorder (ODD) or conduct disorder (CD) (p. 173)	Children without any treatment (p. 173)	Aggression or delinquency or conduct disorder or oppositional defiant disorder or disruptive behavior (p. 173)	Programs presented in peer-reviewed journals (p. 173)	Studies in peer-reviewed journals (p. 172)	1980–2008 (p. 173)

Table 2.2 (continued)

Researchers (Date)	Intervention	Comparison group	Outcome	Design	Searches	Time period
(B4) Wraparound programs						
Suter and Bruns (2009)	Wraparound programs (p. 336)	Studies providing direct comparisons between youth receiving wraparound and those in a control group (p. 336)	Juvenile justice-related outcomes (p. 336)	Studies must have used a control group design (p. 339)	Earlier narrative reviews of wraparound; electronic databases (Web of Science, PsycINFO, and ERIC); manual search of the Journal of Child and Family Studies, Journal of Emotional and Behavioral Disorders, and the annual research conference proceedings of A System of Care for Children's Mental Health: Expanding the Research Base hosted by the University of South Florida, Research and Training Center for Children's Mental Health (p. 339)	January 1986–December 2008 (p. 339)
(C) Family programs						
(C1) General family programs						
Bernazzani and Tremblay (2006)	Parent training	Two targeted the universal population and the remaining five targeted risk groups (p. 25)	Arrests, convictions, probation violations; major delinquent acts (p. 28)	Randomized and nonrandomized controlled trials (p. 23)	PsycINFO, MEDLINE, the Cochrane Library, The Future of Children and potentially relevant review articles (p. 23)	Not specified

Table 2.2 (continued)

Researchers (Date)	Intervention	Comparison group	Outcome	Design	Searches	Time period
Farrington and Welsh (2003)	Family-based programs	Control group that received no treatment, the usual treatment, or some nonfamily treatment	Delinquency or antisocial child behavior (p. 127)	Randomized or well-controlled experiment (p. 129)	(1) Recent reviews (1997–2002) of the literature covering family-based interventions (2) Articles in major journals in criminology and psychopathology in 1997–2002 (3) Youth update (1997–2002): Regular publication abstracts from over 70 journals in epidemiology and interventions for delinquency and childhood antisocial behavior (4) Contacts with leading researchers in the field to solicit recently published or in-press papers. (p. 130)	Up to 2002 (p. 130)

Table 2.2 (continued)

Researchers (Date)	Intervention	Comparison group	Outcome	Design	Searches	Time period
Woolfenden, Williams, & Peat (2002)	Family and parenting interventions (e.g. short-term family intervention, parent training MST, MTFC) (pp. 251–252)	Control groups used including usual intervention controls, wait list controls and no intervention controls (p. 252)	Arrests, academic performance, future employment, etc. (p. 255)	Randomized controlled trials (p. 251)	Cochrane Controlled Trial Register, MEDLINE, EMBASE, CINAHL, PsycInfo, Sociofile, ERIC, and Healthstar; other sources of information were the bibliographies of systematic and nonsystematic reviews and reference lists of articles identified through the search strategy; in order to identify unpublished trials, experts in the field were contacted by letter (p. 251)	1966–1999 (p. 251)
(C2) Home visiting programs						
Bilukha, Hahn, Crosby, Fullilove, Liberman, Moscicki, Snyder, Tuma, Corso, Scholfield, & Briss (2005)	Home visiting studies (p. 17)	Families who were not exposed to the intervention (p. 15)	Violence by the child; violence by the parent; intimate partner violence and child maltreatment (abuse and neglect) (p. 15)	Randomized and nonrandomized experiments and pre-post studies (p. 19)	Online databases: MEDLINE; EMBASE; ERIC; NTIS; PsycINFO; Sociological Abstracts; National Criminal Justice Reference Service (NCJRS) and CINAHL (p. 15)	Before July 2011 (p. 15)

Table 2.2 (continued)

Researchers (Date)	Intervention	Comparison group	Outcome	Design	Searches	Time period
(C3) Multisystemic therapy						
Curtis, Ronan, & Borduin (2004)	Multisystemic therapy (MST), a family- and home-based therapeutic approach (p. 411)	Randomly assigned control groups (p. 412)	23 different outcome measures, including aggression, number of arrests for all crimes, number of arrests for substance abuse crimes, seriousness of arrests, days incarcerated, self-reported delinquency (p. 415)	Randomized controlled studies (p. 412)	Studies listed in the Psychological literature and ERIC databases; recent tables of contents of journals most likely to publish studies on MST were manually searched (p. 412)	From 1986 to 2003 (p. 412)

2 Developmental and Social Prevention

Table 2.2 (continued)

Researchers (Date)	Intervention	Comparison group	Outcome	Design	Searches	Time period
Littell, Popa, & Forsythe (2005)	MST	Studies on juvenile offenders compared MST with individual therapy, usual services in juvenile justice, or outpatient substance abuse services (p. 14)	Behavioral outcomes included antisocial behavior (arrest or conviction of criminal offense), drug use and school attendance; aggression. Psychosocial outcomes included measures of psychiatric symptoms, school performance, peer relations and self-esteem. Family outcomes included living arrangements for children and youth, and quality of family functioning (p. 9).	Randomized controlled trials (p. 15)	Electronic searches of bibliographic databases (including the Cochrane Library, C2-SPECTR, PsycINFO, Science Direct and Sociological Abstracts). Other sources: MEDLINE, EMBASE, CINAHL, PsycINFO, ASSIA, C2-SPECTR, Cambridge Journals, Dissertation Abstracts, ERIC, Family Services Research Center of the Medical University of South Carolina, InfoTrac, Science Direct, Sociological Abstracts, Social Work Abstracts, Web of Knowledge, Government policy sources/search engines (BiblioLine and Google) (p. 10)	1985 to January 2003
Littell (2008)	MST (p. 2)	Individuals not receiving treatment	Out of home placement; self-reported delinquency (p. 11)	Randomized controlled trials (p. 5)	Electronic databases; scanned available reference lists; personal contacts (p. 5)	2005–2008

Table 2.2 (continued)

Researchers (Date)	Intervention	Comparison group	Outcome	Design	Searches	Time period
(C4) Treatment foster care						
MacDonald and Turner (2007)	Treatment foster care (TFC) (p. 3)	Control group could be no-treatment, wait-list control, or regular foster care (p. 9)	Psychosocial and behavioral outcomes, delinquency, placement stability, and discharge status (p. 3)	Randomized controlled trials (p. 15)	Cochrane Controlled Trials Register, MEDLINE, CINAHL, PsycINFO, ASSIA, LILACS, ERIC, Sociological Abstracts, the National Research Register (p. 4)	1872–2007 (p. 4)
(D) School programs						
(D1) General school programs						
Hahn, Fuqua-Whitley, Wethington, Lowy, Crosby, Fullilove, Johnson, Liberman, Moscicki, Price, Snyder, Tuma, Cory, Stone, Mukhopadhaya, Chattopadhyay, Dahlberg, & Task Force on Community Preventive Services (2007)	Universal school-based programs (p. 114)	Comparison group which had not been exposed to programs or had been less exposed (p. 118)	Self- or other reported or observed aggression or violence, including violent crime; aggression or violence as observed by the researcher; conduct disorder; externalizing behavior; acting out; delinquency; school records of suspensions or disciplinary referrals (p. 118)	Experimental and quasi-experimental designs, including pre–post studies	Electronic searches in MEDLINE, EMBASE, ERIC, Applied Social Sciences Index and Abstracts, NTIS, PsycINFO, Sociological Abstracts, NCJRS, and CINAHL (p. 118)	Up to December 2004 (p. 118)

Table 2.2 (continued)

Researchers (Date)	Intervention	Comparison group	Outcome	Design	Searches	Time period
Park-Higgerson, Perumean-Chaney, Bartolucci, Grimley, & Singh (2008)	School-based studies designed to reduce externalizing, aggressive, and violent behavior (p. 465)	Control group (no intervention) (p. 465)	Aggressive and violent behavior (p. 465)	Randomized controlled trials (p. 465)	MEDLINE, PsycINFO, PubMed, Criminal Justice Info, National Institute of Justice, ArticleFirst, VasicBIOSIS, ERIC, and the NCJRS (p. 467)	1970–2004 (p. 467)
Wilson, Gottfredson, & Najaka (2001)	School-based prevention (p. 247)	Comparison group evaluation methodology, including nonequivalent comparison group research designs, and the comparison group was a no-treatment or minimal-treatment condition (p. 251)	Crime, delinquency, theft, violence, substance use, dropout/nonattendance, and other conduct problems (p. 247)	Experimental and quasi-experimental (p. 247)	Computer bibliographic databases (e.g. PsycLit, ERIC, and Sociological Abstracts), and through the references of recent reviews of prevention programs. In some instances, the search of recent reviews resulted in the identification and inclusion of a number of unpublished studies (p. 251)	From 1950 onwards (p. 137)

Table 2.2 (continued)

Researchers (Date)	Intervention	Comparison group	Outcome	Design	Searches	Time period
Wilson and Lipsey (2007)	School-based intervention programs (p. 130)	Intervention and comparison group of students (p. 133)	Aggressive and/or disruptive behaviors (p. 130)	Experimental and quasi-experimental studies (p. 130)	Psychological Abstracts, Dissertation Abstracts International, ERIC, United States Government Printing Office Publications, NCJRS and MEDLINE; Bibliographies of recent meta-analyses and literature reviews were reviewed for eligible studies; comparison of the bibliography with the companion guide to Community Preventive Services (the Community Guide) (p. 133)	1950–2007 (p. 133)

Table 2.2 (continued)

Researchers (Date)	Intervention	Comparison group	Outcome	Design	Searches	Time period
(D2) Antibullying programs						
Farrington and Ttofi (2009)	Evaluations focusing on school bullying (p. 35)	Control group that did not receive intervention (p. 27)	School bullying and victimization (p. 27)	Randomized experiments; intervention-control comparisons with before and after measures of bullying; other intervention-control comparisons and age-cohort designs (p. 27)	(1) Established names in the area of bullying prevention (e.g. Australia, Ken Rigby; England, Peter K. Smith; Finland, Christina Salmivalli; Greece, Eleni Andreou; Spain, Rosario Ortega; Norway, Dan Olweus) (2) Keywords in 18 electronic databases (3) Hand-searching of 35 journals either online or in print, from 1983 until end of May 2009 (4) Information from key researches on bullying and from international colleagues in the Campbell Collaboration (5) Title or abstract of each paper would have to include one of the essential keywords that were searched (p. 33)	1983 up to May 2009 (p. 27)
Ferguson, San Miguel, Kilburn, & Sanchez (2007)	School-based intervention programs (p. 407)	Control group (p. 407)	Bullying behavior or aggression toward peers (p. 407)	Randomized controlled trials (p. 407)	PsycINFO (p. 406)	1995–2006 (p. 406)

Table 2.2 (continued)

Researchers (Date)	Intervention	Comparison group	Outcome	Design	Searches	Time period
Merrell, Gueldner, Ross, & Isava (2008)	School-based intervention (p. 28)	Control group; mixed design with two-groups, pre-post, and wait-list or control groups (pp. 29–30)	Bullying behavior (p. 28)	Experimental or quasi-experimental designs (p. 28)	PsycINFO and ERIC; descriptions of published research studies, dissertation abstracts, and related research documents (p. 28)	1980–2004 (p. 26)
Mishna, Cook, Saini, Wu, & MacFadden (2009)	Programs designed to prevent cyber abuse (p. 3)	No treatment or minimal treatment control group (p. 12)	Cyber abuse of children and adolescents; risky behaviors; knowledge related to cyber abuse; negative impact on psychological state among those victimized by cyber abuse (p. 14)	Experimental and quasi-experimental designs (p. 3)	Psychological Abstracts (PsycINFO, PsycLIT, ClinPsyc-clinical subset); MEDLINE; EMBASE; database of reviews of effectiveness (DARE online); ChildData (child health and welfare); ASSIA; caredata; Social Work Abstracts; Child abuse, Child Welfare and Adoption; Cochrane Collaboration; C2-SPECTR; Social Sciences Abstracts; Social Service Abstracts; Dissertation Abstracts International (DAI). Hand search of Youth and Society; Journal of Interpersonal Violence; Annual Review of Sex Research; Computers in Human Behavior; Computers and Education; Journal of Adolescent Health; Contacted experts in the field and searched grey literature (pp. 3–4)	1999–2009

Table 2.2 (continued)

Researchers (Date)	Intervention	Comparison group	Outcome	Design	Searches	Time period
Smith, Schneider, Smith, & Ananiadou (2004)	Various interventions (e.g. school policy, teacher workshops) (p. 549)	Eight controlled studies, including four with random assignment of either classes or schools to intervention and control conditions; A further six were uncontrolled studies (p. 550)	Quantitative data on victimization and/or bullying in schools (p. 549)	Controlled or uncontrolled group assignment (p. 549)	Online Databases (PsycINFO, ERIC, Dissertation Abstracts)	Up to December 2002 (p. 549)
Vreeman and Carroll (2007)	Types of interventions could be categorized as curriculum (ten studies), multidisciplinary or whole-school interventions (ten studies), social skills groups (four studies), mentoring (one study), and social worker support (one study) (pp. 78–82)	Control groups (p. 79)	Bullying (bullying, victimization, aggressive behavior, and school responses to violence) and outcomes indirectly related to bullying (school achievement, perceived school safety, self-esteem, and knowledge or attitudes towards bullying) (p. 78)	Pretest-posttest, randomized controlled trials, randomized matched pairs, quasi-experimental with time-lagged age cohort (pp. 80–81)	MEDLINE, PsycINFO, EMBASE, ERIC, Cochrane Collaboration, the Physical Education Index, and Sociology: A Sage Full-text Collection searched for the terms bullying and bully (p. 78)	1966–2004 (p. 79)

Table 2.2 (continued)

Researchers (Date)	Intervention	Comparison group	Outcome	Design	Searches	Time period
(D3) School violence programs						
Dymnicki, Weissberg, & Henry (2011)	Universal school-based violence prevention programs (p. 320)	Students who did not receive these prevention programs (p. 320)	Overt aggressive behavior (p. 315)	Randomized designs (p. 320)	Online databases: PsycINFO, Psychological Abstracts, and ERIC; studies cited in a number of violence prevention meta-analyses and additional studies identified by the members of the team (p. 320)	1970–2010 (p. 320)
Howard, Flora, & Griffin (1999)	Classroom, school, home programs (p. 200)	Randomly selected control group, or multiple measurements of panels of youth over time (p. 199)	Knowledge, attitudes, aggressive, bullying, violent, and prosocial behavior (p. 197)	Randomized, non-randomized, quasi-experimental, or pre–post longitudinal designs (p. 199)	MEDLINE and PsycINFO; Colleagues and reference lists	1993–1997 (p. 197)
Mytton, DiGuiseppi, Gough, Taylor, & Logan (2002)	School-based violence prevention programs (p. 752)	No intervention (control or placebo group) (p. 754)	Violent injuries, observed or reported aggressive or violent behaviors, and school or agency responses to aggressive behaviors (p. 752)	Randomized controlled trials (p. 753)	Cochrane Controlled Trials Register, MEDLINE, EMBASE, ERIC, CINAHL, Dissertation Abstracts, IBSS, NCJRS, bibliographies of published reviews, and relevant trials (p. 753)	1987–1999 (p. 753)

Table 2.2 (continued)

Researchers (Date)	Intervention	Comparison group	Outcome	Design	Searches	Time period
(D4) Social information processing programs						
Wilson and Lipsey (2006a, b)	Universal (2006a) and selected/indicated (2006b) school-based social information processing interventions on aggressive behavior. Other treatment components were allowed to be present (e.g. behavioral social skills training, parenting skills training) but the social information processing component needed to be the clear focus of the program (2006a, p. 8; 2006b, p. 8)	Only studies using a control group design were eligible; the intervention and control groups could be randomly or nonrandomly assigned, but if nonrandom, needed to be matched or provide evidence of initial equivalence on key demographic variables. Control groups could represent placebo, wait-list, no treatment or "treatment as usual" (2006a, p. 8; 2006b, p. 9)	Aggressive behavior broadly defined to include violence, aggression, fighting, person crimes, disruptive behavior problems, acting out, conduct disorder, externalizing problems, and so forth (2006a, p. 8; 2006b, p. 9)	Experimental and quasi-experimental (2006a, p. 8; 2006b, p. 9)	Database compiled at the Center for Evaluation Research and Methodology was searched for eligible interventions. In addition, a comprehensive search of bibliographic databases, including Psychological Abstracts, Dissertation Abstracts International, ERIC, the Campbell and Cochrane Collaboration trials registers, US Government Printing Office publications, National Criminal Justice Reference Service, and MEDLINE was conducted (2006a, p. 9; 2006b, p. 9)	Published from the 1970s to the present (i.e. 2006) (2006a, p. 14; 2006b, p. 14)

Table 2.2 (continued)

Researchers (Date)	Intervention	Comparison group	Outcome	Design	Searches	Time period
(D5) Cognitive-behavioral programs						
Robinson, Smith, Miller, & Brownell (1999)	School-based cognitive-behavioral programs to increase self-control (p. 197)	No treatment or traditional behavior therapy (p. 197)	Aggression measured by observation and behavior checklists (p. 197)	Experimental and quasi-experimental (p. 197)	ERIC, PsycLIT, Dissertation Abstracts (p. 197)	1967–1995 (p. 197)
Sukhodolsky, Kassinove, & Gorman (2004)	School-based cognitive-behavioral therapy for anger (39% of studies in clinic or correctional settings) (p. 255)	No treatment or attention control conditions (p. 254)	Measure of anger or aggression	Experimental or quasi-experimental	PsycLIT, MEDLINE, Dissertation Abstracts (p. 253)	1968–1997 (p. 254)

Table 2.3 Results of included reviews

Researchers (Date)	Participants	Number of studies	Number of experiments	Effect size/Significance	Moderators
(A) General prevention programs					
Dekovic, Slagt, Asscher, Boendermaker, Eichelsheim, & Prinzie (2011)	Programs administered from infancy up to 12 years old; outcomes were assessed during adulthood (18 and older). Universal programs or those targeted on at-risk children (p. 535)	9 (meta-analysis) (p. 536)	9 (p. 536)	Effect size on adult criminal offending: OR = 1.26; CI = 1.06–1.50 (p. 532)	Target population; SES; gender; timing (when did it start); duration (length of program in years); intensity (number of hours involved in the program); targeted domain and focus on the program; design; type of control condition; source of information (p. 535 and p. 539)
Manning, Homel, & Smith (2010)	Children aged up to 5; universal programs or those targeted on at-risk children (p. 509)	11 (meta-analysis) (p. 508)	Not defined	Mean effect size was $d = .313$ (p. 506) Deviance: $d = .481$, CI = .266–.707 Criminal Justice: $d = .243$, CI = .146–.342	Duration of the program; program intensity; number of sessions; programs with a follow-through component (p. 513)

Table 2.3 (continued)

Researchers (Date)	Participants	Number of studies	Number of experiments	Effect size/Significance	Moderators
Wilson et al. (2003a)	Between 12 and 21 (p. 10)	305 studies (p. 3)	150 study descriptors (p. 3)	For minority youth, the weighted mean effect size for delinquency outcomes across all treatment modalities was d = .11; for majority youth, the corresponding effect size value was d = .17. Both these values were statistically significant (p. 12)	Pretreatment equivalence of experimental and control groups: Studies in which treatment and control groups were similar prior to treatment produced smaller effect sizes than those in which treatment and control groups were not similar; unpublished technical reports tended to produce smaller effect sizes than published journal articles, books, and dissertations; studies in which the evaluator assumed only a research role tended to produce smaller effect sizes; studies in which control participants received more services as part of treatment as usual control groups resulted in smaller effect sizes; studies in which those collecting outcome data were blind to the group status of participants produced larger effect sizes than those in which data collectors were not blind (p. 15)

Table 2.3 (continued)

Researchers (Date)	Participants	Number of studies	Number of experiments	Effect size/Significance	Moderators
(B) Individual programs					
(B1) Child training programs					
Fossum, Handegå, Martinussen, & Morch (2008)	Children with high disruptive or aggressive behavior; mean age was below 18 (p. 439), from 3.4 to 13.5 (p. 442)	65 studies, 33 with untreated controls (p. 438)	Not defined	Mean d of change in aggression in studies with untreated controls was .62 (CI = .49–.76) (p. 444)	Sample size; studies with younger children; studies applying a behavior therapy intervention; studies providing diagnostic information (p. 444)
Lösel and Beelmann (2006)	Treated youngsters had to be between the ages of 0 and 18 years; universal programs or at-risk samples (p. 35)	55 reports; final database was 89 treatment–control group comparisons (p. 36)	Not defined	For aggressive behavior, $d = .24$ ($p < .05$) at postintervention and $d = .17$ (ns) at follow-up; for delinquent behavior $d = .18$ (post) and .19 (follow-up), both significant (p. 42)	Mode of treatment; treatment dosage; age of children; type of prevention; sample size (p. 42 and following)
(B2) Wilderness challenge programs					
Wilson and Lipsey (2000)	Antisocial or delinquent youth between the ages of 10 and 21 (p. 2)	28 eligible studies (p. 3)	60 effect sizes on outcome variables (p. 3)	Overall mean effect size for delinquent outcomes was $d = .18$, CI = .10–.27 (pp. 1 and 5)	Program length was not related to outcome among short-term programs (up to 6 weeks) but extended programs (over 10 weeks) showed smaller effects overall (p. 1)

Table 2.3 (continued)

Researchers (Date)	Participants	Number of studies	Number of experiments	Effect size/Significance	Moderators
(B3) Programs targeting odd/cd problems					
Grove, Evans, Pastor, & Mack (2008)	Children and adolescents aged up to 18 who have not shown ODD or CD; minimum $N=10$ (p. 173)	45 (p. 174)	Not defined	Total $d=.17$, CI = .10–.24 Property violations: $d=.26$, CI = .05–.46; Aggression: $d=.15$, CI = .03–.26 (p. 177)	Conduct disorder; methods of measuring outcomes; amount of time at follow-up, age and gender of participants, and type of treatment (pp. 171–172)
(B4) Wraparound programs					
Suter and Bruns (2009)	Youth (3–21 years) with social, emotional, or behavioral difficulties (p. 339)	7 (p. 344)	3 (p. 341)	Overall $d=.33$, CI = .14–.53; for juvenile justice outcomes, $d=.21$, CI = −.02–.44 (p. 344)	d smaller in experiments (.17) than in quasi-experimental studies (.46) (p. 344)
(C) Family programs					
(C1) General family programs					
Bernazzani and Tremblay (2006)	Children under the age of 3 at the time intervention was implemented (p. 22)	7 (p. 24)	7	Effect sizes only given for individual evaluations; no weighted mean effect size	Not defined
Farrington and Welsh (2003)	Birth to 17 years old, minimum $N=50$ (p. 129–134)	40 (p. 129)	30 with individuals (p. 133)	For all delinquency outcomes, the weighted mean effect size $d=.321$, CI = .250–.391 (p. 144)	Effects greater in smaller studies but not related to age or year of publication (p. 144)

Table 2.3 (continued)

Researchers (Date)	Participants	Number of studies	Number of experiments	Effect size/Significance	Moderators
Woolfenden, Williams, & Peat (2002)	Aged 10–17 (p. 251)	8 (p. 251)	8	Family interventions significantly reduced the time spent by juvenile delinquents in institutions (weighted mean difference 51.34 days) CI=30.16–72.52. There was also a significant reduction in self-reported delinquency ($d=-.41$, CI=$-.65$ to $-.17$) and in the rate of subsequent arrests ($d=-.56$, CI=$-.03$ to -1.10) (pp. 254–255)	Not defined

(C2) Home visiting programs

Researchers (Date)	Participants	Number of studies	Number of experiments	Effect size/Significance	Moderators
Bilukha, Hahn, Crosby, Fullilove, Liberman, Moscicki, Snyder, Tuma, Corso, Scholfield, & Briss (2005)	Parents; partners; children (p. 17)	Four (on violence by the visited children, two with delinquency outcomes); 22 (on child maltreatment) (p. 17)	18 out of 26 comparisons on child maltreatment were randomized	Median effect size for child maltreatment was -38.9% (interquartile range=-74.1% to $+24.0\%$) (p. 18)	Outcome; visitor type; components; randomization; time of program initiation (p. 19)

Table 2.3 (continued)

Researchers (Date)	Participants	Number of studies	Number of experiments	Effect size/Significance	Moderators
(C3) Multisystemic therapy					
Curtis, Ronan, & Borduin (2004)	Youths from 8.3 to 17.6 years (median = 14.8) (p. 413)	Seven primary outcome studies and four secondary studies (p. 411)	Seven primary outcome studies were randomized	Average effect of MST was $d = .55$, CI = .40–.70 (p. 415); Effect size for ultimate outcomes (criminal activity) .50 (p. 415)	Target population (not significant); difference in study conditions (i.e. efficacy vs. effectiveness conditions). The average effect size achieved in more controlled studies with graduate student therapists ($d = .81$) was compared with the average effect size achieved in community-based studies ($d = .26$). (p. 416)
Littell, Popa, Forsythe (2005)	Youth aged 10–17 (p. 5)	8 (p. 5)	8	Arrest or conviction for a criminal offense: MST cases were less likely to be arrested or convicted (OR = .39) but not significantly so (CI = .14–1.05); Self-reported delinquency: $d = -.21$, CI = -.50–.08), again not significant (p. 20)	Methodological quality, sample characteristics, intensity and duration of MST, comparison conditions, observation periods, and independence of evaluation (p. 23)
Littell (2008)	Youths (p. 8)	5 (p. 6)	5	Self-reported delinquency $d = -.13$ CI = -.33–.07 (p. 11)	Not defined

Table 2.3 (continued)

Researchers (Date)	Participants	Number of studies	Number of experiments	Effect size/Significance	Moderators
(C4) Treatment foster care					
MacDonald and Turner (2007)	Young people up to the age of 18 (p. 4)	5 (p. 3)	5	Criminal referrals: $d=-.54$, CI $=-.31$ to $-.78$; self-reported delinquency: $d=-.15$, CI $=.32$ to $-.61$; but only based on 2 studies (pp. 91–92)	Not defined
(D) School programs					
(D1) General school programs					
Hahn et al. (2007)	Prekindergarten through high school (p. 114)	53 studies of universal school-based programs that met the inclusion criteria (p. 120)	Not defined	The median effect size (relative reduction among students who received the program) was −10.3 % for violence (interquartile range =−1.7% to −50.0%) and −6.7% for bullying (interquartile range −64.8–17.2%) (p. 121)	Intervention strategies; school environments; predominant ethnicity; length of program exposure; time since program end; economic efficiency (pp. 122–123)
Park-Higgerson, Perumean-Chaney, Bartolucci, Grimley, & Sigh (2008)	Grades 1–11 (p. 465)	26 (p. 465)	26	No significant effect of interventions ($d=-.09$, CI $=-.23-.05$) (p. 475)	Not defined
Wilson, Gottfredson, & Najaka (2001)	Students (p. 251)	165 (p. 251)	42 (p. 260)	Effect size for delinquency: $d=.04$, CI $=-.03-.11$ (p. 261)	Effect size is related to methodological quality (weighted correlation equals.10; $p=.07$) (p. 262)
Wilson and Lipsey (2007)	Prekindergarten through grade 12 (p. 133)	249 (p. 135)	158	Aggression $d=.21$, CI $=.17–.25$ (p. 134)	Implementation quality, age and SES of students, type of treatment (pp. 137–139)

Table 2.3 (continued)

Researchers (Date)	Participants	Number of studies	Number of experiments	Effect size/Significance	Moderators
(D2) Antibullying programs					
Farrington and Ttofi (2009)	Kindergarten to high school children (p. 31)	89 in systematic review, 44 in meta-analysis (p. 6)	11 RCTs	Bullying: OR = 1.36, CI = 1.26–1.47 (p. 136)	More intensive programs were more effective, as well as programs including parent meetings, firm disciplinary methods, and improved playground supervision (p. 140)
Ferguson, San Miguel, Kilburn, & Sanchez (2007)	School students (p. 408)	42 (p. 407)	42	Violence: $r = .13$, CI = .05–.20; non-violent bullying $r = .12$, CI = .06–.17; combined $r = .12$, CI = .08–.17 (p. 408)	Moderator variables included (a) grade level of the program implementation, (b) whether the samples were drawn from populations identified as at risk for violence or were part of the general school population and (c) whether the outcome variables clearly used measures of violent behavior or focused on broader measures of bullying behaviors such as teasing (p. 407)
Merrell, Gueldner, Ross, & Isava (2008)	Kindergarten through grade 12 (p. 26)	16 (p. 26)	Not defined	For bullying others, $d = .04$ (p. 37)	Not defined

Table 2.3 (continued)

Researchers (Date)	Participants	Number of studies	Number of experiments	Effect size/Significance	Moderators
Mishna, Cook, Saini, Wu, & MacFadden (2009)	Children aged between 5 and 19 (p. 12)	3 (the I-SAFE, Missing, and HAHASO projects) (p. 23)	0	Cyber bullying only measured in HAHASO project: it decreased in the treatment group ($d=.37$, SE$=.42$), but it decreased even more in the control group ($d=.88$, SE$=.48$) (p. 27)	Not defined
Smith, Schneider, Smith, & Ananiadou (2004)	Grades 1–11 and ages 8–16 (p. 551)	14	4	Best intervention conditions: for bullying, 33% of r values were .10–.29, 50% were .00–.09, 17% were negative (p. 555)	Program components in all studies were shown but not related to effect sizes
Vreeman and Carroll (2007)	Grades 1–10 (p. 80)	26 (p. 79)	10	Reviewers do not provide effect sizes, but refer to specific studies using p values (pp. 80–86)	Not defined
(D3) School violence programs					
Dymnicki, Weissberg, & Henry (2011)	Elementary students (Kindergarten to fifth grade) (p. 320)	26 (p. 320)	Not defined	$d=.11$ (CI$=.06$–.16) (p. 323)	Not defined
Howard, Flora, Griffin (1999)	Grade 1–12 (p. 200)	13 (p. 200)	6	No specific effect sizes are reported, only descriptive information (p. 200)	Not defined

Table 2.3 (continued)

Researchers (Date)	Participants	Number of studies	Number of experiments	Effect size/Significance	Moderators
Mytton, DiGuiseppi, Gough, Taylor, & Logan (2002)	Kindergarten through grade 12 (p. 753)	44 trials (p. 742); 28 trials assessed aggressive behaviors	44	$d = -.36$ (CI = $-.54$ to $-.19$) in favor of a reduction in aggression after intervention (p. 752)	Larger studies reported smaller effects (p. 759); Differences in age group, sex, and training focus contributed to, but did not fully explain the substantial heterogeneity. There were signs of publication bias (p. 760)

(D4) Social information processing programs

| Wilson and Lipsey (2006a) | School-age children (Kindergarten—grade 12) | 73 (p. 13) | 32 | Overall $d = .21$, indicating that children in the treatment groups had significantly lower aggressive behavior than comparison children after participating in universal social information processing programs (p. 16). | Effect sizes were greater if programs were implemented well, with more frequent sessions and low-SES children. Effect sizes were smaller if programs were implemented in routine practice rather than as demonstration programs (p. 22) |

Table 2.3 (continued)

Researchers (Date)	Participants	Number of studies	Number of experiments	Effect size/Significance	Moderators
Wilson and Lipsey (2006b)	School-age children (Kindergarten—grade 12)	47 (p. 13)	40	Overall $d = .26$ ($p = .001$) indicating that children in the treatment groups had significantly lower aggressive behavior than comparison children after participating in selected or indicated social information processing programs (p. 16)	Only two variables were significant in the final model, attrition and special education school, both associated with smaller effect sizes (p. 22)
(D5) Cognitive-behavioral programs					
Robinson, Smith, Miller, & Brownell (1999)	School age children (Kindergarten—grade 12)	23 (p. 197)	Not stated	In 12 studies with aggression outcomes, $d = .64$ (SD = .57). (p. 199)	Date, sample size, and gender were not related to effect size (p. 200)
Sukhodolsky, Kassinove, & Gorman (2004)	Children with a mean age of 7–17 (p. 254)	40 (p. 253)	41 out of 51 comparisons (p. 255)	For 36 comparisons with aggression outcomes, $d = .63$, SD = .35 (p. 258)	d was greater when the control group received no treatment (p. 261)

Table 2.4 Effect sizes

Researchers (date)	Original effect size	Converted effect size	Final effect size (Odds ratio, confidence interval)
(A) General prevention programs			
Deković et al. (2011)	OR = 1.26, CI = 1.06–1.50		OR = 1.26, CI = 1.06–1.50
Manning et al. (2010)	d = .243, CI = .146–.342		OR = 1.55, CI = 1.30–1.86
Wilson et al. (2003)	White: d = .11, CI = .07–.15. Minority: d = .17, CI = .12–.22	Combined d = .133, CI = .102–.164	OR = 1.27, CI = 1.20–1.35
(B) Individual programs			
Fossum et al. (2008)	d = .62, CI = .49–.76		OR = 3.08, CI = 2.43–3.97
Wilson and Lipsey (2000)	d = .18, CI = .10–.27		OR = 1.39, CI = 1.20–1.63
Grove et al. (2008)	Property: d = .26, CI = .05–.46; Aggression: d = .15, CI = .03–.26	Combined d = .175, CI = .062–.278	OR = 1.37, CI = 1.12–1.66
Suter and Bruns (2009)	d = .27, CI = −.04–.58		OR = 1.63, CI = .93–2.86
(C) Family programs			
Farrington and Welsh (2003)	d = .321, CI = .250–.391		OR = 1.79, CI = 1.57–2.03
Woolfenden et al. (2002)	Arrest: d = −.56, CI = −.03 to −1.10; SRD: d = −.41, CI = −.17 to −.65	Combined d = .434, CI = .216–.652	OR = 2.20, CI = 1.48–3.26
Curtis et al. (2004)	d = .50, CI = .35–.65		OR = 2.48, CI = 1.89–3.25
Littell et al. (2005)	Arrest: OR = .39, CI = .14–1.05; SRD: d = −.21, CI = −.50–.08	Arrest: OR = 2.56, CI = .95–7.14; SRD: OR = 1.46, CI = .86–2.48	OR = 1.65, CI = 1.03–2.63
Littell (2008)	d = −.13, (CI = −.33–.07)		OR = 1.27, CI = .88–1.82
MacDonald and Turner (2007)	Crime: d = −.54 (CI = −.31 to −.78); SRD: d = −.15 (CI = −.61–.32)	Combined d = .461, CI = .251–.671	OR = 2.31, CI = 1.58–3.38

Table 2.4 (continued)

Researchers (date)	Original effect size	Converted effect size	Final effect size (Odds ratio, confidence interval)
(D) School programs			
Park-Higgerson et al. (2008)	$d=-.09$, CI $=-.23-.05$		OR $= 1.18$, CI $= .91-1.52$
Wilson et al. (2001)	$d=.04$, CI $=-.03-.11$		OR $= 1.08$, CI $= .95-1.22$
Wilson and Lipsey (2007)	$d=.21$, CI $=.17-.25$		OR $= 1.46$, CI $= 1.36-1.57$
Farrington and Ttofi (2009)	OR $= 1.36$, CI $= 1.26-1.47$		OR $= 1.36$, CI $= 1.26-1.47$
Ferguson et al. (2007)	$r=.12$, CI $=.08-.17$	$d=.24$, CI $=.15-.33$	OR $= 1.55$, CI $= 1.31-1.82$
Dymnicki et al. (2011)	$d=.11$ (CI $=.06-.16$)		OR $= 1.22$, CI $= 1.11-1.34$
Mytton et al. (2002)	$d=-.36$ (CI $=-.19$ to $-.54$)		OR $= 1.92$, CI $= 1.41-2.66$
Robinson et al. (1999)	$d=.57$, SD $=.57$	$d=.57$, CI $=.25-.89$	OR $= 2.81$, CI $= 1.57-5.02$
Sukhodolsky et al. (2004)	$d=.63$, SD $=.35$	$d=.63$, CI $=.52-.74$	OR $= 3.14$, CI $= 2.57-3.83$

However, we did not include later reviews because we have not searched systematically for them.

There are other appraisals of systematic reviews of developmental prevention programs. For example, Lösel, (2012), in a German language article, reviewed 22 meta-analyses of developmental prevention. Some of these are not included in Tables 2.2 and 2.3 because they do not report results for one of our outcomes, but only for antisocial behavior. Ttofi, Eisner, & Bradshaw (2014) discussed six systematic reviews of bullying prevention programs. Five of these (all except Baldry & Farrington, 2007, which was superseded by Farrington & Ttofi, 2009) are included in Tables 2.2 and 2.3. Butler, Chapman, Forman, & Beck (2006) reviewed meta-analyses of cognitive-behavioral treatment programs. Beelmann and Raabe (2009) synthesized meta-analyses on the prevention of antisocial behavior and crime in childhood and adolescence, and Matjasko, Vivolo-Kantor, Massetti, Holland, Holt, & Dela Cruz (2012) reviewed meta-analyses of youth violence prevention programs. And Welsh and Rocque (2014) studied Campbell Collaboration systematic reviews to discover harmful effects of prevention programs.

Farrington and Welsh (2006) published a systematic review of randomized experiments in criminology, updating earlier reviews by Farrington (1983) and Farrington and Welsh (2005). Farrington and Welsh (2006) reviewed 122 policing, prevention, corrections, court, and community experiments published between 1957 and 2004, including 20 prevention experiments. Their main measure of effect size was the percentage reduction in offending in the experimental group compared with the control group. Farrington (2006, 2013) and Farrington, Loeber, & Welsh (2010) also reviewed longitudinal-experimental studies (most of which were concerned with developmental prevention), and Farrington and Welsh (2013) reviewed randomized experiments with a long-term (at least 10 years) follow-up (again, most of which were concerned with developmental prevention).

It is noticeable that reviews conducted under the auspices of the Campbell Collaboration (see, e.g. Farrington, Weisburd, & Gill, 2011) generally have higher methodological quality than other reviews (and the same is true of reviews on medical and health topics conducted under the auspices of the Cochrane Collaboration). Therefore, we note which are Campbell (or Cochrane) reviews.

General Prevention Programs

Deković et al. (2011) aimed to summarize the long-term effects of prevention programs implemented during early and middle childhood (from infancy up to age 12) on later criminal offending during adulthood (age 18 or older). They also reported effects on positive outcomes such as academic attainment, and found nine evaluations. Taken together, the programs were effective in reducing adult offending (OR = 1.26, CI = 1.06–1.50). The effects on positive outcomes were somewhat larger (OR = 1.36, CI = 1.20–1.55). Children who were more at risk and those from low socioeconomic status (SES) families benefited more. Shorter, more intensive programs tended to produce larger effects.

Manning et al. (2010) aimed to investigate the effectiveness of early developmental prevention programs on children aged up to 5 on non-health outcomes in adolescence (including criminal justice outcomes such as arrests, as well as educational success and socio-emotional development). They found 11 evaluations. Only five of these studied criminal justice outcomes, but overall these programs were effective ($d=.243$, CI$=.146-.342$). These d values were transformed into OR values using the equation $\ln(OR) = \dfrac{d}{.5513}$ (Farrington & Ttofi, 2009, p. 81). The largest effect size was on educational success ($d=.528$, CI$=.400-.679$). Generally, longer and more intensive programs tended to be more effective.

Wilson et al. (2003a) were mainly interested in the relative effectiveness of delinquency prevention programs with white compared with minority youth. They analyzed 164 evaluations with predominantly (at least 60%) white youth and 141 evaluations with predominantly (at least 60%) minority youth. About a quarter of the samples were institutionalized. Overall, the programs were effective in reducing delinquency for both white ($d=.11$, CI$=.07-.15$) and minority ($d=.17$, CI$=.12-.22$; estimated from their Fig. 2.1) samples. The programs were also effective in regard to other outcomes such as academic achievement and nonaggressive behavior problems. Wilson et al. (2003a) concluded that programs are equally effective with white and minority youth. However, they seemed to be more effective with delinquent samples than with predelinquent or institutionalized samples. Table 2.4 estimates that the combined effect size was OR$=1.27$ (CI$=1.20-1.35$).

Individual Programs

Child Training Programs

Fossum et al. (2008) aimed to investigate the effectiveness of psychosocial interventions (behavior therapy, cognitive behavior therapy, family therapy, and psychodynamic therapy) on children's aggressive behavior (rated by teachers, although parent ratings correlated $r=.65$ with teacher ratings). They found 65 evaluations, of which 33 had an untreated control group and 32 had either a treated control group or no control group. Focusing only on the 33 controlled evaluations, the weighted mean $d=.62$ (CI$=.49-.76$). The only moderator variable that was significant for these studies was sample size, with smaller studies having larger effect sizes.

The review by Lösel and Beelmann (2006) updated the earlier review by Lösel and Beelmann (2003). They focused on social competence training programs that did not include other elements such as parent or teacher training. They found 55 reports containing 89 randomized treatment–control comparisons. For aggressive behavior, the weighted mean $d=.24$ for immediate follow-up measures (up to two months) and $d=.17$ for longer follow-up measures. For delinquency, $d=.18$ immediately and $d=.19$ later. Unfortunately, CI were not reported for these d values, so they are not shown in Table 2.4. Effect sizes were greater for cognitive-behavioral programs, intensive treatment, older children (age 13 or older), at-risk children, and smaller samples.

Wilderness Challenge Programs

Wilson and Lipsey (2000) evaluated the effectiveness of wilderness challenge programs for delinquent youth. They found 28 eligible evaluations. For delinquent and antisocial outcomes, the programs were effective ($d=.18$, $CI=.10-.27$). The programs also had desirable effects on self-esteem, interpersonal adjustment, and school adjustment. Programs with intensive activities or with a distinct therapeutic component produced the greatest reductions in delinquent behavior.

Programs Targeting ODD or CD Problems

Grove et al. (2008) reviewed evaluations of programs designed to prevent oppositional defiant disorder (ODD) or CD problems, and found 45 evaluations. Eleven evaluations showed that these programs were effective in reducing property violations ($d=.26$, $CI=.05-.46$), while 16 evaluations showed that these programs were effective in reducing aggression ($d=.15$, $CI=.03-.26$). The effects were largest when outcomes were measured using official records. Table 2.4 estimates that the combined effect size was $OR=1.37$ ($CI=1.12-1.66$).

Wraparound Programs

Suter and Bruns (2009) reviewed evaluations of the effectiveness of wraparound programs, and found seven evaluations. They studied juvenile justice outcomes as well as mental health outcomes and school functioning. Five evaluations found a desirable but nonsignificant effect on juvenile justice outcomes ($d=.27$, $CI=-.02-.44$). Generally, the effects were greater in quasi-experimental evaluations than in randomized experiments.

Family Programs

General Family Programs

Bernazzani and Tremblay (2006) aimed to review evaluations of parent training programs implemented up to age 3, and found seven evaluations. They reported on the results in each evaluation, but only two had clearly delinquent outcomes and there was no attempt to calculate a summary effect size.

Farrington and Welsh (2003) reviewed evaluations of the effectiveness of family programs in preventing delinquency or antisocial behavior. They found 40 evaluations, but in many of these the program had additional components (e.g. a daycare, preschool, or school program). They reported that 19 programs found a desirable effect on delinquency ($d=.321$, CI$=.250–.391$). The effects on long-term delinquency outcomes were greater than on short-term delinquency outcomes, and the effects on antisocial behavior outcomes were less than on delinquency outcomes. Generally, smaller studies found larger effects. This review was later updated to some extent by Welsh and Farrington (2006), but they only presented percentage differences in each evaluation, making it difficult to derive weighted mean effect sizes.

Woolfenden et al. (2002), in a Cochrane review, reviewed eight randomized controlled trials of family interventions with children and adolescents. They studied several outcomes including rearrests, self-reported delinquency (SRD), academic performance, and future employment. Based on the five evaluations, there was a desirable effect on rearrests ($d=.56$, CI$=.03–1.10$). There was also a desirable effect on SRD ($d=.41$, CI$=.17–.65$), but this was based on only three of these evaluations. Our estimate of the combined effect size was OR$=2.20$ (CI$=1.48–3.26$) (see Table 2.4).

Home Visiting Programs

Bilukha et al. (2005) aimed to review evaluations of home visiting during pregnancy and the first two years of a child's life. They found 22 studies with child maltreatment outcomes but only two with measures of child delinquency. They presented only percentage change figures. For child maltreatment outcomes, the median percentage change was -38.9% (interquartile range $=-74.1–24.0\%$; a desirable effect in 26 comparisons, including 18 randomized). Effects were greater in nonrandomized studies and with both prenatal and postnatal visiting.

Multisystemic Therapy

Curtis et al. (2004) reviewed evaluations of the effectiveness of multisystemic therapy (MST). They found seven primary outcome evaluations and four secondary analyses of primary outcome evaluations. They studied numerous outcomes and reported that the average effect size of MST was $d=.55$ (CI$=.40–.70$). They also found that the average effect size across criminal outcomes was $d=.50$. They did not give the CI for this d value but, based on the above information, it would be reasonable to assume that it was about .35–.65. They found that effect sizes were greater in tightly controlled "efficacy" studies with closely supervised graduate student therapists than in less controlled "effectiveness" studies.

Littell et al. (2005), in a Campbell review, also reviewed evaluations of the effectiveness of MST, and found eight randomized controlled trials. They studied numerous outcomes. For five evaluations that measured arrest or conviction for a criminal offense, they reported an effect size on the random effects model of OR$=.39$ (CI$=.14–1.05$), noting the substantial heterogeneity of effects. For three evaluations that measured SRD, they reported $d=-.21$ (CI$=-.50$–.08). Neither of these effect sizes was significant. When they were combined, our estimated effect size was OR$=1.65$ (CI$=1.03$–2.63), which was just significant (see Table 2.4). However, as noted above, our method of combining effect sizes assumes that they are independent, but in this case there were two overlapping studies. If the variance was increased to take account of the nonindependence, it is likely that the combined effect size would not be significant. Littell et al. (2005, p. 24) noted that seven of the eight MST evaluations found significant differences on one or more outcome measures, but the average effects on any single outcome measure were not significant. They also noted that previous reviewers had not distinguished intent-to-treat analyses from analyses restricted to program completers.

Littell (2008) then produced a partial update in a PowerPoint presentation, adding five new experiments to her original eight. She extended her analyses of SRD outcomes by adding two intent-to-treat analyses to the original three analyses restricted to program completers. The two new studies had a negligible effect size of $d=-.02$ (CI$=-.31$–.26). Taken together, the effect size of all five experiments with SRD outcomes was $d=-.13$ (CI$=-.33$–.07), which was not significant.

Henggeler, Schoenwald, & Swenson (2006) replied in detail to an article on MST by Littell (2005). Henggeler et al. argued, for example, that Littell had given too much weight to the unpublished report by Leschied and Cunningham (2002) and had focused too much on intent to treat and randomization, ignoring other issues relevant to internal and external validity. Littell (2006) then replied in detail to Henggeler et al. (2006), pointing out, for example, that Henggeler and his colleagues had a significant financial stake in the success of MST.

Treatment Foster Care

MacDonald and Turner (2007), in a Campbell review, aimed to assess the effectiveness of Treatment Foster Care (TFC) on delinquency, behavior problems, psychological functioning, educational outcomes, and mental and physical health. They found five randomized controlled trials. Only two of these had delinquency outcomes, and they combined short-term (up to one year) with long-term (over one year) results. For criminal referrals, $d=-.54$ (CI$=-.31$ to $-.78$); for SRD, $d=-.15$ (CI$=-.61$–.32). Our estimate of the combined effect size was OR$=2.30$ (CI$=1.57$–3.37) (see Table 2.4).

School Programs

General School Programs

Hahn et al. (2007) aimed to review the effectiveness of universal school-based programs for preventing violence and aggressive behavior, but included programs targeting other outcomes such as CD and externalizing behavior. They included pre–post studies with no control condition and their main outcome measure was the percentage reduction in problem behavior. The median reduction was 10.3 % for violence and 6.7 % for bullying, but it is difficult to convert these figures into OR. The effects were similar for black and white children and similar in low-SES and high-SES areas.

Park-Higgerson et al. (2008) reviewed 26 school-based randomized controlled trials that were designed to reduce violent, aggressive, or externalizing behavior. They concluded that, overall, the programs were not significantly effective ($d=-.09$, CI$=-.23–.05$). However, theory-based programs were less effective than non-theory-based programs, universal programs were less effective than single-approach programs, and programs were generally more effective with older children (grade 4 or higher).

Wilson et al. (2001) reviewed 165 evaluations of the effects of school-based prevention programs on crime, delinquency, theft, violence, aggression, and several other outcomes. Over 40 evaluations, the effect size for delinquency was nonsignificant: $d=.04$ (CI$=-.03–.11$). However, these programs were effective in reducing alcohol and drug use, school dropout, nonattendance, and other problem behaviors. Programs including self-control or social competency promotion using cognitive-behavioral and behavioral methods were effective, whereas counseling, social work, and other therapeutic interventions were ineffective. The programs worked best with at-risk populations and older children (in senior high school).

Wilson and Lipsey (2007) reviewed 249 experimental and quasi-experimental evaluations of the effects of school-based prevention programs on aggressive and disruptive behavior. This review was an update of that by Wilson, Lipsey, & Derzon (2003b), but apparently not an update of the review by Wilson et al. (2001), as the authors did not overlap. Wilson and Lipsey (2007) presented results for several outcome measures, including attention problems, school performance, and internalizing problems. For aggressive/disruptive behavior, $d=.21$ (CI$=.17–.25$; estimated from their Fig. 2.1). For universal programs, effect sizes were greater for teacher reports than for self-reports, and greater for low-SES and younger students. For selected programs, effect sizes were greater for higher-risk students, better implemented programs, and individual compared with group treatment.

Antibullying Programs

Farrington and Ttofi (2009; see also Ttofi & Farrington, 2011), in a Campbell review, assessed controlled programs designed to prevent school bullying. They included 89 evaluations in their systematic review, and 44 contained effect size information and could be included in their meta-analyses. They presented effects on bullying perpetration and victimization (being bullied), but in this chapter we focus only on the specific outcome measure of bullying perpetration. The weighted mean effect size was $d=1.36$ (CI$=1.26–1.47$). They investigated numerous program components and design features that were related to the effectiveness of antibullying programs, and concluded that parent training or meetings were the most important program component (see also Axford, Sontalia, Wrigley, Goodwin, Ohlsen, Bjornstad, Barlow, Schrader-McMillan, Coad, & Toft, 2015), followed by playground supervision and the intensity and duration of the program. The programs worked better for older children (age 11 or older: see Ttofi & Farrington, 2012).

Ferguson et al. (2007) also evaluated the effectiveness of school-based antibullying programs. Their outcome measure was bullying or aggression toward peers. They reported a weighted mean effect size of $r=.12$ (CI = .08–.17). When r is small, and in randomized trials with equal numbers in treated and control groups, $d = 2*r$ is a good approximation (see Farrington & Ttofi, 2009, p. 81), and this equation was used (see Table 2.4). Ferguson et al. found that effect sizes were greater for high-risk children ($r=.19$) than for low-risk children ($r=.09$).

Merrell et al. (2008) reviewed 16 evaluations of anti-bullying programs. They investigated a variety of outcome variables, including self-reports of bullying perpetration, being bullied, witnessing bullying (etc.), and teacher and peer reports. They reported d values but not the associated CI. For bullying others, $d=.04$. This was much smaller than the d value for being bullied, which was .27. It is not obvious why these two d values should be so different.

Mishna et al. (2009), in a Campbell review, assessed the effectiveness of programs designed to prevent cyber abuse, including cyber bullying and cyber pornography. Despite screening over 3000 works, only three evaluations were included in their review. Many of the outcomes focused on knowledge of cyber abuse and cyber safety and negative effects of cyber victimization. Only one of the three evaluations (of the HAHASO project) reported effects on cyber bullying. This decreased in the treatment group ($d=.37$, SE = .42), but it decreased even more in the control group ($d=.88$, SE = .48), and the change in the control group was not significantly greater than the change in the treatment group ($z=1.23$).

Smith et al. (2004) reviewed the effectiveness of whole-school antibullying programs. They found 14 evaluations, including eight with control conditions. They used r values to summarize the effect size of the controlled studies but did not calculate weighted mean r values or CI. The average r value for bullying was small ($r=.04$). In the best intervention conditions, they reported that 33% of r values were small (.10–.29), 50% were negligible (.00–.09), and 17% were negative. However, an r value of .1 corresponds approximately to a d value of .2, which in turn corresponds to an OR of 1.44, which is not negligible in our opinion. An r value of .1 would typically correspond to a 10% difference in recidivism probabilities (e.g. from 50 to 40%; see Farrington & Loeber, 1989), which is also not negligible in our opinion.

Vreeman and Carroll (2007) also aimed to assess the effectiveness of school-based interventions to prevent bullying. They identified 26 evaluations with a wide range of outcome measures. They summarized effect sizes for each outcome and each evaluation using only p values; this is the widely discredited "vote-counting" method. They concluded that 13 of the 26 studies showed clear reductions in bullying, but there were no measures in seven studies.

School Violence Programs

Dymnicki et al. (2011) aimed to investigate how elementary school-based violence prevention programs operated to reduce overt aggressive behavior (including fighting and bullying), by studying possible mediators. They used Hedges' g to summarize the effect size; this is very similar to d, differing only in using $(n-1)$ rather than (n) in estimating pooled variances. Therefore, we interpreted g as a d value. Over 26 studies and 36 comparisons, $d=.11$ (CI=.06–.16). Dymnicki et al. then investigated possible mediators, and concluded that social skills, aggressive attitudes, and classroom characteristics (e.g. the prevalence of behavior problems) were mediators.

Howard et al. (1999) aimed to evaluate the effectiveness of school violence prevention programs, and identified 13 evaluations. They measured a variety of outcomes, including aggression, violence, and bullying. Unfortunately, however, they only provided descriptive information on each evaluation (e.g. whether there was a decrease in aggression) and no specific effect sizes.

Mytton et al. (2002, 2006), in a Cochrane review, assessed 44 randomized controlled trials of school-based violence prevention programs. In 28 of these trials, there was an outcome measure of aggressive behavior (including parent and teacher ratings of antisocial behavior). The weighted mean d value was $-.36$ (CI=$-.19$ to $-.54$), indicating that the programs were successful in reducing aggression. Their effectiveness was somewhat greater in secondary schools ($d=-.43$) than in primary schools ($d=-.33$), but these values were not significantly different. The effects were smaller for programs delivered to boys alone, and larger studies found smaller effects.

Social Information Processing

Wilson and Lipsey (2006a) reviewed the effectiveness of universal school-based social information processing interventions in reducing aggressive behavior, while Wilson and Lipsey (2006b) reviewed the effectiveness of these interventions for selected or indicated (i.e. at risk) populations. Both of these reviews were published by the Campbell Collaboration. These reviews target individual risk factors and could have been classified as individual reviews, but we classified them as school-based reviews. The universal review was based on 73 evaluations, while the selected review was based on 47 evaluations. The weighted mean effect size (d) was .21 in the universal review and .26 in the selected review, equivalent to OR of 1.46 and 1.60, respectively. Unfortunately, CI were not reported in either case, so these results are not shown in Table 2.4. Moderator variables were studied in each review (see Table 2.1). For universal programs, the most important moderators were the level of attrition and the nature of the school, with high attrition and special education schools both associated with smaller effect sizes. For selected programs, the most important moderators were implementation quality, frequency of sessions, low-SES children (all positively related to effect size) and whether the program was implemented in routine practice, which was negatively related to effect size.

Cognitive-Behavioral Programs in Schools

Robinson et al. (1999) reviewed 23 evaluations of school-based cognitive-behavioral programs with hyperactivity-impulsivity and aggressive outcomes. These programs also target individual risk factors in school settings. The aggressive outcomes were measured by observation or by behavior checklists completed by teachers and/or students. For 12 studies with aggressive outcomes, the weighted mean $d=.64$, with a standard deviation of .57. This converts into a standard error of .165, so that this d value was significant. Robinson et al. investigated several moderators but did not find that any of them were significantly related to the effect size.

Sukhodolsky et al. (2004) reviewed studies of cognitive-behavioral therapy for anger in children and adolescents, most of which were based in schools. They found 40 studies, with 51 treatment–control comparisons. For 36 comparisons with aggression outcomes (including disruptive behavior), they reported that the mean $d=.63$ with a standard deviation of .35. This converts into a standard error of .058, so that this d value was significant. Sukhodolsky et al. investigated several moderators, but the only significant result was that d was greater when the control group received no treatment.

Conclusions

Main Results

In this chapter, 33 systematic reviews of developmental prevention programs have been summarized: three general reviews, five reviews of individually focused interventions such as child skills training programs, eight reviews of family-based programs, and 17 reviews of school-based programs (four of which were individually focused). It was possible to calculate effect sizes and CI from 22 reviews: three general reviews, four individual reviews, six family reviews, and nine school reviews. Figure 2.1 shows the forest plot.

The good news is that every summary OR effect size was greater than 1, indicating that the program was effective. Furthermore, the effect size was statistically significant in 18 out of 22 cases; all except Suter and Bruns (2009), Littell (2008), Park-Higgerson et al. (2008), and Wilson et al. (2001). The median OR was 1.55 and the interquartile range was from 1.27 to 2.20. It is not possible to carry out a meta-analysis of these OR because they are not all independent; in quite a few cases, the same evaluation was included in more than one systematic review.

With regard to practice these effects are quite large. For example, an OR=1.46 was obtained in the Wilson and Lipsey (2007) review, based on $d=.21$. They help-

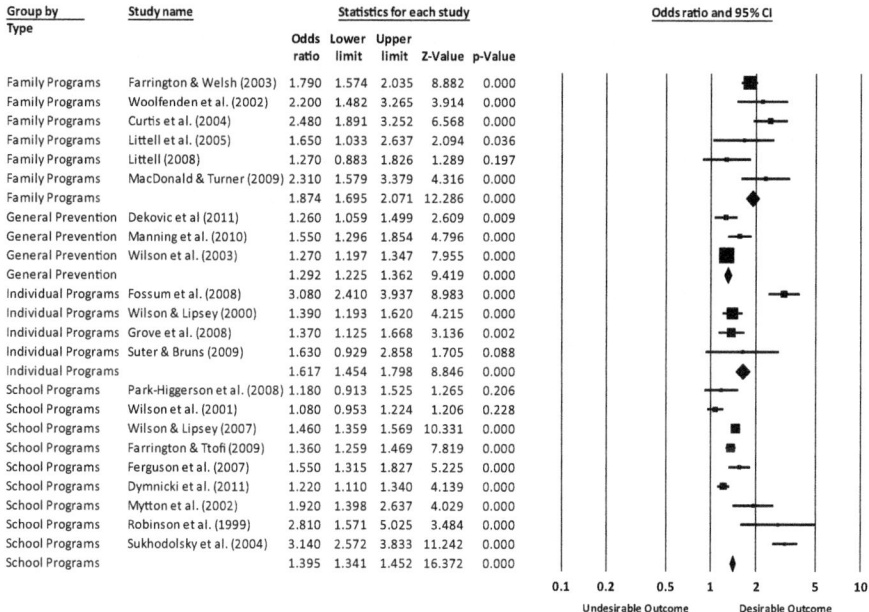

Fig. 2.1 Forest graph for the meta-analyses that provided confidence intervals

fully say (p. 141) that $d=.21$ corresponds to a reduction from a prevalence of 20% to about 15%, or a one-quarter reduction in aggression. Assuming 100 children in the treatment group and 100 children in the control group, and assuming that 20 children in the control group were aggressive, OR=1.55 corresponds to 13.9 children in the treatment group being aggressive, or a reduction in aggression of over 30%. This is not a small effect.

The median OR was 1.27 in the general reviews, 1.37 in the individual reviews, 1.79 in the family reviews, and 1.46 in the school-based reviews. While the number of reviews was too small to draw definitive conclusions, it is possible that the family-based interventions were the most effective.

Discussion

The present assessment of systematic reviews and meta-analyses follows earlier approaches that integrated meta-analyses to provide the most robust evidence on the effectiveness of interventions (e.g. Lipsey & Wilson, 1993; Lösel, 1995). Since then, the importance of developmental prevention has increased greatly in research and practice. We offer the following observations.

Numerous moderators of effect size are important (see the last column of Table 2.3). As the various reviews analyzed different kinds of moderators, a systematic comparison across the studies is not possible. However, the systematic investi-

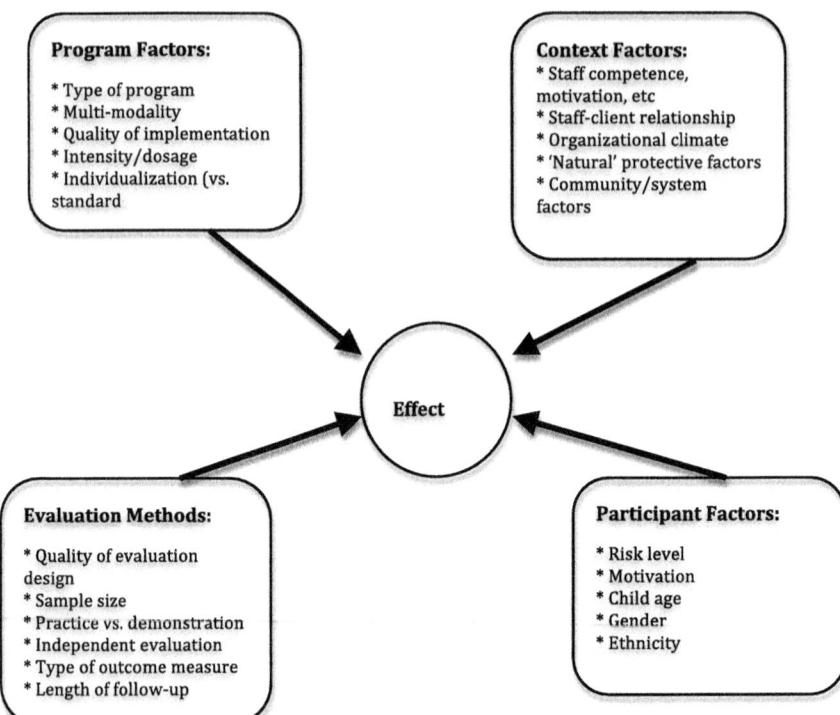

Fig. 2.2 Factors that may influence the effect of developmental and social prevention programs on child behavior problems

gation of moderator effects is a key task for the future because it would help to make developmental prevention programs more effective. As suggested by Lösel (2012), potential moderators can be grouped into four types: (a) program, (b) context, (c) participants, and (d) evaluation method (see Fig. 2.2).

Program Factors As shown in various meta-analyses, the *content* of a prevention program is relevant for its effect (e.g. Fossum et al., 2008; Lösel & Beelmann, 2006; Manning et al., 2010). Many interventions are multimodal, making it difficult to identify the "active ingredient." Effective programs should also aim at targeting *multiple agents* in the children's social system (Curtis et al., 2004; Farrington & Ttofi, 2009). Although manual-based delivery in a structured group format can be more reliable and less expensive, various meta-analyses suggest that a more *individualized approach* that serves the specific needs of a family and a child is particularly promising (Curtis et al., 2004; Nowak & Heinrichs, 2008). Although more intensive programs do not always have larger effects (e.g. Beelmann, Pfost, & Schmitt, 2014; Wilson & Lipsey, 2000), various studies suggest that *intensity/dosage* is an important program characteristic (e.g. Deković et al., 2011; Farrington & Ttofi, 2009; Hahn et al., 2007; Manning et al., 2010). Partially, this issue is confounded with selective/indicated prevention. As in other fields, the *quality (integrity, fidelity) of* *delivery* is important for effective prevention (e.g. Durlak & DuPre, 2008; Wilson & Lipsey, 2007). Therefore, systematic knowledge from implementation science (e.g. Fixsen, Blase, Naoom, & Wallace, 2009) needs to be used in practice.

Context Factors The above reviews rarely addressed specific *staff factors*, but other fields of prevention clearly show that staff competence, motivation, training, and supervision are important in psychosocial interventions (e.g. Durlak & DuPre, 2008; Dusenbury, Brannigan, Falco, & Hansen, 2003; Fixsen et al., 2009). As evaluations of the Nurse-Family-Partnership program have shown, effects may be lower when less qualified staff are delivering the program (Bilukha et al., 2005; Olds, Henderson, Cole, Eckenrode, Kitzman, Luckey, Pettitt, Sidora, Morris, & Powers, 1998). The *staff–client relationship* is relevant for sound program delivery. As psychotherapy research suggests, the quality of the relationship can have as much influence as the type of program (Orlinsky, Grawe, & Parks 1994). A good relationship with participants will also contribute to regular attendance, low dropout, and more consumer satisfaction. Staff features are part of the broader *organizational climate* of the institution that delivers the prevention program. For example, characteristics of the school environment are important moderators of program effectiveness (e.g. Dymnicki & The Multisite Violence Prevention Project, 2014; Farrington & Ttofi, 2009; Hahn et al., 2007). Prevention institutions need systematic (but not too bureaucratic) documentation, staff feedback strategies, an administration that supports the practical work, and close relations to other institutions in the community (Curtis et al., 2004; Fixsen et al., 2009). As with MST, the network can help to counteract problems of an isolated program delivery. Beyond the institutional level, developmental prevention should try to make use of *protective factors* in informal social networks such as the wider family, friends, or neighbors (Lösel & Farrington, 2012).

Participant Factors A replicable moderator of effect size is the *risk level* of the child and the family. Evaluations of indicated prevention tend to show larger effects than universal programs (e.g. Farrington & Welsh, 2003; Weiss, Schmucker, & Lösel, 2015). This is plausible because targeted prevention addresses children or families with stronger needs, whereas universal approaches are delivered to many participants who would not develop serious problems even in the absence of any program. However, as in preventive medicine, universal programs can be implemented more easily and can also reach the groups who are most in need of help (e.g. Coid, 2003; Rose, 1992). Promoting *participant motivation* is one of the biggest challenges in developmental crime prevention. Whereas middle-class mothers are often interested in parenting programs, it is difficult to reach at-risk parents from deprived backgrounds. In routine practice, typical recruitment rates rarely exceed one third of the target population and some ethnic minorities are particularly difficult to recruit (Runkel, Lösel, Stemmler, & Jaursch, 2013; Staudt, 2007). *Ethnicity, child age, and gender* also need to be considered as potential moderators (e.g. Deković et al., 2011; Fossum et al., 2008; Grove et al., 2008; Hahn et al., 2007; Mytton et al., 2002). However, intervention at a younger child age does not generally lead to better effects (e.g. Farrington & Welsh, 2003; Lösel & Beelmann, 2003; Ttofi & Farrington, 2012).

Methodological Factors Various reviews show that methodological characteristics of the outcome evaluation are highly important moderators. With regard to the overall *design quality*, the findings are mixed: some reviews found stronger effects in randomized controlled trial designs and others found stronger effects in weaker designs (e.g. Bilukha et al., 2005; Curtis et al., 2004; Littell et al., 2005; Suter & Bruns, 2009; Wilson et al., 2001, 2003a). There is a clear relation between effect size and *sample size*. Generally, smaller studies show larger effects (e.g. Farrington & Welsh, 2003; Fossum et al., 2008; Lösel & Beelmann, 2003; Mytton et al., 2002; Weiss et al., 2015; Wilson et al., 2003a). This may partly be attributable to publication bias: Significant results in smaller studies may be published while nonsignificant results are not, whereas all results in larger studies are published. However, problems of maintaining program integrity in large studies may also be relevant, suggesting that a broad (e.g. nationwide) roll-out of prevention programs needs a great deal of effort in order to ensure a good quality of delivery. Smaller studies are often carried out as *demonstration/model projects*. Therefore, as in other fields of psychosocial intervention, one should expect lower effectiveness in routine practice than in demonstration projects (e.g. Curtis et al., 2004; Wilson et al., 2003). Also, *self-evaluations* by program developers or deliverers tend to produce larger effects than studies by independent evaluators (e.g. Eisner, 2009; Littell et al., 2005; Wilson et al., 2003). The *kind of outcome measurement* is also related to effect size (e.g. Lösel & Beelmann, 2003; Grove et al., 2008; Nowak & Heinrichs, 2008). As a trend, there are smaller effects with objective measures of child behavior than with proximal measures of attitudes, behavior, and knowledge that are related to the program content. Also, outcome measures that are closer to the intervention (e.g. parent ratings after a parenting program) may show larger effects than more independent outcome measures (e.g. teacher ratings after a parenting program). Also, immediate post-treatment or short *follow-up measurement* tends to show larger effects than outcome measurements after longer follow-up periods (e.g. Grove et al., 2008; Littell et al., 2005; Lösel & Beelmann, 2006).

Research Implications

Clearly, more systematic reviews of developmental prevention are needed. It was noticeable that the Campbell (and Cochrane) reviews were generally of better quality than other reviews. Therefore, all systematic reviews should be carried out according (at least) to the standards of the Campbell Collaboration. In particular, each review should:

- set clear criteria for inclusion and exclusion of studies;
- carry out extensive searches of bibliographic databases (not just Google Scholar), backed up by hand searches of key journals and contacts with key researchers;
- set methodological quality standards for the primary studies, preferably including only randomized controlled trials with pretest measures and setting a minimum sample size for inclusion;

- carefully specify how many reports were found, screened, included, and excluded;
- code and report characteristics of studies (e.g. research design, implementation quality, nature of control condition, number and characteristics of participants, attrition, whether it is a demonstration project or routine practice, whether the treatment developer is also the evaluator) and components of the intervention (including the duration and intensity of the treatment);
- specify effect sizes, weighted mean effect sizes, and CI;
- investigate moderators by studying how the characteristics of studies and intervention components are related to effect sizes (see, e.g. Gardner, Hutchings, & Bywater, 2010; Kaminski et al., 2008).

Ideally, more primary evaluations are needed with high methodological quality (e.g. randomized controlled trials). Ideally, long-term follow-ups are needed to investigate the persistence of effects (Farrington & Welsh, 2013). Ideally, more primary evaluations should include a cost–benefit analysis (see, e.g. Farrington & Koegl, 2015) and systematic reviews should attempt to summarize the results of these cost–benefit analyses.

Policy Implications

In general, developmental prevention is effective, whether targeted on individuals, families, or schools. Therefore, it is justifiable to continue and preferably increase investment in developmental prevention. This chapter has shown that there are numerous more or less well-controlled evaluations of programs that aim to prevent aggression, delinquency, and violence in childhood and youth. The findings are rather variable, but overall very encouraging. In our view, there is less need to develop more and more programs than to further investigate the most promising approaches. To consolidate and advance the current evidence base and ensure quality management in daily practice, it is necessary to take into account many factors, such as characteristics of the program, the context, the target groups, and also the evaluation methodology. Policy-makers should further invest in systematic and large scale approaches to promote the quality of program implementation and sound outcome evaluation. Intervention policies should be sustainable, cross-departmental, independent from lobbyists, and based on realistic expectations about effectiveness. As "early starters" contribute to a large proportion of total offending (e.g. Farrington & Welsh, 2007; Moffitt, 1993), an increased investment in developmental prevention policies would make an important contribution to reducing crime and violence. And this investment would also pay off in financial terms. Typically, the benefits of developmental prevention greatly outweigh the costs (e.g. Aos, Lieb, Mayfield, Miller, & Pennucci, 2004; Welsh, Farrington, & Raffan Gowar, 2015).

Acknowledgment We are very grateful to B. Raffan Gowar for her assistance with literature searches.

References

Aos, S., Lieb, R., Mayfield, J., Miller, M., & Pennucci, A. (2004). *Benefits and costs of prevention and early intervention programs for youth*. Olympia: Washington State Institute for Public Policy.

Axford, N., Sontalia, S., Wrigley, Z., Goodwin, A., Ohlsen, C., Bjornstad, G., Barlow, J., Schrader-McMillan, A., Coad, J., & Toft, A. (2015). *The best start at home: A report on what works to improve the quality of parent-child interactions from conception to age 5*. London: Early Intervention Foundation.

Babcock, J. C., Green, C. E., & Robie, C. (2004). Does batterers' treatment work? A meta-analytic review of domestic violence treatment. *Clinical Psychology Review, 23*, 1023–1053.

Baldry, A. C., & Farrington, D. P. (2007). Effectiveness of programs to prevent school bullying. *Victims and Offenders, 2*, 183–204.

Barlow, J., & Parsons, J. (2009). Group-based parent-training programmes for improving emotional and behavioural adjustment in 0–3 year old children. *The Cochrane Library, 2009*, 1.

Barlow, J., Parsons, J., & Stewart-Brown, S. (2005). Preventing emotional and behavioural problems: The effectiveness of parenting programmes with children less than 3 years of age. *Child Care, Health & Development, 31*, 33–42.

Beelmann, A., & Raabe, T. (2009). The effects of preventing antisocial behavior and crime in childhood and adolescence: Results and implications of research reviews and meta-analyses. *European Journal of Developmental Science, 3*, 260–281.

Beelmann, A., Pfingsten, U., & Lösel, F. (1994). Effects of training social competence in children: A meta-analysis of recent evaluation studies. *Journal of Clinical Child Psychology, 23*, 260–271.

Beelmann, A., Pfost, M., & Schmitt, C. (2014). Prävention und Gesundheitsförderung bei Kindern und Jugendlichen. Eine Meta-Analyse der deutschsprachigen Wirksamkeitsforschung. [Prevention and health promotion in children and youth: A meta-analysis of outcome evaluations in German-speaking countries]. *Zeitschrift für Gesundheitspsychologie, 22*, 1–14.

Bennett, D. S., & Gibbons, T. A. (2000). Efficacy of child cognitive-behavioral interventions for antisocial behavior: A meta-analysis. *Child & Family Behavior Therapy, 22*, 1–15.

Bernazzani, O., & Tremblay, R. E. (2006). Early parent training. In B. C. Welsh & D. P. Farrington (Eds.), *Preventing crime: What works for children, offenders, victims and places* (pp. 21–32). Dordrecht: Springer.

Bilukha, O., Hahn, R. A., Crosby, A., Fullilove, M. T., Liberman, A., Moscicki, E., Snyder, S., Tuma, F., Corso, P., Scholfield, A., & Briss, P. A. (2005). The effectiveness of early childhood home visitation in preventing violence: A systematic review. *American Journal of Preventive Medicine, 28*, 11–39.

Brestan, E. V., & Eyberg, S. M. (1998). Effective psychosocial treatments of conduct-disordered children and adolescents: 29 years, 82 studies, and 5272 kids. *Journal of Clinical Child Psychology, 27*, 180–189.

Butler, A. C., Chapman, J. E., Forman, E. M., & Beck, A. T. (2006). The empirical status of cognitive-behavioral therapy: A review of meta-analyses. *Clinical Psychology Review, 26*, 17–31.

Coid, J. W. (2003). Formulating strategies for the primary prevention of adult antisocial behaviour: "high risk" or "population" strategies? In D. P. Farrington & J. W. Coid (Eds.), *Prevention of adult antisocial behavior* (pp. 32–78). Cambridge: Cambridge University Press.

Cooper, H., Charlton, K., Valentine, J. C., & Muhlenbruck, L. (2000). Making the most of summer school: A meta-analytic and narrative review. *Monographs of the Society for Research in Child Development, 65*(1), 1–117.

Curtis, N. M., Ronan, K. R., & Borduin, C. M. (2004). Multisystemic treatment: A meta-analysis of outcome studies. *Journal of Family Psychology, 18*, 411–419.

De Graaf, I. M., Speetjens, P., Smit, F., De Wolff, M., & Tavecchio, L. (2008). Effectiveness of the Triple P Positive Parenting Program on behavioral problems in children: A meta-analysis. *Behavior Modification, 32*, 714–735.

Deković, M., Slagt, M. I., Asscher, J. J., Boendermaker, L., Eichelsheim, V. I., & Prinzie, P. (2011). Effects of early prevention programs on adult criminal offending: A meta-analysis. *Clinical Psychology Review, 31*, 532–544.

DiGuiseppe, & Tafrate, R. C. (2003). Anger treatments for adults: A meta-analytic review. *Clinical Psychology: Science and Practice, 10*, 70–84.

Dretzke, J., Davenport, C., Frew, E., Barlow, J., Stewart-Brown, S., Bayliss, S., Taylor, R.S., Sandercock, J., & Hyde, C. (2009). The clinical effectiveness of different parenting programmes for children with conduct problems: A systematic review of randomised controlled trials. *Child and Adolescent Psychiatry Mental Health, 3*, 7.

Durlak, J. A., & DuPre, E. P. (2008). Implementation matters: A review of research on the influence of implementation on program outcomes and the factors affecting implementation. *American Journal of Community Psychology, 41*, 327–350.

Durlak, J. A., Fuhrman, T., & Lampman, C. (1991). Effectiveness of cognitive-behavior therapy for maladaptive children: A meta-analysis. *Psychological Bulletin, 110*, 204–214.

Durlak, J. A., Weissberg, R. P., & Pachan, M. (2010). A meta-analysis of after-school programs that seek to promote personal and social skills in children and adolescents. *American Journal of Community Psychology, 45*, 294–309.

Durlak, J. A., Weissberg, R. P., Dymnicki, A. B., Taylor, R. D., & Schellinger, K. P. (2011). The impact of enhancing students' social and emotional learning: A meta-analysis of school-based universal interventions. *Child Development, 82*, 405–432.

Dusenbury, L., Brannigan, R., Falco, M., & Hansen, W. (2003). A review of research on fidelity of implementation: Implications for drug abuse prevention in school settings. *Health Education Research, 18*, 237–256.

Dymnicki, A. B., & The Multisite Violence Prevention Project. (2014). Moderating effects of school climate on outcomes for the Multisite Violence Prevention Project universal program. *Journal of Research on Adolescence, 24*, 383–398.

Dymnicki, A. B., Weissberg, R. P., & Henry, D. B. (2011). Understanding how programs work to prevent overt aggressive behaviors: A meta-analysis of mediators of elementary school–based programs. *Journal of School Violence, 10*, 315–337.

Eisner, M. (2009). No effects in independent prevention trials: Can we reject the cynical view? *Journal of Experimental Criminology, 5*, 163–183.

Evans, C. B. R., Fraser, M. W., & Cotter, K. L. (2014). The effectiveness of school-based bullying prevention programs: A systematic review. *Aggression and Violent Behavior, 19*, 532–544.

Eyberg, S. M., Nelson, M. M., & Boggs, S. R. (2008). Evidence-based psychosocial treatments for children and adolescents with disruptive behavior. *Journal of Clinical Child & Adolescent Psychology, 37*, 215–237.

Fabiano, G. A., Pelham, W. E., Coles, E. K., Gnagy, E. M., Chronis-Tuscano, A., & O'Connor, B. C. (2009). A meta-analysis of behavioral treatments for attention-deficit/hyperactivity disorder. *Clinical Psychology Review, 29*, 129–140.

Faggiano, F., Vigna-Taglianti, F., Burkhart, G., Bohrn, K., Cuomo, L., Gregori, D., Panella, M., Scatigna, M., Siliquini, R., Varona, L., van der Kreeft, P., Vassara, M., Wiborg, G., & Galanti, M.R., & the EU-Dap Study Group (2010). The effectiveness of a school-based substance abuse prevention program: 18-month follow-up of the EU-Dap cluster randomized controlled trial. *Drug and Alcohol Dependence, 2010*, 256–264.

Farahmand, F. K., Grant, K. E., Polo, A. J., & Duffy, S. N. (2011). School-based mental health and behavioral programs for low-income, urban youth: A systematic and meta-analytic review. *Clinical Psychology: Science and Practice, 18*, 372–390.

Farrington, D. P. (1983). Randomized experiments on crime and justice. In M. Tonry & N. Morris (Eds.), *Crime and justice: An annual review of research* (Vol. 4, pp. 257–308). Chicago: University of Chicago Press.

Farrington, D. P., & Loeber, R. (1989). Relative improvement over chance (RIOC) and phi as measures of predictive efficiency and strength of association in 2 × 2 tables. *Journal of Quantitative Criminology, 5*(3), 201–213.

Farrington, D. P. (2006). Key longitudinal-experimental studies in criminology. *Journal of Experimental Criminology, 2,* 121–141.

Farrington, D. P. (2013). Longitudinal and experimental research in criminology. In M. Tonry (Ed.), *Crime and Justice in America 1975–2025* (pp. 453–527). Chicago: University of Chicago Press.

Farrington, D. P., & Ttofi, M. M. (2009). School-based programs to reduce bullying and victimization. *Campbell Systematic Reviews, 5*(6). http://www.campbellcollaboration.org/lib/project/77/.

Farrington, D. P., & Welsh, B. C. (2003). Family-based prevention of offending: A meta-analysis. *Australian and New Zealand Journal of Criminology, 36,* 127–151.

Farrington, D. P., & Welsh, B. C. (2005). Randomized experiments in criminology: What have we learned in the last two decades? *Journal of Experimental Criminology, 1,* 9–38.

Farrington, D. P., & Welsh, B. C. (2006). A half-century of randomized experiments on crime and justice. In M. Tonry (Ed.), *Crime and justice, vol. 34* (pp. 55–132). Chicago: University of Chicago Press.

Farrington, D. P., & Welsh, B. C. (2007). *Saving children from a life of crime: Early risk factors and effective interventions.* New York: Oxford University Press.

Farrington, D. P., & Welsh, B. C. (2013). Randomized experiments in criminology: What has been learned from long-term follow-ups? In B. C. Welsh, A. A. Braga, & G. J. N. Bruinsma (Eds.), *Experimental criminology: Prospects for advancing science and public policy* (pp. 111–140). New York: Cambridge University Press.

Farrington, D. P., Loeber, R., & Welsh, B. C. (2010). Longitudinal-experimental studies. In A. R. Piquero & D. Weisburd (Eds.), *Handbook of quantitative criminology* (pp. 503–518). New York: Springer.

Farrington, D. P., & Koegl, C. J. (2015). Monetary benefits and costs of the Stop Now And Plan Program for boys aged 6–11, based on the prevention of later offending. *Journal of Quantitative Criminology, 31*(1), 263–287.

Farrington, D. P., Weisburd, D. L., & Gill, C. E. (2011). The Campbell Collaboration Crime and Justice Group: A decade of progress. In C. J. Smith, S. X. Zhang, & R. Barberet (Eds.), *Routledge handbook of international criminology* (pp. 53–63). New York: Routledge.

Ferguson, C. J., San Miguel, C., Kilburn, J. C., & Sanchez, P. (2007). The effectiveness of school-based anti-bullying programs: A meta-analytic review. *Criminal Justice Review, 32,* 401–414.

Fisher, H., Montgomery, P., & Gardner, F. (2008a). Cognitive-behavioural interventions for preventing youth gang involvement for children and young people (7–16): A systematic review. *Campbell Systematic Reviews, 4*(7). http://www.campbellcollaboration.org/lib/project/39/.

Fisher, H., Montgomery, P., & Gardner, F. (2008b). Opportunities provision for preventing youth gang involvement for children and young people (7–16): A systematic review. *Campbell Systematic Reviews, 4*(8). http://www.campbellcollaboration.org/lib/project/40/.

Fixsen, D. L., Blase, K. A., Naoom, S. F., & Wallace, F. (2009). Core implementation components. *Research on Social Work, 19,* 531–540.

Forness, S. R., & Kavale, K. A. (1996). Treating social skill deficits in children with learning disabilities: A meta-analysis of the research. *Learning Disability Quarterly, 19,* 2–13.

Fossum, S., Handega, B. H., Martinussen, M., & Morch, W. T. (2008). Psychosocial interventions for disruptive and aggressive behaviour in children and adolescents: A meta-analysis. *European Child & Adolescent Psychiatry, 17,* 438–451.

Furlong, M., McGilloway, S., Bywater, T., Hutchings, J., Smith, S. M., & Donnelly, M. (2012). Behavioural and cognitive-behavioural group-based parenting programmes for early-onset conduct problems in children aged 3–12 years. *Campbell Systematic Reviews, 8*(12). http://www.campbellcollaboration.org/lib/project/251/.

Gansle, K. A. (2005). The effectiveness of school-based anger interventions and programs: A meta-analysis. *Journal of School Psychology, 43,* 321–341.

Gardner, F., Hutchings, J., & Bywater, T. (2010). Who benefits and how does it work? Moderators and mediators of outcome in a randomised trial of parenting interventions in multiple 'Sure Start' services. *Journal of Clinical Child and Adolescent Psychology, 39,* 568–580.

Garrard, W. M., & Lipsey, M. W. (2007). Conflict resolution education and antisocial behavior in U.S. schools: A meta-analysis. *Conflict Resolution Quarterly, 25*, 9–38.

Garrett, C. J. (1985). Effects of residential treatment on adjudicated delinquents: A meta-analysis. *Journal of Research on Crime and Delinquency, 22*, 287–308.

Gilliam, W. S., & Zigler, E. F. (2000). A critical meta-analysis of all evaluations of state-funded preschool from 1977 to 1998: Implications for policy, service delivery, and program implementation. *Early Childhood Research Quarterly, 15*, 441–473.

Gottfredson, D., & Wilson, D. (2003). Characteristics of effective school-based substance abuse prevention. *Prevention Science, 4*, 27–38.

Grove, A., Evans, S., Pastor, D., & Mack, M. (2008). A meta-analytic examination of follow-up studies designed to prevent the primary symptoms of oppositional defiant and conduct disorders. *Aggression and Violent Behavior, 13*, 169–184.

Hahn, R., Fuqua-Whitley, D., Wethington, H., Lowy, J., Crosby, A., Fullilove, M., Johnson, R., Liberman, A., Moscicki, E., Price, L. S., Snyder, S., Tuma, F., Cory, S., Stone, G., Mukhopadhaya, K., Chattopadhyay, S., Dahlberg, L., & Task Force on Community Preventive Services (2007). Effectiveness of universal school-based programs to prevent violent and aggressive behavior: A systematic review. *American Journal of Preventive Medicine, 33*, 114–129.

Hawkins, D. J., Brown, E. C., Oesterle, S., Arthur, M. W., Abbott, R. D., & Catalano, R. F. (2008). Early effects of Communities That Care on targeted risks and initiation of delinquent behavior and substance use. *Journal of Adolescent Health, 43*, 15–22.

Henggeler, S. W., Schoenwald, S. K., & Swenson, C. C. (2006). Methodological critique and meta-analysis as Trojan horse. *Children and Youth Services Review, 28*, 447–457.

Henggeler, S. W., Schoenwald, S. K., Borduin, C. M., Rowland, M. D., & Cunningham, P. B. (2009). *Multisystemic treatment of antisocial behavior in children and adolescents* (2nd edn.). New York: Guilford Press.

Howard, K. A., Flora, J., & Griffin, M. (1999). Violence-prevention programs in schools: State of science and implications for future research. *Applied and Preventive Psychology, 8*, 197–215.

Huey, S. J. Jr., & Polo, A. J. (2008). Evidence-based psychosocial treatments for ethnic minority youth. *Journal of Clinical Child & Adolescent Psychology, 37*, 262–301.

Kaminski, W., Valle, L. A., Filene, J. H., & Boyle, C. L. (2008). A meta-analytic review of components associated with parent training program effectiveness. *Journal of Abnormal Child Psychology, 36*, 567–589.

Lauer, P. A., Akiba, M., Wilkerson, S. B., Apthorp, H. S., Snow, D., & Martin-Glenn, M. L. (2006). Out-of-school time programs: A meta-analysis of effects for at-risk students. *Review of Educational Research, 76*, 275–313.

Leen, E., Sorbring, E., Mawer, M., Holdsworth, E., Helsing, B., & Bowen, E. (2013). Prevalence, dynamic risk factors and the efficacy of primary interventions for adolescent dating violence: An international review. *Aggression and Violent Behavior, 18*, 159–174.

Leschied, A. W., & Cunningham, A. (2002). *Seeking effective interventions for serious young offenders: Interim results of a four-year randomized study of multisystemic therapy in Ontario, Canada.* London: Centre for Children & Families in Justice.

Lipsey, M. W. (2009). The primary factors that characterize effective interventions with juvenile offenders: A meta-analytic overview. *Victims and Offenders, 4*, 124–147.

Lipsey, M. W., & Wilson, D. B. (1993). The efficacy of psychological, educational, and behavioral treatment: Confirmation from meta-analysis. *American Psychologist, 48*, 1181–1209.

Littell, J. H. (2005). Lessons from a systematic review of effects of multisystemic therapy. *Children and Youth Services Review, 27*, 445–463.

Littell, J. H. (2006). The case for Multisystemic Therapy: Evidence or orthodoxy? *Children and Youth Services Review, 28*, 458–472.

Littell, J. H. (2008). *Systematic review of Multisystemic Therapy: An update.* www.campbellcollaboration.org/artman2/.../Littell_MST_update.pdf.

Littell, J. H., Popa, M., & Forsythe, B. (2005). Multisystemic Therapy for social, emotional, and behavioral problems in youth aged 10–17: A systematic review. *Campbell Systematic Reviews, 1*(1). http://www.campbellcollaboration.org/lib/project/5/.

Littell, J. H., Winswold, A., Bjorndal, A., & Hammerstrom, K. T. (2007). *Functional family therapy for families of youth (age 11–18) with behaviour problems.* Protocol in the Cochrane Library, 2009, Issue 4, www.thecochranelibrary.com.

Lösel, F. (1995). The efficacy of correctional treatment: A review and synthesis of recent meta-evaluations. In J. McGuire (Ed.), *What works: Effective methods to reduce re-offending* (pp. 79–111). Chichester: Wiley.

Lösel, F. (2012). Entwicklungsbezogene Prävention von Gewalt und Kriminalität: Ansätze und Wirkungen [Developmental prevention of violence and crime. Approaches and effects]. *Forensische Psychiatrie, Psychologie und Kriminologie, 6*, 71–84.

Lösel, F., & Beelmann, A. (2003). Effects of child skills training in preventing antisocial behavior: A systematic review of randomized evaluations. *Annals of the American Academy of Political and Social Science, 587*, 84–109.

Lösel, F., & Beelmann, A. (2006). Child social skills training. In B. C. Welsh & D. P. Farrington (Eds.), *Preventing crime: What works for children, offenders, victims, and places* (pp. 33–54). Dordrecht: Springer.

Lösel, F., & Bender, D. (2012). Child social skills training in the prevention of antisocial development and crime. In D. P. Farrington & B. C. Welsh (Eds.), *Handbook of crime prevention* (pp. 102–129). Oxford: Oxford University Press.

Lösel, F., & Farrington, D. P. (2012). Direct protective and buffering protective factors in the development of youth violence. *American Journal of Preventive Medicine, 43*(2 S1), 8–23.

Luke, N., & Banerjee, R. (2012). Differentiated associations between childhood maltreatment experiences and social understanding: A meta-analysis and systematic review. *Developmental Review, 33*, 1–28.

Lundahl, B., Risser, H. J., & Lovejoy, M. C. (2006). A meta-analysis of parent training: Moderators and follow-up effects. *Clinical Psychology Review, 26*, 86–104.

MacDonald, G., & Turner, W. (2007). Treatment foster care for improving outcomes in children and young people. *Campbell Systematic Reviews, 4*(9). http://www.campbellcollaboration.org/lib/project/32/.

Maggin, D. M., Chafouleas, S. M., Goddard, K. M., & Johnson, A. H. (2011). A systematic evaluation of token economies as a classroom management tool for students with challenging behavior. *Journal of School Psychology, 49*, 529–554.

Maggin, D. M., Johnson, A. H., Chafouleas, S. M., Roberto, L. M., & Bergren, M. (2012). A systematic evidence review of school-based group contingency interventions for students with challenging behavior. *Journal of School Psychology, 50*, 625–654.

Manning, M., Homel, R., & Smith, C. (2010). A meta-analysis of the effects of early developmental prevention programs in at-risk populations on non-health outcomes in adolescence. *Children and Youth Services Review, 32*, 506–519.

Matjasko, J. L., Vivolo-Kantor, A. M., Massetti, G. M., Holland, K. M., Holt, M. K., & Dela Cruz, J. (2012). A systematic meta-review of evaluations of youth violence prevention programs: Common and divergent findings from 25 years of meta-analyses and systematic reviews. *Aggression and Violent Behavior, 17*, 240–252.

Maughan, D. R., Christiansen, E., Jenson, W. R, Olympia, D., & Clark, E. (2005). Behavioral parent training as a treatment for externalizing behaviors. *School Psychology Review, 34*, 267–286.

McCart, M. R., Priester, P. E., Davies, W. H., & Azen, R. (2006). Differential effectiveness of behavioral parent-training and cognitive-behavioral therapy for antisocial youth: A meta-analysis. *Journal of Abnormal Child Psychology, 34*, 527–543.

Merrell, K. W., Gueldner, B. A., Ross, S. W., & Isava, D. M. (2008). How effective are school bullying intervention programs? A meta-analysis of intervention research. *School Psychology Quarterly, 23*, 26–42.

Mishna, F., Cook, C., Saini, M., Wu, M.-J., & MacFadden, R. (2009). Interventions for children, youth, and parents to prevent and reduce cyber abuse. *Campbell Systematic Reviews, 5*(2). http://www.campbellcollaboration.org/lib/project/75/.

Moffitt, T. E. (1993). Adolescence-limited and life-course-persistent antisocial behavior: A developmental taxonomy. *Psychological Review, 100*, 674–701.

Montgomery, P., Bjornstad, G., & Dennis, J. (2007). Media-based behavioural treatments for behavioural problems in children (Review). *Evidence-Based Child Health: A Cochrane Review Journal, 2*, 1154–1190.

Mytton, J. A., DiGuiseppi, C., Gough, D. A., Taylor, R. S., & Logan, S. (2002). School-based violence prevention programs: Systematic review of secondary prevention trials. *Archives of Pediatric and Adolescent Medicine, 156*, 752–762.

Mytton, J. A., DiGuiseppi, C., Gough, D., Taylor, R., & Logan, S. (2006). School-based secondary prevention programs for preventing violence. *Cochrane Database of Systematic Reviews, 19*(3), CD004606.

Nowak, A. E., & Heinrichs, N. (2008). A comprehensive meta-analysis of Triple P-Positive Parenting Program using hierarchical linear modeling: Effectiveness and moderating variables. *Clinical Child and Family Psychology Review, 11*, 114–144.

Olds, D. L., Henderson, C. R., Cole, R., Eckenrode, J., Kitzman, H., Luckey, D., Pettitt, L., Sidora, K., Morris, P., & Powers, J. (1998). Long-term effects of nurse home visitation on children's criminal and antisocial behavior. *Journal of the American Medical Association, 280*, 1238–1244.

Orlinsky, D. E., Grawe, K., & Parks, B. K. (1994). Process and outcome in psychotherapy. In A. E. Bergin & S. L. Garfield (Eds.), *Handbook of psychotherapy and behavior change* (4th edn., pp. 270–376). New York: Wiley.

Park-Higgerson, H.-K., Perumean-Chaney, S. E., Bartolucci, A. A., Grimley, D. M., & Singh, K. P. (2008). The evaluation of school-based violence prevention programs: A meta-analysis. *Journal of School Health, 78*, 465–479.

Payton, J., Weissberg, R. P., Durlak, J. A., Dymnicki, A. B., Taylor, R. D., Schellinger, K. B., & Pachan, M. (2008). *The positive impact of social and emotional learning for kindergarten to eighth-grade students: Findings from three scientific reviews*. Chicago: Collaborative for Academic, Social, and Emotional Learning.

Piquero, A. R., Farrington, D. P., Welsh, B. C., Tremblay, R. E., & Jennings, W. G. (2008). Effects of early family/parent training programs on antisocial behavior and delinquency. *Campbell Systematic Reviews, 4*(11). http://www.campbellcollaboration.org/lib/project/43/.

Prout, S. M., & Prout, H. T. (1998). A Meta-analysis of school-based studies of counseling and psychotherapy: An update. *Journal of School Psychology, 36*, 121–136.

Reddy, L. A., Newman, E., De Thomas, C. A., & Chun, V. (2009). Effectiveness of school-based prevention and intervention programs for children and adolescents with emotional disturbance: A meta-analysis. *Journal of School Psychology, 47*, 77–99.

Reyno, S., & McGrath, P. J. (2005). Predictors of parent training efficacy for child externalizing behavior problems: A meta-analytic review. *Journal of Child Psychology and Psychiatry, 47*, 99–111.

Robinson, T. R., Smith, S. W., Miller, M. D., & Brownell, M. T. (1999). Cognitive behavior modification of hyperactivity-impulsivity and aggression: A meta-analysis of school-based studies. *Journal of Educational Psychology, 91*, 195–203.

Rose, G. (1992). *The strategy of preventive medicine*. Oxford: Oxford Medical Publications.

Runkel, D., Lösel, F., Stemmler, M., & Jaursch, S. (2013). Preventing social behavior problems in children from deprived migrant families: Evaluation of a child and parent training in Europe. (revise and resubmit).

Serketich, W. J., & Dumas, J. E. (1996). The effectiveness of behavioral parent training to modify antisocial behavior in children: A meta-analysis. *Behavior Therapy, 27*, 171–186.

Shadish, W. R., & Baldwin, S. A. (2003). Meta-analysis of MFT interventions. *Journal of Marital and Family Therapy, 29*, 547–570.

Smith, J. D., Schneider, B. H., Smith, P. K., & Ananiadou, K. (2004). The effectiveness of whole-school antibullying programs: A synthesis of evaluation research. *School Psychology Review, 33*, 548–561.

Solomon, B. G., Klein, S. A., Hintze, J. M., Cressey, J. M., & Peller, S. L. (2012). A meta-analysis of school-wide positive behavior support: An exploratory study using single-case synthesis. *Psychology in the Schools, 49*, 105–121.

Stanton, D. M., & Shadish, W. R. (1997). Outcome, attrition, and family-couples treatment for drug abuse: A meta-analysis and review of the controlled, comparative studies. *Psychological Bulletin, 122*, 170–191.

Staudt, M. (2007). Treatment engagement with caregivers of at-risk children: Gaps in research and conceptualization. *Journal of Child and Family Studies, 16*, 183–196.

Stoltz, S., Londen, M., Deković, M., Orobio de Castro, B., & Prinzie, P. (2012). Effectiveness of individually delivered indicated school-based interventions on externalizing behavior. *International Journal of Behavioral Development, 36*, 381–388.

Sukhodolsky, D. G., Kassinove, H., & Gorman, B. S. (2004). Cognitive-behavioral therapy for anger in children and adolescents: A meta-analysis. *Aggression and Violent Behavior, 9*, 247–269.

Suter, J. C., & Bruns, E. J. (2009). Effectiveness of the wraparound process for children with emotional and behavioral disorders: A meta-analysis. *Clinical Child and Family Psychology Review, 12*, 336–351.

Thomas, M., & Zimmer-Gembeck, M. J. (2007). Behavioral outcomes of parent-child interaction therapy and Triple P-Positive Parenting Program: A review and meta-analysis. *Journal of Abnormal Child Psychology, 35*, 475–495.

Tong, L. S. J., & Farrington, D. P. (2006). How effective is the Reasoning and Rehabilitation programme in reducing offending? A meta-analysis of evaluations in four countries. *Psychology, Crime and Law, 12*, 3–24.

Tong, L. S. J., & Farrington, D. P. (2008). Effectiveness of "Reasoning and rehabilitation" in reducing reoffending. *Psicothema, 20*(1), 20–28.

Ttofi, M. M., & Farrington, D. P. (2011). Effectiveness of school-based programs to reduce bullying: A systematic and meta-analytic review. *Journal of Experimental Criminology, 7*, 27–56.

Ttofi, M. M., & Farrington, D. P. (2012). Bullying prevention programs: The importance of peer intervention, disciplinary methods, and age variations. *Journal of Experimental Criminology, 8*, 443–462.

Ttofi, M. M., Eisner, M., & Bradshaw, C. P. (2014). Bullying prevention: Assessing existing meta-evaluations. In G. J. N. Bruinsma & D. L. Weisburd (Eds.), *Encyclopedia of criminology and criminal justice* (pp. 231–242). New York: Springer.

Vreeman, R. C., & Carroll, A. C. (2007). A systematic review of school-based interventions to prevent bullying. *Archives of Pediatrics and Adolescent Medicine, 161*, 78–88.

Walker, D. F., McGovern, S. K., Poey, E. L., & Otis, K. E. (2008). Treatment effectiveness for male adolescent sexual offenders: A meta-analysis and review. *Journal of Child Sexual Abuse, 13*, 281–293.

Weiss, M., Schmucker, M., & Lösel, F. (2015). Meta-Analyse zur Wirkung familien-bezogener Präventionsmaßnahmen in Deutschland [Meta-analysis on the effects of family-oriented prevention programs in Germany]. *Zeitschrift für Klinische Psychologie und Psychotherapie, 44*, 27–44.

Weisz, J. R., Jensen-Doss, A., & Hawley, K. M. (2006). Evidence-based youth psychotherapies versus usual clinical care: A meta-analysis of direct comparisons. *American Psychologist, 61*, 671–689.

Welsh, B. C., & Farrington, D. P. (2006). Effectiveness of family-based programs to prevent delinquency and later offending. *Psicothema, 18*, 596–602.

Welsh, B. C., & Rocque, M. (2014). When crime prevention harms: A review of systematic reviews. *Journal of Experimental Criminology, 10*, 245–266.

Welsh, B. C., Farrington, D. P., & Raffan Gowar, B. (2015). Benefit-cost analysis of crime prevention programs. In M. Tonry (Ed.) *Crime and justice: An annual review of research* (Vol. 44, pp. 447–516). Chicago: University of Chicago Press.

Wilson, D. B., Gottfredson, D. C., & Najaka, S. S. (2001). School-based prevention of problem behaviors: A meta-analysis. *Journal of Quantitative Criminology, 17*, 247–272.

Wilson, P., Rush, R., Hussey, S., Puckering, C., Sim, F., Allely, C. S., Doku, P., McConnachie, A., & Gillberg, C. (2012). How evidence-based is an 'evidence-based parenting program'? A PRISMA systematic review and meta-analysis of Triple P. *BMC Medicine, 10*, 130.

Wilson, S. J., & Lipsey, M. W. (2000). Wilderness challenge programs for delinquent youth: A meta-analysis of outcome evaluations. *Evaluation and Program Planning, 23*, 1–12.

Wilson, S. J., & Lipsey, M. W. (2006a). The effects of school-based social information processing interventions on aggressive behavior: Part I: Universal programs. *Campbell Systematic Reviews, 2*(5). http://www.campbellcollaboration.org/lib/project/14/.

Wilson, S. J., & Lipsey, M. W. (2006b). The effects of school-based social information processing interventions on aggressive behavior: Part II: Selected/indicated pull-out programs. *Campbell Systematic Reviews, 2*(6). http://www.campbellcollaboration.org/lib/project/15/.

Wilson, S. J., & Lipsey, M. W. (2007). School-based interventions for aggressive and disruptive behavior: Update of a meta-analysis. *American Journal of Preventive Medicine, 33*, 130–143.

Wilson, S. J., Lipsey, M. W., & Soydan, H. (2003a). Are mainstream programs for juvenile delinquency less effective with minority youth than majority youth? A meta-analysis of outcomes research. *Research on Social Work Practice, 13*, 3–26.

Wilson, S. J., Lipsey, M. W., & Derzon, J. H. (2003b). The effects of school based intervention programs on aggressive behavior: A meta-analysis. *Journal of Consulting and Clinical Psychology, 71*, 136–149.

Woolfenden, S. R., Williams, K., & Peat, J. K. (2002). Family and parenting interventions for conduct disorder and delinquency: A meta-analysis of randomized controlled trials. *Archives of Disease in Childhood, 86*, 251–256.

Chapter 3
Community Interventions

Charlotte Gill

Crime and crime prevention at the community level have been of interest to criminologists since the early twentieth century. Sherman (1997) described the community as the center of crime prevention efforts, the foundation on which other social institutions such as families, schools, labor markets, and agents of formal social control function. Community-based crime prevention embraces a number of diverse strategies, from civic engagement and empowerment in response to crime and disorder issues at the neighborhood level, to interventions for at-risk youth and community correctional and reentry services for adjudicated offenders.

Strong meta-analytic evidence indicates that community-based treatment programs for at-risk or adjudicated individuals, especially juveniles, are more effective than those offered in secure settings (e.g., Lipsey, 1992, 1995, 2009). Such programs are particularly effective when they engage informal rather than formal sources of social control within the community, such as the family (Greenwood, 2008; Shelden, 1999). However, the primary mechanisms of effectiveness underlying these programs operate at the individual level. The community is simply the location in which the intervention occurs. We know much less about crime prevention programs that seek to directly leverage resources. Prior reviews of such programs indicate few promising studies and a lack of rigorous evidence (Welsh & Hoshi, 2006), and the evidence for some community corrections strategies, such as intensive supervision probation (ISP), is mixed at best (Gill, 2010; MacKenzie, 2006; Petersilia & Turner, 1993).

The goal of this chapter is to take stock of what has been learned from systematic reviews of primary and secondary community-based crime prevention initiatives. Primary prevention programs are community-based efforts to stop crime at its source, for example, a neighborhood watch program that engages local residents with the police in an effort to identify and reduce problematic conditions or behaviors. Primary prevention programs may also be delivered at the level of the individual rather than neighborhood (or other geographic places); for example, after-school

---

C. Gill (✉)
George Mason University, Fairfax, VA, USA
e-mail: cgill9@gmu.edu

programs designed to provide supervision for youth, or mentoring programs that bring young people at high risk for delinquency into prosocial relationships with community members. Secondary prevention programs are community-based efforts to supervise, rehabilitate, and prevent recidivism among convicted offenders, as either an alternative to incarceration or a period of postrelease supervision.

The chapter begins with a brief review of the key theories underlying community-based crime prevention. Welsh and Hoshi (2006) argue that "there is little agreement in the academic literature on the definition of community prevention and the types of programs that fall within it." This lack of clarity makes it particularly important to consider the theoretical bases and potential causal mechanisms. In this chapter, I make the case for multiple definitions of community-based crime prevention based on the focus of intervention (primary or secondary), the target or unit of analysis (places or people), and the theoretical mechanism for effectiveness. Returning to theoretical principles may help identify common features of effective programs and assist policymakers in developing future interventions, even when the actual strategies identified in the literature are too disparate to draw conclusions about effectiveness.

The next part of the chapter summarizes the findings of systematic reviews of primary and secondary community-based interventions. Following the Maryland Report framework (Sherman et al., 1997), the findings are categorized into "what works," "what doesn't," and "what's promising," within the three realms of community interventions described previously. The chapter concludes with a summary of the contribution systematic reviews on community interventions have made to the field, including what has been learned and where gaps remain in our knowledge, and a commentary on future directions for systematic review and community crime prevention research more generally.

Community-Based Crime Prevention

The definition and role of the community vary greatly across different crime prevention contexts. The community can be the target or focus of an intervention, whereby community resources are mobilized to promote social cohesion and guardianship, tackle disorder and deterioration in neighborhoods, or work with agents of formal social control to improve trust and relationships. The community can also be the physical setting in which supervision and services are provided to individuals who are at risk of criminal involvement or who have already committed an offense. In these contexts, the community, both in the abstract sense of a place's "social fabric" and the actual people within it, can act either as a source of resources and support (for example, mentorship and activities, or a setting in which prosocial institutions and ties can be formed and maintained) or as a source of deterrence and surveillance, in which the appeal of remaining in the community rather than being incarcerated is intended to discourage offenders from recidivating. These varied roles suggest that a number of diverse theoretical mechanisms may underlie effective community-based crime prevention programs.

Place-based primary prevention programs conceptualize the community and its representatives as direct actors and the basis for problem solving, ideas that are rooted in the theoretical tradition of social ecology. Sociologists and criminologists have long understood the role of the community in regulating behavior, and recognize that crime rates at places vary according to their structural and social features (*see* reviews by Bursik & Grasmick, 1993; Weisburd, 2012). Community effects on crime have been explained by factors including the nature of social ties and interactions, norms and collective efficacy, institutional resources, anomie, and routine activities.

Social problems cluster in communities when structural conditions such as poverty, unemployment, rapid social change, and population turnover produce breakdowns in informal social controls driven by family disruption and reduced social cohesion (e.g., Morenoff, Sampson, & Raudenbush, 2001; Sampson, 1987; Sampson, Raudenbush, & Earls, 1997; Sampson, Morenoff, & Gannon-Rowley, 2002; Shaw & McKay, 1942; Sutherland, 1947). These breakdowns in turn may manifest as signs of physical disorder and community deterioration, which can attract more serious crime and leave residents fearful and subsequently creates a spiral of increasing disorder and eroding social control: the "broken windows" principle (Wilson & Kelling, 1982; *see also* Skogan, 1986). These effects may be reversed when community resources are mobilized for crime prevention through collective action. Sampson et al. (1997) noted that this "collective efficacy" can mediate the effects of concentrated poverty and population transition, such that residents bonded together by a common sense of purpose can produce crime reductions in highly disorganized areas.

Routine activities and opportunity theories are closely integrated with ideas about social ecology, because they emphasize that crime opportunities at places arise under similar environmental and social conditions (*see* Weisburd, 2012). Thus, place-based prevention efforts may also emphasize increased guardianship, deterrence of offenders, and/or reducing the vulnerability of targets at crime places within the community (e.g., Cohen & Felson, 1979). Increased guardianship in particular is closely related to social cohesion and collective efficacy. Concerned citizens with a stake in the success of their communities and neighborhoods, and who are engaged with their neighbors and fellow residents, may be expected to look out for each other and take action when something seems amiss.

In primary and secondary efforts to prevent crime at the individual level, the community is not necessarily mobilized but provides the setting for intervention. Crime prevention is facilitated through the imposition of social controls, which can be formal or informal and supportive or restrictive. Person-based primary prevention programs seek to prevent individuals (most often young people) becoming delinquent in the first place by emphasizing positive social bonds and attachments to social institutions (Hirschi, 1969). Social control theory posits that youth who are strongly bonded to legitimate social institutions, such as the family, school, or nondelinquent peer groups (i.e., have a "stake in conformity"; Toby, 1957), and are involved in prosocial activities will internalize conventional beliefs and goals, such as educational attainment and job prospects (Hagan, 1993), and thus be less likely to engage in delinquency. These social institutions are thus an integral part of the child's community, exerting informal social controls to support and encourage positive behavior and providing a supportive context for intervention and supervision (Shelden, 1999).

Conversely, social learning theories (Akers, 1973; Sutherland, 1947) and routine activities theory support a link between unstructured socializing by youth in unsupervised places and juvenile delinquency rates at those places (Osgood, Wilson, O'Malley, Bachman, & Johnston, 1996; Weisburd, Morris, & Groff, 2009). Thus, prevention programs that provide participants with opportunities for involvement in positive pursuits through recreational activities and after-school programs supervised by community members provide guardianship and may directly remove opportunities for delinquency, especially when they are targeted at key juvenile crime times (Gottfredson, Gottfredson, & Weisman, 2001).

Allowing pre-adjudicated delinquents or convicted offenders to remain in the community as an alternative to a custodial sentence (i.e., diversion from prosecution or community sanctions like probation and community service) is also intended to promote and maintain social bonds. Both the physical removal from the community and the stigma of incarceration can break an individual's ties to positive community and family influences (Lowenkamp & Latessa, 2004) and prevent participation in conventional activities and treatment (MacKenzie & Brame, 2001). Even secondary prevention programs for convicted and incarcerated offenders can be oriented toward community and social ties, such as reentry programs focusing on developing job skills and obtaining housing. Restorative justice conferencing and victim–offender mediation involve bringing together an offender (who may or may not have been convicted, but must have accepted responsibility for the offense), their victim, supporters of each, and sometimes community leaders or representatives who can attest to the more general social harm caused by the offense, to discuss the harm and how it can be dealt with. A key component of most restorative justice conferences is the reintegration of the offender into the community. Rituals of forgiveness and reintegration are intended to create and reinforce positive social bonds and enhance the offender's stake in conformity (e.g., Braithwaite, 1989).

Labeling theory is an additional theoretical principle underpinning diversion programs and secondary prevention programs that allow convicted offenders to remain in the community. Young people in particular tend to respond better to services provided outside the formal criminal justice system, and can be harmed by formal processing (Lundman, 1993; Petrosino, Turpin-Petrosino, & Guckenburg, 2010). The processes of court adjudication, punishment, incarceration, and obtaining a criminal record create a stigmatizing or "labeling" effect, which in turn is hypothesized to result in social exclusion, marginalization from family and friends, increased scrutiny from the justice system, and ultimately the reinforcement of delinquent behavior (Becker, 1963; Lemert, 1951; Schur, 1973). While community sanctions for convicted offenders do not remove stigmatizing labels, they at least reduce the potential for marginalization because the individual is not completely removed from positive community influences.

Secondary prevention programs and strategies for convicted offenders also involve more formal and restrictive elements of social control. Some community-based sanctions, such as intensive probation and electronic monitoring, are rooted in principles of deterrence, surveillance, and control. These strategies, which center on close and frequent (or constant, in the case of some electronic monitoring schemes) surveillance, give offenders the opportunity to remain in the community on the understanding that they are being constantly monitored, further offending will be detected, and swift, certain, and severe consequences will result. The most serious consequence of failure to comply is loss of liberty. In this way, the community setting is an incentive, a strong deterrent against failure. Consistent with classical deterrence theory, the benefit of remaining in one's community is assumed to outweigh any benefit of committing a further crime (e.g., Zimring & Hawkins, 1973).

Methodology

This review synthesizes existing systematic reviews of evidence on the effectiveness of community-based interventions that fall into the three categories described earlier: place-based primary prevention, person-based primary prevention, and secondary prevention. Systematic reviews were eligible for inclusion in this chapter if they examined:

1. A primary prevention intervention, strategy, or policy to stop crime at its source through a community-based effort; or
2. A primary prevention intervention, strategy, or policy in a community setting to reduce the risk of crime in an at-risk population; or
3. A secondary prevention intervention, strategy, or policy to supervise or rehabilitate convicted offenders in the community.

Since these categories are extremely broad, several limitations were imposed to ensure that the reviews identified fell within the theoretical framework above. Although correctional and preventive treatment programs (for example, Reasoning and Rehabilitation, cognitive behavioral therapy, or programs for specialized populations like sex offenders) could fall under category (2) or (3), these types of programs were excluded. Many correctional programs are discussed in Chap. 7 of this volume, and in general they do not fit the theoretical framework because they are geared toward within-individual change, rather than changing, enhancing, or maintaining the individual's relationship with the community.

Reviews of programs delivered within distinct social institutions (such as school or family-based programs) were also excluded. This chapter takes a broad view of community as a collectivity of social institutions that shape the behavior and experiences of individuals or groups. Programs delivered within specific institutions such as schools may have a different dynamic in terms of shaping behavior because of the distinct nature of the school environment (for example, control and structure of time and activities; the fact that students are to a greater extent a "captive audience"). In addition, family-based programs often address problems and risk factors within the specific family, rather than focusing on family as a social institution. Finally, these types of programs are discussed in Chap. 2.

Reviews were also excluded if they did not include a systematic search or clear inclusion and exclusion criteria for studies. Inclusion/exclusion criteria had to ensure that only rigorous studies were included: At minimum, all the studies in the review had to include a nonequivalent comparison group (rigorous designs without traditional comparison groups, such as multiple time series or regression discontinuity designs, were also acceptable). Reviews had to examine at least one crime-related outcome measure. Reviews that included community- and noncommunity-based strategies were required to report findings separately so that noncommunity strategies could be excluded from this review. Finally, reviews had to include at least two studies to be eligible, but were not required to include a quantitative meta-analysis.

Search Strategy

Most reviews discussed here were identified through the Campbell Collaboration's online library.[1] I screened the titles of all completed and in-progress reviews registered with Campbell's Crime and Justice and Social Welfare Groups. This search identified five completed systematic reviews and four in-progress reviews. I obtained draft final reports for three of the four in-progress reports, some of which have since been published (Tolan et al., 2013; Gill & Hyatt, in progress—some findings are available in Gill, 2010; Strang, Sherman, Mayo-Wilson, Woods, & Ariel, 2013). A further three reviews (Braga & Weisburd, 2012a, b; Gill, Weisburd, Bennett, Telep, & Vitter, in progress—since published as Gill, Weisburd, Telep, Vitter, & Bennett, 2014; Heidemann, Soydan, & Xie, in progress) were excluded.[2] The Cochrane Collaboration Library[3] was also examined for completed systematic reviews in public health, but no relevant reviews were found.

I also searched several online databases to identify non-Campbell Collaboration systematic reviews, using the broad search string *community AND crime AND ("systematic review" OR "meta analysis")*:[4]

1. Criminal Justice Abstracts
2. Criminal Justice Periodicals Index[5]
3. Google Scholar[5,6]

---

[1] http://www.campbellcollaboration.org/library.php.
[2] See Table 3.3 for a full list of excluded reviews and the reasons for exclusion.
[3] http://www.cochrane.org/cochrane-reviews/.
[4] The search string was modified as needed to meet the specific requirements of each database.
[5] Because these two databases produced an unmanageable number of hits, I only examined the first 500, sorted by relevance.
[6] Google Scholar does not support the Boolean OR operator, so two separate searches were performed (*community crime "systematic review"; community crime "meta analysis"*). The first 500 hits for each search were reviewed.

4. JSTOR
5. Sociological Abstracts

I screened each title for relevance, resulting in a total of 155 downloads (including duplicates). Title and abstract screening of these downloads produced a sample of 16 unique documents for review (excluding journal article versions of Campbell reviews). Of these, six were eligible, five were ineligible, and five were not systematic reviews but contained relevant information. Along with the Campbell Collaboration reviews, this yielded a total of 15 systematic reviews that were eligible for inclusion in this chapter.[7]

Results

A brief discussion of the focus and findings of each eligible review is given as follows. Further details about the reviews can be found in Tables 3.1 and 3.2.

Place-Based Primary Prevention

Neighborhood Watch Bennett, Holloway, and Farrington (2008) examined the effectiveness of neighborhood watch programs intended to increase the involvement of citizens in crime prevention. They found 43 independent evaluations, of which 18 contained data sufficient for a meta-analysis. The review concludes that neighborhood watch is effective at reducing crime, with the meta-analysis suggesting a crime reduction effect of between 16 and 26%. However, most of the included studies had methodological limitations. Control groups were rarely equivalent.

Community Strategies to Prevent Gun Violence Makarios and Pratt (2012) investigated a range of techniques to identify what works in reducing gun violence and reported findings separately by program type, allowing noncommunity interventions to be excluded in this chapter. They identified 44 studies of community programs, including 30 "high-quality" studies. These programs focused on developing community partnerships and coordinating local resources to address gun violence. They included pulling levers strategies such as Operation Ceasefire (Braga, Kennedy, Waring, & Piehl, 2001), in which community workers, social institutions, and social control agencies collaborated to discourage gang members from engaging in violence. The review found a moderate, statistically significant benefit of community-based gun prevention programs.

A Campbell Collaboration systematic review on broken windows policing, which will include studies of strategies in which the community works in collabo-

---

[7] One review (Makarios & Pratt, 2012) is listed twice in the results section because it included separate analyses of two different eligible strategies; however, it is the same report.

Table 3.1 Characteristics of included reviews

Researchers (date)	Intervention	Comparison group	Outcome	Design	Searches	Time period
Place-based primary prevention						
Bennett et al. (2008)	Neighborhood watch	Geographic area in which neighborhood watch was not operating	Crimes against residents; Crimes against dwellings; Other crimes in watch area (e.g., street crimes)	At minimum, pre-post measures of crime in 1+ experimental unit and 1+ nonequivalent control unit	Online databases, literature reviews, lists of references, and bibliographies, contact with experts	1977–1994 (included studies)
Makarios & Pratt (2012)	Community-oriented strategies for preventing gun violence (review also includes noncommunity-based interventions, but results are reported separately)	Geographic areas where/days or times when programs did not operate	Gun crime rates	All research designs included, but results are broken out by research quality. "High-quality" study results reported here ("high quality" is not defined)	Online databases, lists of references	1983–2005 (included studies—including non-community programs)
Person-based primary prevention						
Jolliffe and Farrington (2008)	Mentoring	Any condition that did not include mentoring (including no treatment, treatment as usual, placebo)	Any quantitative offending outcome	Randomized experiments; quasi-experiments with equivalent or nonequivalent comparison group	Rapid evidence assessment of online databases, websites, and research registers, hand searches of journals, contact with experts	1979–2008
Fisher et al. (2008)	Opportunities provision for gang prevention	No intervention	Gang-related delinquent behavior	Randomized experiments or quasi-random allocation	Online databases, hand searches of journals, contact with experts	Earliest—2007

Table 3.1 (continued)

Researchers (date)	Intervention	Comparison group	Outcome	Design	Searches	Time period
Petrosino et al. (2010)	Diversion (compared to formal processing)	Diversion (doing nothing) or diversion with services is the control group—this review focuses on formal processing	Any crime outcome (official record, self-report, or victim report)	Randomized experiments or quasi-random assignment	Online databases, existing reviews	1973–2008
Tolan et al. (2013)	Mentoring	Any condition that did not include mentoring or other interventions (i.e. no treatment, waiting list, treatment as usual, placebo)	Juvenile delinquency and precursors of delinquency (self-report or official)	Randomized experiments or quasi-experiments with equivalent comparison group	Online databases, existing reviews	1976–2010 (included studies)
Secondary prevention						
Latimer et al. (2005)	Restorative justice/direct victim–offender mediation	Individuals who did not participate in a restorative justice program	General recidivism (also victim and offender satisfaction, restitution compliance)	Randomized experiments, quasi-experiments with equivalent or nonequivalent comparison group	Online databases, websites, hand searches of journal, bibliographies of identified studies, contact with experts	1980–2005
Renzema and Mayo-Wilson (2005)	Electronic monitoring	Individuals receiving traditional or intensive probation or parole, incarceration, or an intervention other than parole or incarceration	General recidivism and technical violation	Randomized experiments, quasi-experiments with equivalent comparison group (matching or historical matching)	Online databases, reference lists and conference reports, government agencies, contact with experts and equipment producers	1986–2002

Table 3.1 (continued)

Researchers (date)	Intervention	Comparison group	Outcome	Design	Searches	Time period
Visher et al. (2006)	Ex-offender employment programs	Ex-offenders receiving treatment as usual or no treatment, including waiting lists	General recidivism	Randomized experiments, quasi-experiments with equivalent or nonequivalent comparison group	Online databases, annotated biographies, reference lists, contact with experts	1970–2005
Villettaz et al. (2006)	Noncustodial sentences (compared to custodial sentences)	Convicted individuals (adults and juveniles) sentenced to a period of confinement in a closed institution	General recidivism (arrests, conviction, reincarceration, self-report)	Randomized experiments, quasi-experiments with equivalent comparison group	Online databases, library catalogues, bibliographies, contact with experts	1960–2003
Cheliotis (2008)	Temporary home leave/work release	Individuals not receiving the program	Recidivism (reconviction, return to custody)	Randomized experiments, quasi-experiments with equivalent control group	Online databases, existing reviews, bibliographies, contact with experts	Earliest–Feb 2005
Makarios & Pratt (2012)	Probation-based strategies for preventing gun violence (review also includes noncommunity-based interventions, but results are reported separately)	Geographic areas where/days or times when programs did not operate	Gun crime rates	All research designs included, but results are broken out by research quality. "High quality" study results reported here ("high quality" is not defined)	Online databases, lists of references	1983–2005 (included studies—including non-community programs)
Marsh et al. (2009)	Custody vs. community service/supervision	Convicted individuals receiving a standard prison sentence	General recidivism (offending, arrest, conviction, incarceration)	Randomized experiments, quasi-experiments with equivalent control group	Online databases	1996–2005 (most recent included study)

Table 3.1 (continued)

Researchers (date)	Intervention	Comparison group	Outcome	Design	Searches	Time period
Gill & Hyatt (in progress); Gill (2010)	Intensive supervision probation (ISP)	Standard probation or parole supervision, or existing ISP program that was less intensive	General recidivism (arrests and convictions), technical violations	Randomized experiments, quasi-experiments with equivalent control group	Online databases, search engines, reference lists	Earliest—2009
Strang et al. (2013)	Restorative justice	Individuals not receiving restorative justice, regular prosecution procedures, or other diversion/victim-offender mediation	Repeat offending (including severity of repeat offending), victim outcomes	Randomized experiments, quasi-experiments with equivalent control group	Online databases, reference lists, conference reports, contact with experts	1997–2005 (includes supplemental reports from 2007 and 2008)

Table 3.2 Findings of included reviews

Researchers (date)	Participants	Number of studies	Number of experiments	Effect size/significance	Moderators
Place-based primary prevention					
Bennett et al. (2008)	Geographic areas where neighborhood watch programs were implemented	43 (systematic review) 18 (meta-analysis)	0	*Mean effect* Odds ratio = 1.36*** (favors program) Confidence interval (CI) = 1.15–1.61	Type of comparison area (matched or non-matched), type of data (police vs. survey), type of scheme (just neighborhood watch vs. neighborhood watch with additional components), size of scheme area, year of publication, type of publication, country
Makarios and Pratt (2012)	Geographic areas in which programs operated	30 (high quality only)	Not reported	$r = -0.238$ $z(r) = -0.251*$ (favors program) *There was insufficient data to convert this effect size to an odds ratio for Fig. 1.*	None
Person-based primary prevention					
Jolliffe and Farrington (2008)	Offenders who had committed chargeable offenses	18	7	*Mean effect* Odds ratio = 1.46** (favors program) CI = 1.14–1.86 Original effect size (ES) *presented in report* Standardized mean difference = 0.208** (favors program) CI = 0.07–0.34	Year of publication, mean age of sample, proportion male/white, sample size, quality assessment, length of follow-up, duration of mentoring, total time mentored, program fidelity

Table 3.2 (continued)

Researchers (date)	Participants	Number of studies	Number of experiments	Effect size/significance	Moderators
Fisher et al. (2008)	Children and young people aged 7–16 who were not involved in a gang	0	N/A	N/A	N/A
Petrosino et al. (2010)	Juvenile delinquents (17 and younger) who have not yet been officially adjudicated for current offense	29	29	*Mean effect, processing vs. diversion* Odds ratio = 1.10 (favors program) CI = 0.89–1.36	Type of comparison group, research team from Michigan State University, studies pre-post 1990, published vs. unpublished, extent of prior offending record
				Mean effect, processing vs. diversion with services Odds ratio = 1.35 (favors program) CI = 0.94–1.92	
				Original ES presented in report *Processing vs. diversion* Standardized mean difference (standard error) = −0.051 (0.06) (favors diversion) CI = −0.169–0.067	
				Processing vs. diversion with services Standardized mean difference (standard error) = −0.164 (0.10; favors diversion) CI = −0.386–0.059	
				Standard error of standardized mean difference estimated by this author	

Table 3.2 (continued)

Researchers (date)	Participants	Number of studies	Number of experiments	Effect size/significance	Moderators
Tolan et al. (2013)	Youth involved in or at risk for juvenile delinquency	46 (25 studies examined delinquency) Note: mean effect for delinquency is the same as mean effect for all outcomes, including aggression, drug use and school achievement)	27	*Mean effect* Odds ratio = 1.49*** (favors program) CI = 1.22–1.82 *Original ES presented in report* Sample size weighted mean effect size, delinquency Standardized mean difference (standard error) = 0.22 (favors program) CI = 0.11–0.33	Selectivity in inclusion, attention to modeling/identification promotion, emotional support, advocacy, and teaching, stand-alone mentoring vs. mentoring with major or minor add-ons, motivation of mentors in participating, quality of work and fidelity
Secondary prevention					
Latimer et al. (2005)	Adult and juvenile offenders who participated in a face-to-face restorative justice conference or victim–offender mediation program	35 (66 effect sizes)	Not reported	Phi coefficient for recidivism (standard deviation) = 0.07 (0.13) CI = 0.02–0.12 N = 32 studies *There was insufficient data to convert this effect size to an odds ratio for Fig. 1*	Random assignment status (results not reported), offender age, publication source, restorative justice model, entry point, control/comparison group type
Renzema and Mayo-Wilson (2005)	Moderate to high-risk adult offenders (18+) being monitored by any technology that records offender location or presence of prohibited substance in the body and transmits data to a central location	3	0	*Mean effect* Odds ratio = 1.04 (favors program) CI = 0.77–1.42 *Original ES presented in report* Fixed effects odds ratio = 0.96 (CI = 0.71–1.31) Odds ratio below 1 favored program	None

Table 3.2 (continued)

Researchers (date)	Participants	Number of studies	Number of experiments	Effect size/significance	Moderators
Visher et al. (2006)	Ex-offenders participating in programs delivered in a non-custodial setting	8 (10 independent effect sizes)	2	*Mean effect* Odds ratio = 1.03 (favors program) CI = 0.99–1.07 *Original ES presented in report* Logged odds ratio (standard error) = 0.03 (0.02; positive favors program) CI = −0.01–0.07	Conviction status of subjects
Villettaz et al. (2006)	Convicted individuals (adults and juveniles) sentenced to sanctions not involving confinement in a closed institution (including fines or probation)	23	5 (only these 5 were included in the meta-analysis)	*Mean effect* Random effects full information maximum likelihood odds ratio = 1.08 (positive favors non-custodial sentences) CI = 0.93–1.25	None
Cheliotis (2008)	Prisoners released on temporary license (unescorted/minimally supervised home leave, work release)	23 (5 home leave, 12 work release, 6 therapeutic community work release)	4 (0 home leave, 3 work release, 1 therapeutic community work release)	No meta-analysis conducted Author concludes home leave and work release can be effective in decreasing return to custody and post-release arrest rates. Work release as part of a therapeutic community intervention was more effective than basic work release programs	None
Makarios and Pratt (2012)	Geographic areas in which programs operated	4 (high quality only)	Not reported	$r = -0.325$ $z(r) = -0.340*$ (favors program) *There was insufficient data to convert this effect size to an odds ratio for Fig. 1*	None

Table 3.2 (continued)

Researchers (date)	Participants	Number of studies	Number of experiments	Effect size/significance	Moderators
Marsh et al. (2009)	Individuals receiving an alternative (non-prison) sentence This chapter focuses on community service, community supervision, and surveillance (excluding surveillance with drug treatment)	50 (41 adults, 9 juveniles) Includes studies comparing custody to interventions other than community sentences (residential or institutional programs, prison with services) 7 studies examined community service/supervision/surveillance/reparation	Not reported	No meta-analysis conducted for community-related comparisons. Individual studies favored community sentence in all adult studies and victim reparation with juveniles. Community supervision had no effect for juveniles	None
Gill & Hyatt (in progress); Gill (2010)	Juvenile and adult probationers of moderate to high risk placed in high-intensity probation supervision	47	38	*Mean effect, recidivism, RCTs* Random effect odds ratio = 1.03 (favors program) CI = 0.89–1.20 *Mean effect, recidivism, non-RCTs* Random effect odds ratio = 1.49* (favors program) CI = 1.04–2.13 *Mean effect, technical violations, RCTs* Random effect odds ratio = 0.65 (favors control) CI = 0.42–1.01 *Mean effect, technical violations, non-RCTs* Random effect odds ratio = 0.78 (favors control) CI = 0.52–1.16	Type of publication, research timeframe, study location, program type, caseload reduction, contact frequency increase, drug test requirement increase, supervision philosophy, control group type, target population, target offense type, age/gender of sample, offender risk level

3 Community Interventions

Table 3.2 (continued)

Researchers (date)	Participants	Number of studies	Number of experiments	Effect size/significance	Moderators
Strang et al. (2013)	Individuals (adults and juveniles) attending a face-to-face restorative justice conference	10	10	*Mean effect, recidivism* Odds ratio = 1.33*** (favors program) CI = 1.13–1.56 *Original ES presented in report Recidivism* Standardized mean difference (standard error) = −0.155 (0.046)*** (favors program) CI = −0.246— 0.064	Crime type, adult vs. juvenile offender, RJ as supplement or substitute to conventional justice, outcome type, time at risk

*$p \leq .05$; **$p \leq .01$; ***$p \leq .001$

ration with the police to deal with conditions of disorder that may be precursors to more serious types of crime, is currently in development (Braga & Welsh, in progress). This review, recently published by Braga, Welsh, and Schnell (2015), is discussed in Chap. 5.

Person-Based Primary Prevention

Mentoring Two systematic reviews of mentoring interventions were identified (Jolliffe & Farrington, 2008; Tolan et al., 2013). Both reviews identified many of the same studies, although Jolliffe and Farrington conducted a rapid evidence assessment over a shorter time frame, so they included fewer studies. Both reports conclude that mentoring is a promising approach for reducing youth delinquency. Jolliffe and Farrington's conclusion, based on 18 studies, was more cautious, as they noted that studies of higher methodological quality yielded less positive results than weaker studies; however, Tolan et al. found over a larger sample of 46 studies that randomized controlled trials had larger effect sizes than other designs.

Opportunities Provision for Gang Prevention Fisher, Montgomery, and Gardner (2008) examined opportunities provision for preventing youth gang involvement for children and young people (aged 7–16) who had no previous involvement in gang membership. These programs provide tutoring, job training, development, placement, and other interventions designed to increase educational or economic opportunities and reduce social exclusion and anomie. However, the reviewers found no rigorous evaluations and simply concluded that primary research on these programs is needed.

Diversion from Formal Processing for Juveniles Petrosino et al. (2010) examined the effect of formal system processing on juvenile delinquency compared with diversion. The authors' moderator analysis comparing formal processing to "diversion" (i.e., doing nothing) and "diversion with services" is the focus of this chapter. The authors conclude that juveniles who were formally processed fared worse than those who were simply diverted, and worse still than those who were diverted to services.

Secondary Prevention

Custodial vs. Noncustodial Sentences Two systematic reviews investigated the impact on recidivism of being sentenced to a noncustodial sanction compared with incarceration. Villettaz, Killias, and Zoder (2006) took a broad view of noncustodial sentences, including fines as well as community service and supervision. Marsh, Fox, and Sarmah (2009) focused specifically on comparing standard prison (without additional services, treatment or programs) to community service, supervision, and surveillance as well as some other custodial programs. They present separate meta-analyses for each comparison type, but there is no meta-analysis of prison compared to community sentences or supervision because each category contained only one study. Consequently, no quantitative findings from this review are presented in this chapter. The authors conclude that in most cases community sentences appeared more effective than prison for adults but results were mixed for juveniles. Villettaz et al. (2006) identified 23 studies, of which five were included in a meta-analysis. Most studies found that noncustodial sanctions produced greater reductions in reoffending than custodial sanctions, but their meta-analysis results were nonsignificant and they identified numerous shortcomings in the methodology of the included studies.

Temporary Home Leave/Work Release Cheliotis (2008) examined the effectiveness of temporary home leave and work release schemes for prisoners. The author finds that both home leave and work release schemes are effective at decreasing reincarceration and postrelease arrest rates, and that work release programs additionally reduce reconviction rates and enhance employment prospects for ex-offenders. He also examined six studies of the same therapeutic community work release program for substance abusers. The additional therapeutic community element appeared to enhance the effectiveness of work release. Note that this systematic review did not include a quantitative meta-analysis.

Employment Programs for Ex-Offenders Visher, Winterfield, and Coggeshall (2006) examined the effectiveness of noncustodial employment programs for preventing recidivism among ex-offenders. The programs they studied were designed to increase employment prospects through educational and vocational training, job training, or job placement. The systematic review included eight randomized controlled trials of such programs for older youth (age 16–17) and adults. No significant effects on rearrest were identified, but the authors note that the studies in this area are old and highly heterogeneous.

Intensive Supervision Probation Gill and Hyatt (in progress; *see also* Gill, 2010) examined the effectiveness of ISP, in which high-risk probationers or parolees are placed into smaller caseloads and/or have more frequent contact with their probation officer. On the basis of 47 studies, of which 38 were randomized controlled trials, the authors conclude that intensive probation has no effect on recidivism and increases technical violations relative to regular probation supervision. However, quasi-experiments indicated a marginally significant crime reduction and a smaller increase in technical violations compared with randomized controlled trials. Some of the more promising studies focused on behavioral management, incentive systems, and focused deterrence, although this finding should be viewed with caution because of the much smaller number of quasi-experiments and the weaker research designs.

Probation-Based Strategies to Prevent Gun Violence Makarios and Pratt (2012) also considered probation-based strategies in the same broad review of gun violence described above. They identified four "high-quality" studies of probation programs of enhanced supervision strategies that targeted gun offenders through increased frequency of contact with probation officers, police, and social workers, including home visits and service brokerage. Probation-based strategies had the strongest favorable mean effect size over all the strategies they reviewed, but the authors urge caution because only four studies were included.

Electronic Monitoring Renzema and Mayo-Wilson (2005) examined the effects of electronic monitoring on the recidivism of moderate- to high-risk offenders. A future Campbell Collaboration systematic review will also assess this intervention (Ariel & Taylor, in progress). Renzema and Mayo-Wilson found just three eligible studies comparing electronic monitoring (tracking devices or substance use detection) to traditional probation/parole, incarceration, or other interventions. The meta-analysis indicated no effect. The authors note the low quality of matched-sample evaluations of this strategy and a general lack of research relative to the extent of use of electronic monitoring.

Restorative Justice/Victim–Offender Mediation Restorative justice conferencing and victim–offender mediation are similar strategies involving a facilitated or mediated interaction between all the parties to an offense, in which the harm and how to deal with it are discussed. Victim–offender mediation differs from restorative justice conferencing in that the mediator plays a more active role, community members are not always involved, and sometimes the victims and offenders do not meet face-to-face. For this chapter, reviews of restorative justice programs that did not include a face-to-face component were excluded because they do not necessarily embody the same theoretical principles of social bonding and reintegration involved in face-to-face meetings. Two eligible reviews were identified: one on restorative justice conferencing (Strang et al., 2013) and one that examined both conferencing and face-to-face victim–offender mediation (Latimer, Dowden, & Muise, 2005). Both reviews indicate favorable effects of restorative justice on recidivism compared with traditional court or diversion practices. Programs also improved outcomes for victims and increased offender compliance with restitution.

What Works in Community Interventions?

Figure 3.1 shows a forest plot of the main effect sizes from each study that included a meta-analysis, standardized as odds ratios where OR > 1 indicates that the result favored the community-based program.[8] This is purely a visual tool. A meta-analysis of the systematic review findings would not have been appropriate given overlap of primary studies across reviews and the highly disparate range of interventions. Note that two studies (Latimer et al., 2005; Makarios & Pratt, 2012) reported effects

---

[8] Comprehensive Meta-Analysis software was used to convert the effect sizes to odds ratios and produce the forest plot. Where studies reported odds ratios where OR < 1 indicated a favorable effect, the direction was flipped by taking the inverse of the odds ratio and its confidence intervals. Tables 3.1 and 3.2 report the odds ratio effect size as well as each effect size in the same format and direction in which it is reported in the original review.

3 Community Interventions

	Odds ratio	Statistics for each study				Odds ratio and 95% CI
		Lower limit	Upper limit	Z-Value	p-Value	
1. Place-Based Primary						
Neighborhood Watch	1.360	1.149	1.609	3.582	0.000	
2. Person-Based Primary						
Mentoring (Tolan)	1.490	1.221	1.819	3.920	0.000	
Mentoring (Jolliffe)	1.458	1.142	1.863	3.020	0.003	
Diversion with Services	1.346	0.944	1.921	1.640	0.101	
Diversion	1.097	0.886	1.358	0.850	0.395	
3. Secondary						
ISP (Recidivism QE)	1.493	1.044	2.133	2.198	0.028	
Restorative Justice	1.325	1.125	1.560	3.370	0.001	
Community Sentences (Killias)	1.080	0.932	1.252	1.020	0.308	
Electronic Monitoring	1.042	0.767	1.415	0.261	0.794	
ISP (Recidivism RCT)	1.031	0.887	1.198	0.398	0.690	
Employment Programs	1.030	0.991	1.072	1.500	0.134	
ISP (Tech Viol QE)	0.775	0.516	1.164	-1.227	0.220	
ISP (Tech Viol RCT)	0.649	0.418	1.009	-1.920	0.055	

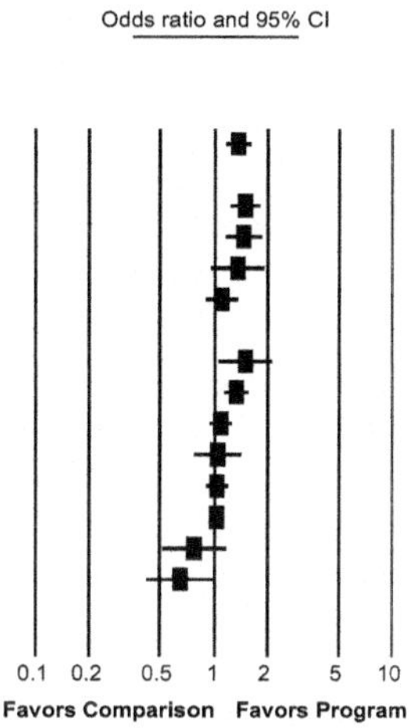

QE Quasi-experiment, *RCT* Randomized controlled trial

Fig. 3.1 Forest plot of mean effect sizes for crime outcomes

as correlation coefficients but did not provide sufficient information in the reports to convert them into odds ratios. These effect sizes are reported in the tables but are not displayed in the forest plot.[9]

What Works?

Figure 3.1 indicates that of the person-based primary prevention reviews, mentoring of youth showed the strongest effects on crime. Jolliffe and Farrington (2008) and Tolan et al. (2013) reported moderate, statistically significant odds ratios (OR) of 1.49 ($p<.001$) and 1.46 ($p\leq.003$), respectively. Restorative justice (Strang et al., 2013) was the only secondary prevention program to show a favorable, statistically significant effect drawn from a sample of highly rigorous experiments (OR = 1.33, $p\leq.001$). Latimer et al. (2005) also found positive, significant effects for restorative justice, although that review included some weaker studies that were excluded by Strang et al. Finally, although it is not shown in Fig. 3.1, the effect size for community-based programs to prevent gun violence (Makarios & Pratt, 2012), which included

---

[9] There were several other cases in which insufficient information was given in the report to convert the effect size to an odds ratio (for example, the standard error of the standardized mean difference (SMD) was missing). These cases were all handled using one of the following methods, in order of preference: (1) if the sample sizes for each study, separated by treatment and control groups, were provided, the SMD and total sample size for treatment and control were used to estimate the odds ratio; (2) if the sample sizes were not provided, but the z-score and confidence intervals for the SMD were available, I used these values to estimate the standard error of the SMD assuming an alpha level of 0.05; (3) if the z-score was not reported but a *p* value was available, I estimated the z-score associated with the *p* value using Stata (assuming an alpha level of 0.05) and proceeded as (2).

some of the same evaluations as the focused deterrence review that was excluded (Braga & Weisburd, 2012a; b), was also moderate and statistically significant (*see* Table 3.2).

I return to the theoretical principles of community-based programs set out in the first part of this chapter to attempt to draw some comparisons between this disparate set of effective interventions. It appears that the mechanisms of effectiveness underlying the most effective of these community programs across all three dimensions are efforts to enhance informal and supportive social controls and reintegration, and maintain or repair social bonds. Both mentoring and restorative justice programs seek to connect at-risk youth or offenders back to prosocial influences in the community, whether through building supportive relationships with positive role models and supporters or reaffirming the individual's bond to conventional society and place in the community.

However, the lack of effectiveness of other interventions that are intended to operate on the same principles, such as diversion, community-based sanctions, and reentry services such as employment programs, casts doubt on the prominence of informal social control as the chief mechanism of effectiveness in community-based programs. One factor that distinguishes restorative justice and mentoring from diversion and community-based sanctions is that the latter include a very broad range of strategies, from doing nothing to providing needed services. Conversely, mentoring and restorative justice are highly specific and targeted interventions that involve one-on-one interactions and building personal relationships. It is possible that the key mechanism of effectiveness in community-based programs that emphasize informal social control and bonding is the proactive effort to connect the individual to the community on a one-to-one basis, rather than simply placing the individual in the community without setting a clear path to internalizing or restoring conventional values and relationships.

The positive effects of community-based gun prevention initiatives also suggest that deterrence can be an effective crime prevention mechanism when it is appropriately implemented. As noted earlier, many of the studies included in this review fit the focused deterrence framework, which involves implementing a menu of highly specific, targeted sanctions aimed at stopping offending behavior. Community resources, police, and probation efforts are leveraged to directly communicate to offenders about the reasons for the sanctions (Braga & Weisburd, 2012a, b). This idea is consistent with research in policing (Lum, Koper, & Telep, 2011; Weisburd & Eck, 2004) and correctional treatment (Andrews, Bonta, & Hoge, 1990; Gendreau, Goggin, & Fulton, 2001; Lowenkamp, Latessa, & Holsinger, 2006) suggesting that interventions should be implemented at a high level of focus—whether at small places or with high-risk individuals—and incorporate specific risk factors.

What's Promising?

Among the place-based programs, neighborhood watch schemes (Bennett et al., 2008) show some promise. Although the review found a moderate, statistically significant favorable effect for the programs (OR = 1.36, $p < .001$), the methodological quality of the studies included in the review was generally low, so the findings do not conclusively indicate that the program is effective. In general, weaker studies tend to show better effects than more rigorously designed studies (Weisburd, Lum, & Petrosino, 2001).

For primary prevention with individuals, diversion with services for juveniles shows promise when compared with formal juvenile justice system programming (Petrosino et al., 2010). The review found a moderate, positive effect but it was not statistically significant at $\alpha = 0.05$ (OR = 1.35, $p \leq .101$). However, the finding is based on rigorous experiments. Diversion with services was distinctly more effective than simple diversion (i.e., doing nothing) when compared with formal processing. Given the discussion earlier, it is likely that a wide range of services were included in these studies and some (particularly those that are highly focused and targeted) were more promising than others, making it difficult to identify an overall effect.

Among the secondary prevention studies, temporary home leave and work release appear to be promising strategies (Cheliotis, 2008), although many of the studies were methodologically weaker and the author did not attempt to estimate a quantitative effect size. The review of ISP (Gill, 2010; Gill & Hyatt, in progress) reported effects for randomized controlled trials and quasi-experiments separately and found a moderate, statistically significant crime reduction effect for programs evaluated using rigorous quasi-experiments (OR = 1.49, $p \leq .028$). Although this finding contradicts the meta-analysis of experiments and is based on a smaller number of studies with slightly weaker designs, the authors note that several of the programs in the quasi-experiment analysis incorporated features of behavioral management and focused deterrence, rather than simply increased surveillance and greater frequency of contact with probation officers. This is supported by the moderate, statistically significant effect reported by Makarios and Pratt (2012) in their meta-analysis of probation-based programs to prevent gun violence, which examines programs based on similar principles, although that analysis is also based on a very small number of studies.

The mechanisms underlying the promising programs reflect those seen in those that "worked." Informal social control and maintenance of bonds to conventional social institutions are key elements of diversion and temporary home leave or work release, although the content of the individually targeted services provided in diversion programs is also likely to be a key factor of the success of those schemes, as discussed earlier. Cheliotis (2008) also noted that work release appeared most effective when combined with treatment in a therapeutic community, although this finding was based on a limited number of studies.

Elements of the focused deterrence framework also appear in some more recent intensive probation efforts that were reviewed by Gill and Hyatt (in progress) and Gill (2010). These programs focus on service brokerage and case planning, behavioral incentives and rewards, behavioral contracts and offender accountability (e.g., Taxman, Yancey, & Bilanin, 2006). For example, the Hawaii HOPE experiment (Hawken & Kleiman, 2009) was a deterrence-based probation scheme that combined drug testing and swift and certain sanctions for failure with treatment and positive reinforcement.

The promise of neighborhood watch indicates that elements of collective efficacy, social cohesion, routine activities, and informal social control at the community level as well as the individual level may also drive promising place-based prevention strategies. Although this chapter includes only one systematic review focused on an intervention of this type, the endurance of the theoretical tradition in this area suggests that these principles could also influence the development of other place-based programs. Weisburd (2012) provided empirical evidence that a lack of collective efficacy and social disorganization are strongly associated with the location of chronic high-crime hot spots and calls for the development of social interventions at small places.

What Shows Little or No Effect?

All of the primary prevention programs targeted at places or individuals were generally effective or promising. Systematic reviews showing little or no effect were concentrated within the secondary prevention category. Ex-offender employment programs (Visher et al., 2006) had no effect on recidivism (OR=1.03, $p \leq .134$). Electronic monitoring programs (Renzema & Mayo-Wilson, 2005) also had no effect on recidivism compared with traditional or intensive probation or incarceration (OR=1.04, $p \leq .794$), although only three studies were included in the review. ISP (Gill, 2010; Gill & Hyatt, in progress) was ineffective against recidivism across 38 randomized controlled trials (OR=1.03, $p \leq .690$) and produced the only backfire effects across all the reviews: a marginally significant increase in technical violations for the treatment group in the randomized experiments reviewed (RCTs: OR=.65, $p \leq .055$; quasi-experiments: OR=0.78, $p \leq .220$).

The common feature across most of these ineffective programs is the underlying basis of formal social control, general deterrence, and surveillance. Unlike the more promising versions of enhanced probation, which embodied elements of focused deterrence, most of the intensive probation programs assessed by randomized controlled trials adhered to a surveillance and control model of supervision. Probation officers were required to maintain a closer and more frequent watch over their clients, but they were not always equipped with the knowledge of how to improve the quality of the increased contact (e.g., Clear & Hardyman, 1990). Bonta, Rugge, Scott, Bourgon, and Yessine (2008) found in a qualitative study of supervision that some probation officers spent too much time on enforcement, not enough time on service delivery, did not account for criminogenic need or risk, and did not know how to effect behavior change—many of the features described in the more successful strategies. As noted above, the potential crime-suppressing elements of the community, such as positive social controls, are not necessarily leveraged simply by placing an offender in the community and assuming that the desire to remain there will act as a sufficient deterrent to recidivism. The more successful community programs suggest that a targeted and focused approach may be required.

The lack of effectiveness of employment programs for ex-offenders is more surprising, because this type of program appears to embody some of the more promising mechanisms of effectiveness described earlier, such as reinforcing bonds with conventional social institutions (i.e., the workplace). However, the authors suggest that the failure to find an effect was more an issue with the available evaluations than the programs themselves. First, the studies they included in their review assessed a highly diverse range of strategies and were not comparable with each other. They also note that most of the studies were more than 10 years old at the time of the review and that the participants were not representative of ex-prisoners at the present time. Newer programs should be developed and evaluated in this area. The findings of this chapter tentatively suggest that the focus should be on building relationships and long-term job prospects and enhancing social support through employment, as well as practical skills and education.

What's Uncertain? What's Missing?

This review highlights a number of challenges to drawing conclusions about the overall effectiveness of community-based programs. Two reviews examining the general effectiveness of sanctions delivered in a community setting compared with incarceration produced contradictory results. Villettaz et al. (2006), based on a meta-analysis of four randomized controlled trials and a natural experiment, found a very small, nonsignificant reduction in recidivism for individuals receiving noncustodial sentences (OR = 1.08, $p \leq .308$). Marsh et al. (2009) concluded that community sentences were more effective at reducing recidivism compared with standard incarceration, especially for adults, but found more mixed results for juveniles. However, their review did not include a meta-analysis across all studies, and in many cases, there was only one study for each type of community sentence.

Both of these reviews covered a very broad range of sentences, from community service, supervision, and treatment, to fines and victim restitution. As discussed earlier, it may not be possible to detect an effect when the types of intervention are highly heterogeneous. Future reviews in this area should use moderator analyses or separate analyses, as Marsh et al. (2009) used, although the Marsh et al. review gave such a fine-grained breakdown of the different treatment components that there were insufficient studies in each category to meta-analyze. The overall availability of primary research is a barrier to conducting more detailed analyses. Marsh et al. (2009) restricted the time frame of their search, but Villettaz et al. (2006) were also unable to include a moderator analysis because they only deemed five of their 23 studies to be of sufficient methodological quality to quantitatively combine.

This review also highlights a number of areas for which no knowledge from systematic reviews is available. The wide scope of programs that could be categorized as community-based prevention precludes a comprehensive discussion of the gaps in the literature, but the following discussion summarizes the main theoretical dimensions that have not yet been reviewed. It is important to keep in mind that a potential reason for the lack of systematic reviews may result from a lack of primary studies in these areas: On average, the reviews identified here each contain more than 21 studies examining community-based interventions, and the number that was suitable for inclusion in a quantitative meta-analysis is much lower.

The lack of systematic reviews on place-based primary prevention was surprising, given the long-standing theoretical tradition supporting the community's active role in crime prevention and the emerging role of collective efficacy and community trust in social institutions as a foundation for prevention efforts. One reason for the absence of studies in this area may be the fact that many place-based community crime prevention evaluations primarily involve police-led strategies (for example, community-oriented policing, some problem-oriented policing programs, strategies to increase legitimacy, and many street-level focused deterrence programs), systematic reviews of which are covered in Chap. 5 and are therefore not considered here. However, no systematic reviews have looked at community mobilization and engagement in general, or with social institutions other than the police, to prevent crime.

There is also a dearth of studies on the supervision of youth. While some of the person-based studies considered here focused on preventing crime among youth who are already at high risk of delinquency, there are no systematic reviews looking at general supervision and constructive activities provided in the community. Only one review even attempted to examine a similar type of program (providing educational and vocational opportunities for children at risk of gang involvement), and it was an "empty review"—no evaluations were identified (Fisher et al., 2008). It would also be important for systematic reviews to cover this type of program to assess whether strategies that bring together at-risk or delinquent youth could increase crime, even when prosocial activities and opportunities to strengthen social bonds are offered, due to deviant peer contagion, whereby delinquent values are reinforced by other similarly situated youth (Andrews, 1989; Dishion & Dodge, 2006; Dishion, McCord, & Poulin, 1999).

Among the secondary prevention programs, there was very little attention in the systematic review literature to reentry issues, with the exception of Visher et al. (2006). Reentry is a crucial issue in contemporary criminology. In 2010, releases from state and federal prisons in the USA exceeded admissions for the first time since records began (Guerino, Harrison, & Sabol, 2011). Many corrections agencies have specialist teams that focus on reentry issues. Yet there is very little high-quality evaluation research on reentry programs and strategies, and consequently even fewer high-quality systematic reviews. One problem with systematic reviews in this area is that many different strategies could be classified as "reentry," including treatment as well as practical assistance and services. Offenders returning to the community have diverse needs across all of these domains. Individualized treatment issues are often confounded with community-based practical services and reintegration in studies and systematic reviews (e.g., Heidemann et al., in progress; Table 3.3), but the mechanisms underlying them are different. It is not possible to tell whether the community element or the individual psychological or behavioral element drives effectiveness. Before systematic reviews of community-based

Table 3.3 Excluded reviews

Researchers (date)	Intervention	Reason for exclusion
Williams-Hayes (2002)	Restorative justice	No screening for methodological quality; appeared to include studies without controls. Compared two different types of restorative justice conference
Umbreit, Coates, and Vos (2002)	Restorative justice	No systematic review methods, inclusion/exclusion criteria, or assessment of methodological quality reported
Nugent, Williams, and Umbreit (2004)	Victim–offender mediation (restorative justice) for juveniles	Almost identical paper to Bradshaw, Roseborough, and Umbreit (2006). Uses nonstandard meta-analysis methodology and includes refusers in study comparison groups
Bradshaw et al. (2006)	Direct victim–offender mediation for juveniles	Almost identical paper to Nugent et al. (2004). Refusers are included in study comparison groups. Reports effect size (possibly standardized mean difference) but inconsistencies in paper
Limbos et al. (2007)	Interventions to prevent youth violence	Combines community interventions with treatment, school-based programs, and legislative changes; no screening for methodological quality
Heidemann et al. (in progress)	Reentry programs for women	Included programs included treatment as well as services/supervision; not all provided in community setting
Gill et al. (in progress; 2014)	Community-oriented policing	Editorial decision: discussed in Chap. 5
Braga and Weisburd (2012a, b)	Focused deterrence	Editorial decision: discussed in Chap. 5

reentry services can be completed, more primary studies are needed that can disentangle the effects of individualized treatment versus practical support and community reintegration elements.

A key challenge to measuring the effectiveness of community-based crime prevention is the lack of definition of "community." As discussed earlier, there is no agreement in the academic literature about the definition of "community prevention" (Welsh & Hoshi, 2006), and this chapter's attempt to construct a framework around key theoretical principles is only one way of going about developing such a definition. The present approach is also limited because many of the theories discussed earlier have been developed in the context of US society and may not be transferable to other countries or cultural contexts.

It is rare that primary studies or even systematic reviews explicate the theoretical mechanisms by which interventions are hypothesized to work. For example, should reentry programs primarily be concerned with community reintegration or individualized treatment, and which approach has the greatest preventive effect? Is mentoring effective because it helps young people form positive social bonds, or does it simply keep them constructively occupied and under frequent adult guardianship? Is diversion more effective than formal processing because it reduces labeling and stigma and keeps individuals connected to the community, or is it a question of providing the right services? Which elements of noncustodial sentences can make them more effective than prison? These are all fundamental questions in assessing the effectiveness of community-based interventions, but the answers are not yet available. Although systematic reviews lend themselves best to answering broad questions about "what works?" they should not dismiss rigorous qualitative and mixed-methods studies that help to answer the rest of that question—"for whom, and why?"

Conclusion and Future Directions

This chapter summarized the findings of 14 systematic reviews of community-based crime prevention interventions, covering 15 different efforts to stop crime at its source at places and with individuals as well as community sentences and reintegrative services for convicted offenders. The discussion reveals a number of lessons for current practice and further development in this area, as well as a number of challenges that can be addressed going forward.

Overall, the findings of this chapter suggest that community-based interventions can be effective whether the community is simply the setting for the intervention, or directly involved or targeted in the prevention effort. Practitioners and policymakers working to develop community interventions might find better effects by focusing on programs and strategies that seek to develop and maintain social bonds and restore offenders' connections to the community, including family members, prosocial peers, and social institutions such as school and work. Highly focused programs that leverage community and criminal justice resources to deter potential or convicted offenders from committing crime through a system of incentives, behavioral management, and frequent but supportive contact also appear to show promise for both individuals and places. Conversely, strategies that leverage the community only as a "Sword of Damocles" to threaten loss of liberty for infractions appear to be ineffective, as do general deterrence efforts that focus on surveillance and control but not social support and rewards for good behavior.

This review suggests that the community as a setting for crime prevention efforts is much more widely studied than the community as a direct actor or facilitator of crime prevention. The latter has received much less attention than the former, and secondary prevention has been more widely studied than primary prevention efforts with at-risk individuals, particularly youth. Yet many of the secondary prevention efforts showed little or no effect on recidivism, while primary prevention programs seem to be more effective, especially when the community is directly engaged and/or young people are targeted. As we have seen, this is in line with the strong theoretical tradition that places the community at the center of problem solving efforts and social capital building, as well as our understanding of concentrations of crime in space and time, and among specific age groups.

While there is a clear gap in the literature around reentry services for convicted offenders, this review suggests that future program development should focus on efforts to stop crime at its source. The lack of evidence for effectiveness of secondary prevention programs suggests that it may be too late to draw on community resources once an offender has already been convicted, unless the intervention is highly focused and provides immediate and direct strategies to repair harm and restore social bonds, as in restorative justice programs, or provides direct practical assistance rather than indirect services that may never result in an actual benefit (for example, job placement rather than job training). As Cheliotis (2008, p. 153n) notes, terms like "reentry" and "reintegration" are "potentially misleading, for they largely assume that prisoners, albeit socio-economically disadvantaged in their vast majority, were once integrated into the community." The real benefit in community-based crime prevention may be in working to strengthen collective efficacy and social bonds before at-risk individuals drift too far away from conventional values.

Due to small samples of studies within systematic reviews, many methodological limitations reported in those that are included, and a lack of a clear definition of the community and the specifics of its role in crime prevention, it is difficult to say with any certainty how effective the above strategies could be. It may be that the community should not be seen as a setting or a direct actor in crime prevention efforts at all. At the beginning of this chapter, I noted that Sherman (1997) characterized the community as "the central institution for crime prevention, the stage on which all other institutions perform." The role of the community may then be indirect, rather than as a resource that can be directly leveraged. Programs that enhance legitimacy, collective efficacy, and community engagement and foster social supports for those at risk may not directly impact crime in the short term, but may set the foundation for longer-term crime control gains. This is the conclusion of the Campbell Collaboration systematic review on community-oriented policing (Gill et al., in progress; Gill, Weisburd, & Telep et al., 2014), which found only a small impact on crime but positive effects on citizen satisfaction and legitimacy in programs where the community collaborated directly with the police to identify and tackle crime problems. The authors speculate that community engagement produces legitimacy, which may be a prerequisite for crime control.

What is clear from this review is that there is still a great deal more to be learned about what works in community-based interventions. This is an extremely broad area covering a broad and diverse range of potential prevention strategies, yet only 14 rigorous systematic reviews were found. Some of the reviews contained a substantial number of studies, but others were limited in scope or even empty. Before we can draw conclusions about "what we have learned" or "what works," we need to go back to basics and develop many more primary research studies. These studies need to focus on operationalizing the concept of "community"—what is community? What should its role in crime prevention be? Which theories underpin effective community mobilization? And most importantly, they need to be based on the most rigorous methods possible—both quantitative and qualitative—to bring us closer to a firm understanding not just of what works, but also how, when, where, and for whom.

References

Akers, R. (1973). *Deviant behavior: A social learning approach.* Belmont: Wadsworth.

Andrews, D. A. (1989). Recidivism is predictable and can be influenced: Using risk assessments to reduce recidivism. *Forum on Corrections Research, 1*(2), 11–17.

Andrews, D. A., Bonta, J., & Hoge, R. D. (1990). Classification for effective rehabilitation: Rediscovering psychology. *Criminal Justice and Behavior, 17,* 19–52.

Ariel, B., & Taylor, F. (in progress). Electronic monitoring of offenders: A systematic review of its effect on recidivism in the criminal justice system. *Campbell Systematic Reviews.*

Becker, H. S. (1963). *Outsiders: Studies in the sociology of deviance.* New York: Free Press.

Bennett, T., Holloway, K., & Farrington, D. (2008). The effectiveness of neighborhood watch. *Campbell Systematic Reviews, 4*(18). http://campbellcollaboration.org/lib/project/50/.

Bonta, J., Rugge, T., Scott, T.-L., Bourgon, G., & Yessine, A. K. (2008). Exploring the black box of community supervision. *Journal of Offender Rehabilitation, 47,* 248–270.

Bradshaw, W., Roseborough, D., & Umbreit, M. S. (2006). The effect of victim offender mediation on juvenile offender recidivism: A meta-analysis. *Conflict Resolution Quarterly, 24*(1), 87–98.

Braga, A. A., & Weisburd, D. L. (2012a). The effects of focused deterrence strategies on crime: A systematic review and meta-analysis of the empirical evidence. *Journal of Research in Crime and Delinquency, 49*(3), 323–358.

Braga, A. A., & Weisburd, D. L. (2012b). The effects of "pulling levers" focused deterrence strategies on crime. *Campbell Systematic Reviews, 8*(6). http://campbellcollaboration.org/lib/project/96/.

Braga, A. A., & Welsh, B. C. (in progress). Broken windows policing to reduce crime. *Campbell Systematic Reviews.*

Braga, A. A., Kennedy, D. M., Waring, E. J., & Piehl, A. M. (2001). Problem-oriented policing, deterrence, and youth violence: An evaluation of Boston's Operation Ceasefire. *Journal of Research in Crime and Delinquency, 38,* 195–225.

Braga, A. A., Welsh, B. C., & Schnell, C. (2015). Can policing disorder reduce crime? A systematic review and meta-analysis. *Journal of Research in Crime and Delinquency, 52,* 567–588.

Braithwaite, J. B. (1989). *Crime, shame, and reintegration.* Cambridge: Cambridge University Press.

Bursik, R. J., & Grasmick, H. G. (1993). *Neighborhoods and crime: The dimensions of effective community control.* New York: Lexington Books.

Cheliotis, L. (2008). Reconsidering the effectiveness of temporary release: A systematic review. *Aggression and Violent Behavior, 13,* 153–168.

Clear, T. R., & Hardyman, P. L. (1990). The new intensive supervision movement. *Crime and Delinquency, 36,* 42–60.

Cohen, L. E., & Felson, M. (1979). Social change and crime rate trends: A routine activity approach. *American Sociological Review, 44,* 588–608.

Dishion, T. J., & Dodge, K. A. (2006). Deviant peer contagion in interventions and programs: An ecological framework for understanding influence mechanisms. In K. A. Dodge, T. J. Dishion, & J. E. Lansford (Eds.), *Deviant peer influences in programs for youth: Problems and solutions* (pp. 14–43). New York: Guilford.

Dishion, T. J., McCord, J., & Poulin, F. (1999). When interventions harm: Peer groups and problem behavior. *American Psychologist, 54,* 755–764.

Fisher, H., Montgomery, P., & Gardner, F. (2008). Opportunities provision for preventing youth gang involvement for children and young people (7–16). *Campbell Systematic Reviews, 4*(8). Retrieved from http://campbellcollaboration.org/lib/project/40/.

Gendreau, P., Goggin, C., & Fulton, B. (2001). Intensive supervision in probation and parole settings. In C. R. Hollin (Ed.), *Handbook of offender assessment and treatment* (pp. 195–204). Chichester: Wiley.

Gill, C. (2010). The effects of sanction intensity on criminal conduct: A randomized low-intensity probation experiment. Unpublished Ph.D. dissertation. Philadelphia, PA: University of Pennsylvania, Department of Criminology. http://repository.upenn.edu/edissertations/121.

Gill, C. E., & Hyatt, J. (in progress). Probation intensity effects on probationers' criminal conduct. *Campbell Systematic Reviews.*

Gill, C. E., Weisburd, D., Bennett, T., Telep, C. W., & Vitter, Z. (in progress). Community-oriented policing to reduce crime, disorder, and fear and increase legitimacy and citizen satisfaction in neighborhoods. *Campbell Systematic Reviews.*

Gill, C., Weisburd, D., Telep, C. W., Vitter, Z., & Bennett, T. (2014). Community-oriented policing to reduce crime, disorder and fear and increase satisfaction and legitimacy among citizens: A systematic review. *Journal of Experimental Criminology, 10*(4), 399–428.

Gottfredson, D. C., Gottfredson, G. D., & Weisman, S. A. (2001). The timing of delinquent behavior and its implications for after-school programs. *Criminology and Public Policy, 1*(1), 61–86.

Greenwood, P. (2008). Prevention and intervention programs for juvenile offenders. *The Future of Children, 18*(2), 185–206. http://futureofchildren.org/futureofchildren/publications/docs/18_02_09.pdf.

Guerino, P., Harrison, P., & Sabol, W. (2011). *Prisoners in 2010.* Washington, DC: U.S. Department of Justice, Bureau of Justice Statistics.

Hagan, J. (1993). The social embeddedness of crime and unemployment. *Criminology, 31*(4), 465–491.

Hawken, A., & Kleiman, M. (2009). Managing drug involved probationers with swift and certain sanctions: Evaluating Hawaii's HOPE. NCJ 229023. http://www.ncjrs.gov/pdffiles1/nij/grants/229023.pdf.

Heidemann, G., Soydan, H., & Xie, B. (in progress). Reentry programs for formerly incarcerated women. *Campbell Systematic Reviews.*

Hirschi, T. (1969). *Causes of delinquency.* Berkeley: University of California Press.

Jolliffe, D., & Farrington, D. P. (2008). *The influence of mentoring on reoffending.* Stockholm: Swedish National Council for Crime Prevention.

Latimer, J., Dowden, C., & Muise, D. (2005). The effectiveness of restorative justice practices: A meta-analysis. *The Prison Journal, 85*(2), 127–144.

Lemert, E. (1951). *Social pathology.* New York: McGraw-Hill.

Limbos, M. A., Chan, L. S., Warf, C., Schneir, A., Iverson, E., Shekelle, P., & Kipke, M. D. (2007). Effectiveness of interventions to prevent youth violence: A systematic review. *American Journal of Preventive Medicine, 33*(1), 65–74.

Lipsey, M. W. (1992). Juvenile delinquency treatment: A meta-analytic inquiry into the variability of effects. In T. D. Cook, H. Cooper, D. S. Cordray, H. Hartmann, L. V. Hedges, R. J. Light, T. A. Louis, & F. Mosteller (Eds.), *Meta-analysis for explanation: A casebook* (pp. 83–127). New York: Russell Sage Foundation.

Lipsey, M. W. (1995). What do we learn from 400 research studies on the effectiveness of treatment with juvenile delinquents? In J. McGuire (Ed.), *What works? Reducing reoffending—Guidelines from research and practice* (pp. 63–78). New York: Wiley.

Lipsey, M. W. (2009). The primary factors that characterize effective interventions with juvenile offenders: A meta-analytic overview. *Victims and Offenders, 4*(2), 124–147.

Lowenkamp, C. T., & Latessa, E. J. (2004). *Understanding the risk principle: How and why correctional interventions can harm low-risk offenders. Topics in Community Corrections* (pp. 3–8). Washington, DC: U.S. Department of Justice, National Institute of Corrections. http://www.nicic.org/pubs/2004/period266.pdf.

Lowenkamp, C. T., Latessa, E. J., & Holsinger, A. M. (2006). The risk principle in action: What have we learned from 13,676 offenders and 97 correctional programs? *Crime and Delinquency, 52*(1), 77–93.

Lum, C., Koper, C., & Telep, C. W. (2011). The evidence-based policing matrix. *Journal of Experimental Criminology, 7,* 3–26.

Lundman, R. J. (1993). *Prevention and control of juvenile delinquency* (2nd ed.). New York: Oxford University Press.

MacKenzie, D. L. (2006). *What works in corrections.* New York: Cambridge University Press.

MacKenzie, D. L., & Brame, R. (2001). Community supervision, prosocial activities, and recidivism. *Justice Quarterly, 18,* 429–448.

Makarios, M. D., & Pratt, T. (2012). The effectiveness of policies and programs that attempt to reduce firearm violence: A meta-analysis. *Crime and Delinquency, 58*(2), 222–244.

Marsh, K., Fox, C., & Sarmah, R. (2009). Is custody an effective sentencing option for the U.K.? Evidence from a meta-analysis of existing studies. *Probation Journal, 56*(2), 129–151.

Morenoff, J. D., Sampson, R. J., & Raudenbush, S. W. (2001). Neighborhood inequality, collective efficacy, and the spatial dynamics of urban violence. *Criminology, 39*(3), 517–558.

Nugent, W. R., Williams, M., & Umbreit, M. S. (2004). Participation in victim-offender mediation and the prevalence of subsequent delinquent behavior: A meta-analysis. *Research on Social Work Practice, 14*(6), 408–416.

Osgood, D. W., Wilson, J. K., O'Malley, P. M., Bachman, J. G., & Johnston, L. D. (1996). Routine activities and individual deviant behavior. *American Sociological Review, 61*, 635–655.

Petersilia, J., & Turner, S. (1993). Intensive probation and parole. *Crime and Justice, 17*, 281–335.

Petrosino, A., Turpin-Petrosino, C., & Guckenburg, S. (2010). Formal system processing of juveniles: Effects on delinquency. *Campbell Systematic Reviews, 6*(1). Retrieved from http://campbellcollaboration.org/lib/project/81/.

Renzema, M., & Mayo-Wilson, E. (2005). Can electronic monitoring reduce crime for moderate to high-risk offenders? *Journal of Experimental Criminology, 1*, 215–237.

Sampson, R. J. (1987). Urban black violence: The effect of male joblessness and family disruption. *American Journal of Sociology, 93*(2), 348–382.

Sampson, R. J., Raudenbush, S. W., & Earls, F. (1997). Neighborhoods and violent crime: A multilevel study of collective efficacy. *Science, 277*, 918–924.

Sampson, R. J., Morenoff, J. D., & Gannon-Rowley, T. (2002). Assessing 'neighborhood effects:' Social processes and new directions in research. *Annual Review of Sociology, 28*, 443–478.

Schur, E. (1973). *Radical nonintervention: Rethinking the delinquency problem*. Englewood Cliffs: Prentice-Hall.

Shaw, C. R., & McKay, H. D. (1942). *Juvenile delinquency and urban areas*. Chicago: University of Chicago Press.

Shelden, R. G. (1999). Detention diversion advocacy: An evaluation. *Juvenile justice bulletin*. Washington, DC: U.S. Department of Justice, Office of Juvenile Justice and Delinquency Prevention.

Sherman, L. W. (1997). Communities and crime prevention. In L. W. Sherman, D. Gottfredson, D. MacKenzie, J. Eck, P. Reuter, & S. Bushway (Eds.) *Preventing crime: What works, what doesn't, what's promising*. Washington, DC: United States Department of Justice, National Institute of Justice. http://ncjrs.gov/works.

Sherman, L. W., Gottfredson, D., MacKenzie, D., Eck, J., Reuter, P., & Bushway, S. (1997). *Preventing crime: What works, what doesn't, what's promising*. Washington, DC: United States Department of Justice, National Institute of Justice. http://ncjrs.gov/works.

Skogan, W. (1986). Fear of crime and neighborhood change. *Crime and Justice, 8*, 203–229.

Strang, H., Sherman, L. W., Mayo-Wilson, E., Woods, D. J., & Ariel, B. (2013). Restorative justice conferencing (RJC): Effects of face-to-face meetings on offenders and victims. *Campbell Systematic Reviews, 9*(12). http://www.campbellcollaboration.org/lib/project/63/.

Sutherland, E. H. (1947). *Principles of criminology* (4th ed.). Philadelphia: Lipppincott.

Taxman, F. S., Yancey, C., & Bilanin, J. E. (2006). *Proactive community supervision in Maryland: Changing offender outcomes*. Towson: Maryland Department of Public Safety and Correctional Services. http://www.dpscs.state.md.us/publications/pdfs/PCS_Evaluation_Feb06.pdf.

Toby, J. (1957). Social disorganization and the stake in conformity: Complementary factors in the predatory behavior of hoodlums. *Journal of Criminal Law, Criminology, and Police Science, 48*, 12–17.

Tolan, P., Henry, D., Schoeny, M., Bass, A., Lovegrove, P., & Nichols, E. (2013). Mentoring interventions to affect juvenile delinquency and associated problems. *Campbell Systematic Reviews, 9*(10). Retrieved from http://www.campbellcollaboration.org/lib/project/48/.

Umbreit, M. S., Coates, R. B., & Vos, B. (2002). *The impact of restorative justice conferencing: A review of 63 empirical studies in 5 countries*. Minnesota: Center for Restorative Justice and

Peacemaking, University of Minnesota. http://www.cehd.umn.edu/ssw/rjp/resources/rj_dialogue_resources/Restorative_Group_Conferencing/Impact_RJC_Review_63_Studies.pdf.
Villettaz, P., Killias, M., & Zoder, I. (2006). The effects of custodial vs. non-custodial sentences on re-offending: A systematic review of the state of knowledge. *Campbell Systematic Reviews, 13,* 1–73. http://campbellcollaboration.org/lib/project/22/.
Visher, C. A., Winterfield, L., & Coggeshall, M. B. (2006). Systematic review of non-custodial employment programs: Impact on recidivism rates of ex-offenders. *Campbell Systematic Reviews, 2*(1). http://campbellcollaboration.org/lib/project/10/.
Weisburd, D. (2012). Bringing social context back into the equation: The importance of social characteristics of places in the prevention of crime. *Criminology and Public Policy, 11*(2), 317–326.
Weisburd, D., & Eck, J. E. (2004). What can police do to reduce crime, disorder, and fear? *Annals of the American Academy of Political and Social Science, 593,* 42–65.
Weisburd, D., Lum, C. M., & Petrosino, A. (2001). Does research design affect study outcomes in criminal justice? *Annals of the American Academy of Political and Social Science, 578,* 50–70.
Weisburd, D., Morris, N. A., & Groff, E. R. (2009). Hot spots of juvenile crime: A longitudinal study of arrest incidents at street segments in Seattle, Washington. *Journal of Quantitative Criminology, 25,* 443–467.
Welsh, B. C., & Hoshi, A. (2006). Communities and crime prevention. In L. W. Sherman, D. P. Farrington, B. C. Welsh, & D. L. MacKenzie (Eds.), *Evidence-based crime prevention* (revised edition). New York: Routledge.
Williams-Hayes, M. M. (2002). *The effectiveness of victim-offender mediation and family group conferencing: A meta-analysis.* Unpublished Ph.D. dissertation. Knoxville, TN: University of Tennessee, Knoxville.
Wilson, J. Q., & Kelling, G. L. (1982). Broken windows: The police and neighborhood safety. *Atlantic Monthly, 249,* 29–38.
Zimring, F., & Hawkins, G. (1973). *Deterrence: The legal threat in crime control.* Chicago: University of Chicago Press.

Chapter 4
Situational Prevention

Kate J. Bowers and Shane D. Johnson

Theories of criminality focus their explanation of crime at the level of the individual, considering factors that predispose an individual to commit crime (e.g., Yochelson & Samenow, 1976), or social influences that might encourage them to do so (Merton, 1938). In contrast, influenced by the finding that the timing and location of crime events are far from random (e.g., Shaw & McKay, 1942), opportunity theories of crime focus on the crime event and how the immediate environment within which offenders may find themselves affects the probability of crime occurrence (e.g., Clarke & Cornish, 1985). In this chapter, we focus on the impact on crime of *situational crime prevention* (SCP) interventions for which the rationale can be found in theories of opportunity. In what follows, we begin with a brief discussion of the theories concerned and a definition of SCP. This is followed by individual summaries of the findings of seven systematic reviews assessing the effectiveness of SCP measures, our own analysis of trends that can be identified by pooling the evidence, and finally, a discussion of what else could usefully be done to improve the current body of evidence.

According to rational choice theory, when making event-level decisions as to whether to offend or not, offenders consider the costs, benefits, and the effort associated with particular options (Clarke & Cornish, 1985). Decision-making is proposed to maximize utility, but is also assumed to be bounded insofar as offenders will base their decisions on information as it is perceived (which may differ from the reality), and decision-making will be affected by previous choices and their outcomes. Thus, offender decision-making may not appear rational to a casual observer.

K. J. Bowers (✉)
Department of Security and Crime Science, University College London,
35 Tavistock Square, London, WC1H 9EZ, UK
e-mail: k.bowers@ucl.ac.uk

S. D. Johnson
Department of Security and Crime Science, University College London,
35 Tavistock Square, London, WC1H 9EZ, UK
e-mail: shane.johnson@ucl.ac.uk

Routine activity theory suggests that for a direct predatory crime to occur, a motivated offender and a suitable target must converge in space and time, in the absence of a capable guardian (Cohen & Felson, 1979). What represents a suitable target may vary from one offender to the next, depending upon their capabilities and experience. Moreover, the likelihood with which the three elements will be found at the same place at the same time is proposed to be a function of the routine activity patterns of those concerned. Some conditions will increase the likelihood of their convergence, others will not. The point of central importance is that changes in the volume of crime are predicted to be a function of such convergence, even if the population of offenders (potential targets, and so on) remains stable.

Crime pattern theory (Brantingham & Brantingham, 1993) makes more explicit how people's routine activity patterns affect the timing and location of crime events, and provides a formal framework for representing concepts. For example, people's routine activity patterns are defined in terms of routine nodes of activity (e.g., the home and place of work) and the paths that connect them (e.g., the street network). To elaborate, as a consequence of traveling to and from routine activity nodes, people develop awareness spaces or mental maps of the places they know. In the case of offenders, it is in the zones that their awareness spaces intersect with opportunities for crime that they are capable of exploiting that crimes are anticipated to be most likely to occur. In line with this and rational choice theory, research consistently demonstrates that, despite the many and varied choices available to them, offenders tend to commit crimes close to their place of residence, and at places with which they are familiar (e.g., Rengert & Wasilchick, 2000).

One implication of opportunity theories of crime is that the manipulation of features of those environments that are known to be conducive to crime should impact on crime. This is what SCP interventions seek to do. Cornish and Clarke (2003) identified 25 techniques of SCP that form five more general categories that seek to:

- Increase the *effort* associated with committing an offence (through hardening targets, controlling access, screening exits, deflecting offenders, and controlling tools and weapons)
- Increase the *risk* associated with committing an offence (by extending guardianship, assisting natural surveillance, reducing anonymity, using place managers, and strengthening formal surveillance)
- Reduce the *benefits* of such action (by concealing targets, removing targets, identifying property, disrupting markets, and denying benefits)
- *Reduce provocations* that might otherwise precipitate crime (by reducing frustrations, avoiding disputes, reducing arousal, neutralizing peer pressure, and discouraging imitation)
- *Remove excuses* that offenders might otherwise use to justify criminal action (by setting rules, posting instructions, alerting consciences, assisting compliance, and controlling drugs and alcohol)

In practice, SCP schemes often involve some combination of techniques and in some cases, changing offender perceptions of one or more of the first three categories shown earlier may in isolation represent an intervention. While affecting offender perception may seem unlikely to impact upon levels of crime, this would be predicted by rational choice theory, and research (Smith et al., 2002; Johnson & Bowers, 2003) suggests that it is not unusual for reductions in crime associated with SCP interventions to be observed prior to the actual implementation of the interventions involved.

SCP is hardly a new idea, with the Great Wall of China, the tradition of building castles at elevated locations, and the practice of concealing cash on the person rather than leaving it on table tops in public places, reflecting humankind's appreciation of how the physical characteristics of the environment can affect the actions of an adversary. However, a formal framework for thinking about SCP in its various forms is relatively new (e.g., Clarke, 1983). Moreover, in their more contemporary form, SCP strategies often involve the alleviation of vulnerabilities in the built environment or manufactured products, or ways of changing the behavior of potential offenders, victims, and guardians, so as to reduce the likelihood of crime occurrence.

It was not until the 1970s that SCP interventions were truly embraced as a recognized method of reducing crime. Since then hundreds of evaluations of SCP interventions have been published, and Guerette (2009) provides an excellent summary of the trends in such evaluations over time. These have varied in methodological adequacy but nevertheless there now exists a fairly substantial cumulative body of knowledge. Not surprisingly then, a number of reviews have been conducted to synthesize knowledge and to estimate the typical effects of interventions. Eck (2006) provides a review of situational approaches to prevention in public and private settings and concludes that nuisance abatement and improved street lighting were particularly effective approaches of this type.

In the current review, we examine what has been learned as a consequence of systematic reviews of SCP interventions. In order to be confident that we had found all relevant reviews, we conducted searches for studies in a number of ways. The two most significant search locations were the Campbell Collaboration Web site[1] (and other information from the Campbell Collaboration) and the POPCenter Web site[2]. The former contains reviews conducted under the explicitly stated, transparent method adopted and documented by the Campbell Collaboration, and the latter is a practitioner-oriented resource that contains an expansive collection of evidence on the effectiveness of various situational prevention approaches. We also searched a number of electronic databases available through the University College London (UCL)MetaLib system (which is a meta-database enabling the search of a large number of individual electronic bibliographic databases and electronic journals) and undertook a Google Scholar as well as a more general Google search. In all cases, we used relevant search terms and allowed for different spellings and phrasing of key concepts (e.g., we searched on both "situational crime prevention" and "SCP"). Since SCP is a phrase that is used to describe a broad range of more specific approaches, we also completed searches on individual strategies that are commonly used. For example, we used terms such as "CCTV," "surveillance," "CPTED," "alley-gating," "entry control," "target hardening," and "lighting" as well as more specific phrases such as "repeat victimization" and "neighborhood watch."

---

[1] http://www.campbellcollaboration.org/. Accessed 15 June 2012.

[2] http://www.popcenter.org/. Accessed 15 June 2012.

Furthermore, we conducted broader searches focusing on reducing certain types of crime, for instance "burglary reduction" and "reducing car theft."

In this chapter, we mainly consider seven systematic reviews that have examined the impact on crime of improvements to street lighting (Welsh & Farrington, 2008a), closed-circuit television cameras (CCTV; Welsh & Farrington, 2008b), repeat victimization (RV) strategies (Grove et al., 2012), public area surveillance (Welsh et al., 2010), neighborhood watch (NW) schemes (Bennett et al., 2008), counterterrorism measures (Lum et al., 2006), and designated driver initiatives (Ditter et al., 2005). While not all Campbell Collaboration reviews, all follow the procedures laid out in Campbell Collaboration guidelines. That is, in all reviews the search terms used, the databases employed, and the specific inclusion and exclusion criteria are explicitly stated. See Table 4.1 for a summary of the features of these reviews.

Two of the reviews mentioned earlier are of relevance to the debate on SCP effectiveness but are not included in the quantitative analysis that we present here for a variety of reasons. First is the review of the effectiveness of counterterrorism strategies mentioned by Lum et al. (2006). This reviews a wide range of different strategies of which those with a situational element form a part. Of particular relevance are the use of metal detectors in airports and the fortification of embassies against attacks. The reported outcomes such as a decline in the number of terrorist attacks are dissimilar to many of the other outcomes discussed in this chapter and it was not possible to convert the effect-sizes to comparable odds ratios, as the outcome measure is unstandardized[3]. Second is the systematic review of the effectiveness of designated driver programs for reducing alcohol-impaired driving conducted by Ditter et al. (2005). This study relied on a small number of studies, and while some interesting trends were identified it did not contain a quantitative meta-analysis or the information necessary to produce effect sizes.

In addition, while the individual effect sizes from the Welsh et al. (2011) review of public area surveillance are included in our later analysis, no formal mean effect size was calculated due to insufficient numbers of cases. Table 4.2 provides details of the overall conclusions of the systematic reviews in terms of effectiveness along with details of the number of evaluations included and the moderators considered in the analysis. Figure 4.1 summarizes the mean effect sizes for the studies where this information was available and for which it was possible to represent the outcome as an odds ratio.

A final review referred to in this chapter summarizes the evidence concerning the displacement (or, rather, lack thereof) of crime to other places as a result of SCP activity (Johnson et al. 2011). This concept is more fully defined later in this chapter but the review is not included in the quantitative analysis here or in Table 4.2 or Fig. 4.1 because the outcome considered in that review is not a direct measure of effectiveness of the SCP measures.

In Sect. 2, we define and discuss each type of intervention, justifying its inclusion here and summarizing the findings of the respective systematic reviews. In Sect. 3, we examine trends observed across (rather than within) the studies and present some novel analyses. In Sect. 4, we draw some general conclusions, consider

---

[3] The authors would like to thank David B. Wilson for a very helpful discussion on this issue.

Table 4.1 Summary features of the systematic reviews

Researcher, date	Intervention	Comparison group	Outcome	Design	Searches
Ditter et al. (2005)	Designated driver programs	The study looked at change in the frequency of designated driver selection over time	The main outcome was self-reports of frequency of designated driver selection before drinking begins	Quasi-experimental (100%)	Systematic with defined databases, search terms, and inclusion/exclusion criteria
Lum et al. (2006) (metal detectors in airports and the protection of embassies and diplomats only)	Counterterrorism strategies	The studies used a time series design following introduction of policies and controls for other factors	Terrorist incidents. For metal detectors, the main outcome was reduction in hijacking	Quasi-experimental (100%)	Systematic using Campbell guidelines; with defined databases, search terms, and inclusion/exclusion criteria
Bennett et al. (2008)	Neighborhood watch	Matched and nonmatched comparison areas, adjacent census tracts, the remainder of the subdivision, nearby police beats, or the city as a whole depending upon the study design	All crime (6%) Burglary (94%)	Quasi-experimental (100%)	Systematic using Campbell guidelines; with defined databases, search terms, and inclusion/exclusion criteria
Welsh & Farrington (2008a)	Street lighting	Surrounding areas, blocks, streets, parking garages, beats or markets depending on study design	All crime (62%) Calls for service (8%) Burglary, assault, and vehicle theft (8%) Burglary, assault, and robbery (8%)	Quasi-experimental (100%)	Systematic using Campbell guidelines; with defined databases, search terms, and inclusion/exclusion criteria
Welsh & Farrington (2009a)	CCTV	Beats, streets, commercial areas, circular zones, town centers, or adjacent areas depending on study design	All crime (66%) Calls for service (7%) Robbery (7%) Theft (12%) Violent crime (7%)	Quasi-experimental (100%)	Systematic using Campbell guidelines; with defined databases, search terms, and inclusion/exclusion criteria

Table 4.1 (continued)

Researcher, date	Intervention	Comparison group	Outcome	Design	Searches
Welsh et al. (2010)	Public area surveillance	Surrounding or adjacent police sectors, municipalities, patrol divisions, neighborhoods, parking lots, subway stations, flats or cities depending upon study design	Vehicle theft (36%) All crime (27%) Violent crime (18%) Property crime (18%)	Quasi-experimental (100%)	Systematic with defined databases, search terms, and inclusion/exclusion criteria
Grove et al. (2012)	Repeat victimization strategies	Hotspots, patrol sectors, nonresidential repeat victims, businesses, nonadjacent areas, remainder of larger area containing action area, or female undergraduates depending on study design	Burglary (74%) Commercial burglary (11%) Sexual assault (15%)	Quasi-experimental (85%) RCT (7%) Unknown (7%)	Systematic using Campbell guidelines; with defined databases, search terms, and inclusion/exclusion criteria

Table 4.2 Effect sizes of the systematic reviews

Researcher, date	Intervention	Time period of studies	No of studies	Mean effect size	Moderators
Ditter et al. (2005)	Designated driver programs	1005–1998	7 designated driver interventions in bars	No formal mean effect size given. Across the studies, the median increase in number of designated drivers per night is 0.9 (interquartile range 0.3–3.2 drivers)	Study design
Lum et al. (2006) (metal detectors in airports and the protection of embassies and diplomats only)	Counterterrorism strategies	1978–2000 (metal detectors) 1988–2000 (protection of embassies/diplomats)	16 (metal detectors) 19 (protection of embassies/diplomats)	Weighted mean effect of a reduction of 6.3 hijackings (CI: −8.79, −3.14). Statistically significant decrease. Weighted mean effect size of a reduction of 0.45 incidents (CI: −2.17, 1.27). Not statistically significant	Type of outcome (hijacking vs. nonhijacking incidents) Type of outcome
Bennett et al. (2008)	Neighborhood watch	1977–1994	18	Odds ratio (random effects) = 1.36, (CI: 1.15, 1.61) (fixed effects) = 1.19 (CI: 1.13, 1.24) Modest significant effect	Size of scheme Type of scheme
Welsh & Farrington (2008a)	Street lighting	1974–1999	13	Relative effect size = 1.27 (CI:1.09, 1.47) Significant effect	Country of study Type of outcome
Welsh & Farrington (2008b)	CCTV	1978–2007	41	Relative effect size = 1.19 (CI: 1.08, 1.32) Modest significant effect	Context (town center; public housing; car park; public transport; other) Type of crime
Welsh et al. (2010)	Public area surveillance	1991–2005	12 (5 on security guards, 2 on place managers, and 5 on defensible space)	No formal effect sizes given due to small numbers. The authors conclude that there is fairly strong evidence that street closures/barricades are effective but less conclusive statements can be made about security guards/ place managers	Type of surveillance: Security guards Place managers Defensible space
Grove et al. (2012)	Repeat victimization strategies	1994–2005	27	Odds ratio = 1.18 (CI: 1.07, 1.32) Modest significant effect	Tactics of scheme Effectiveness of intervention Crime type

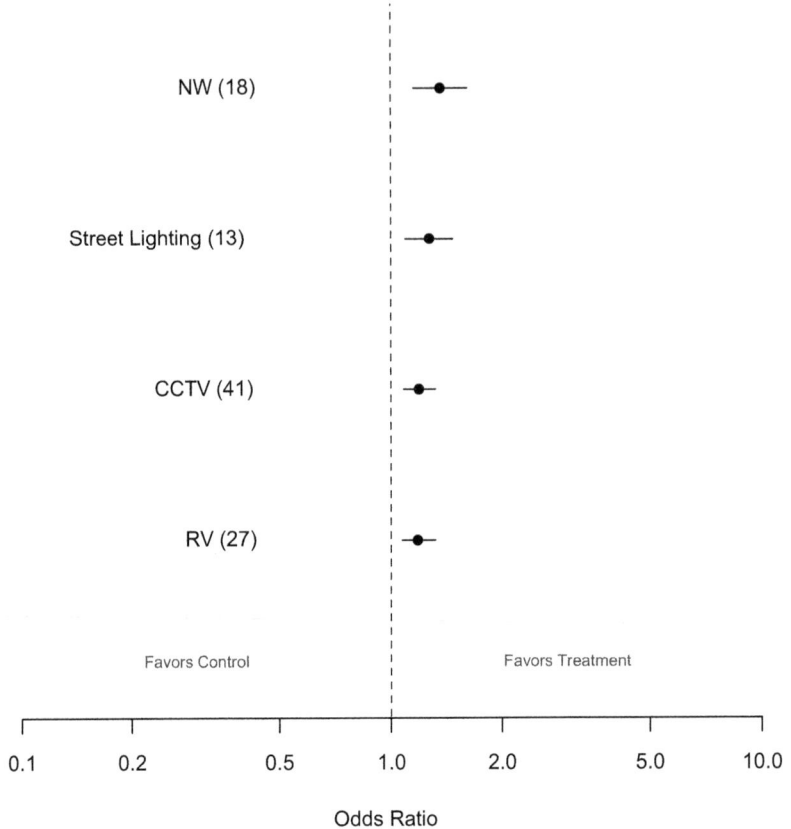

Fig. 4.1 Mean effect sizes, as odds ratios, for the systematic reviews with sufficient information provided (sample sizes shown in parentheses)

issues associated with the evaluation of SCP interventions, and suggest future priorities for evaluation research of this kind.

The Impact of Specific Interventions

Street Lighting

Street lighting interventions involve the installation of new street lighting in areas previously unlit, or the improvement of existing lighting so as to provide elevated levels of illumination during the hours of darkness. The systematic review by Welsh and Farrington (2008a) found that improved street lighting reduced crime by 21% in areas receiving intervention compared to control areas with no improvement.

Importantly, the review also found that improved street lighting does not just affect crime committed under cover of darkness; it also demonstrated a significant effect of these interventions during the daytime.

This highlights the importance of considering the mechanism through which lighting reduces crime. Perhaps the most obvious theory is that lighting increases natural surveillance—this is one of the 25 SCP techniques discussed by Cornish and Clarke (2003). Increasing the probability (or perceived probability) that an offender may be seen increases the risk associated with undertaking an offence. Greater visibility might also increase the on-street population at night, in turn increasing levels of natural guardianship. However, this does not adequately explain the reduction in crime during the daytime. Welsh and Farrington therefore propose that a further mechanism is an increase in community pride in the area. This in turn is likely to increase informal social control and ultimately lead to a reduction in crime through greater community involvement. Future research may usefully test this hypothesis.

The street lighting meta-analysis, which included 13 studies and 13 associated effect sizes, also looked at the effect of some mediating factors. For example, the positive effect of street lighting appeared to be greater in the UK than in the USA.

CCTV

CCTV interventions involve the installation of cameras at locations thought to suffer from insufficient surveillance, and at which the provision of formal surveillance might deter offenders or help to detect crime. The mechanisms through which CCTV might reduce crime therefore fit in to the general SCP strategy of increasing the risk (actual or perceived) to the offender.

The systematic review conducted by Welsh and Farrington (2008b) was based on 44 evaluations (the meta-analysis used 20 studies with 41 distinct effect sizes) of the effects of CCTV on levels of crime in public places. The interventions evaluated varied in terms of their context—some were located in car parks, others were in town centers, whereas still others focused on public transport or were located in areas of public housing. They also varied in terms of the type of crime that they were intended to reduce; some focused on property crime, others on violence, and others still on a combination of these.

Overall the review found that CCTV appeared to be a promising approach showing a modest but significant desirable effect on crime. However, this depended very much on the context and the type of crime addressed. In particular, CCTV was found to be effective at reducing vehicle crime, but was not effective at preventing violence and assault. It was found to be particularly effective at reducing vehicle crime within the context of car parks, demonstrating a reduction of 50% in the problem.

It is therefore apparent that CCTV should not be used as a one-size-fits-all solution and care needs to be taken in considering the particular circumstances in which to implement such measures. For example, it is useful to explore reasons why CCTV might be particularly effective in car parks. In these situations, camera coverage is often high and other security measures coexist along with CCTV (such as better lighting and security guards). These factors are likely to contribute to the success of these schemes.

Public Area Surveillance

CCTV is one form of surveillance that may influence the likelihood of crime occurrence in public places, but it is not the only one. Other forms include the natural surveillance provided by an ambient population, which might be enhanced through environmental design, formal surveillance provided by security guards, or surveillance provided by place managers. These other forms of surveillance are also part of the situational approach to crime reduction, aimed at increasing offender perceptions of the risks associated with crime (Welsh et al., 2010). Security guards have a well-established role in providing surveillance to reduce crime in public places and are often seen to perform a private policing function. Place managers are individuals that are responsible for overseeing security issues through surveillance in specific settings as part of their employment (Eck, 1995). Examples include bus drivers, car park attendants, or train conductors.

The term "natural surveillance" is generally taken to refer to the public's ability to monitor their surroundings as part of their daily activities. Natural surveillance can be improved through a number of situational strategies. Many of these involve manipulation of the design of the environment to encourage or ease natural monitoring. These ideas are incorporated in Crime Prevention Through Environmental Design (CPTED) practices (Jeffery, 1971) which include the redesign of walkways, the removal of items that obscure lines of site such as bushes, and the closure or addition of barricades to streets. Such interventions are often based on the "defensible space" approach proposed by Newman (1972). That is, the public are more likely to act as guardians against crime if they feel ownership of their local area, have the ability to monitor those spaces, and are encouraged to use the space.

A systematic review of the effectiveness of public area surveillance in reducing crime was conducted by Welsh et al. (2010). The research actually comprised three systematic reviews that focused on the impacts of security guards, place managers, and defensible space, respectively. However, the effects of these types of interventions were reported together given the similarity of their themes. In total, 12 studies were identified that met the inclusion criteria and were of sufficient methodological quality. Of these, five evaluated the impact on crime of security guards, five evaluated interventions that focused on enhancing defensible space (in particular street closures), and two considered the effectiveness of place managers. As the numbers were low, the authors did not conduct a formal meta-analysis. However, consideration of the evidence showed generally encouraging results. This was particularly true in the case of street closures and the use of barricades where fairly strong evidence suggested that they were effective in preventing crimes in inner-city neighborhoods. The results were less unequivocal regarding the impact on crime of security guards and place managers, although this was at least in part due to the low number of studies available.

Neighborhood Watch

Neighborhood watch schemes are a situational measure because they attempt to increase the risk associated with offending by increasing levels of surveillance and hence the likelihood that offenders will be deterred from offending or be detected as a consequence of intelligence gathered. The principle behind these schemes is that a structured approach to having residents keeping watch of other houses and property or scanning for unusual events should increase the risk to offenders. Publicity is also often associated with this kind of scheme, and this might deter potential offenders by increasing their perceived risks of being apprehended. Similarly, a neighbor's attempts to increase signs of occupancy when a house is left vacant might increase an offender's perception of risk in a neighborhood.

Neighborhood watch schemes became popular in the 1980s and many streets in the UK and the USA in particular participate. A systematic review that used evidence from 12 evaluation studies, producing 18 effect sizes, was conducted by Bennett et al. (2008) and found that these approaches reduce crime by 16–26%. The meta-analysis focused mainly on volumes of residential burglary and ensured that there was a post-implementation period of at least 1 year. A moderator analysis demonstrated that the size and type of scheme did not appear to affect the size of the effect. Thus, on the basis of this review it would appear that small stand-alone schemes work as well as large, multifaceted ones.

Repeat Victimization Strategies

Research consistently demonstrates that one of the best predictors of future victimization risk is prior victimization (Pease, 1998). Accordingly, RV strategies aim to focus preventative effort on those who have previously been victimized on at least one previous occasion. Theoretically, this should be effective as it ensures limited resources are directed to those people or places where they are most likely to have an impact. Moreover, research shows that when RV occurs it takes place swiftly after an antecedent event (e.g., Johnson et al., 1997), which suggests that the targeting of prior victims immediately after a victimization is most likely to be effective. This is useful insofar as it helps to prioritize not just where but when resources should be deployed. RV strategies enable the victim to tool up against crime in a number of ways; for example, through increasing the risks to offenders (e.g., CCTV or surveillance), increasing the effort (e.g., target hardening doors and windows), or through reducing rewards (e.g., securing or removing expensive goods). RV strategies are undeniably situational and can be used as a framework for effective implementation of SCP interventions and hence we feel they warrant inclusion in this review.

A very recent review of RV strategies, conducted using Campbell guidelines, was undertaken by Grove et al. (2012). The review used evidence from 31 studies (21 were included in the meta-analysis constituting 27 effect sizes) that evaluated efforts to prevent RV. Most of these aimed to prevent residential burglary, but those addressing commercial burglary, domestic violence, and sexual assault were also considered. The results of the review suggested that overall RV strategies were effective at reducing victimization; relative to appropriate comparison groups, crime decreased by one sixth for the intervention groups. Moderator analysis suggests that these strategies are particularly effective for burglary but have limited effectiveness for sexual assaults.

The RV review also (fairly atypically) considered particular tactics and implementation issues in more detail. For example, it was found that SCP tactics appear to be most effective, and that advice and education provided to victims (a more passive approach) was found to be least effective. Furthermore, the review suggested that the effectiveness of a program was highly related to the effectiveness of its implementation.

SCP Counterterrorism Strategies

Situational prevention can also be applied in the context of counterterrorism (Clarke & Newman, 2006). In their review, Lum et al. (2006) examined the impacts of a range of approaches to counterterrorism, including those that may be classified as focusing on the prevention, detection, management, and responses to terrorism. In the prevention category, they examined interventions that are situational in nature and we therefore limit the discussion here to those. However, it should be acknowledged that this is only one part of a review that covered a wider range of interventions.

In the review, a total of seven studies were identified that satisfied the study inclusion criteria. In all, 86 effect sizes were reported and the authors found no evidence of a consistent positive effect of counterterrorism policy. For the subcategories that we would consider as situational approaches, metal detectors in airports appeared to in general be a promising intervention; with 16 reported effect sizes showing a weighted mean effect of a reduction of 6.3 events—a statistically significant decrease. However, the authors note a distinction between outcomes; metal detectors appeared to be effective at reducing hijackings in particular; they note that for nonhijacking outcomes (e.g., bombings, hostage taking, or armed attacks), there was actually a significant increase in the numbers of events. They raise the possibility that this is caused by potential displacement in the types of attacks undertaken.

The second relevant subcategory was the fortification of embassies and protection of diplomats. For this subcategory, there were 19 individual effect sizes. The overall weighted mean effect size of 0.45 was not statistically significant, indicating that the findings did not support the suggestion that these types of approaches were effective at reducing terrorist attacks. From a situational perspective, the first of the two approaches (the fortification of embassies) in this subcategory is arguably the most relevant. However, in the review mean effect sizes for these two different types of approaches (fortification of embassies and the protection of diplomats) are not reported separately.

Designated Driver Initiatives

The initiatives reviewed by Ditter et al. (2005) aimed to reduce alcohol-related crashes by encouraging the nomination of a designated driver. Two types of scheme were considered; campaigns aimed at the general public, and interventions that were implemented in drinking establishments and that provided incentives for people to act as a designated driver. There was some variation in the way the incentive programs operated, in some cases, designated drivers were offered free admission and soft drinks and in others free food. In some cases abstinence was a requirement, in others it was not.

Both of these interventions draw on the philosophy of SCP. In the case of the former, the campaigns aim to remove excuses for the type of undesirable activity targeted. However, the rather general approach, which is not immediately directed at a specific target audience at the time that they might engage in illegal activity (or just before), is less likely to be effective than a more focused campaign (Johnson & Bowers, 2003). With respect to the latter, incentives that might appeal to a rational actor are encountered at the point (in time) that they make a choice and so the effects may be more direct.

Using a systematic search, the authors found nine evaluations that reported a quantifiable outcome and met the minimum standard of quality for both the design and execution of the research. A number of types of outcome were used including the self-reported frequency of designated driver selection: observation of identified designated drivers in drinking establishments and self-reports of being an alcohol-impaired driver or a passenger of one. None of the studies used frequency or seriousness of crashes as an outcome.

One single study of the impact of campaigns aimed at the general population showed no change in any of the key outcomes. The authors conclude that there is insufficient evidence to gauge the effectiveness of these types of interventions. The authors of the review found some small effects for the more focused schemes, with modest increases in the number of designated drivers being (self)-reported. Overall, however, the authors conclude that as yet there is insufficient evidence to assess the effectiveness of these specific types of interventions.

Summary

Across the systematic reviews presented here it appears that there is good reason to be optimistic about the effectiveness of situational approaches to reducing crime problems. Before moving on to discuss the conclusions that can be made by assessing this evidence as a whole, three points are worth making. First, a number of outliers, duplicates, and discrepancies become evident when looking at what is included within and between the reviews. For example, in the RV review, it was noted that the studies that focused on sexual assaults provided treatment to individuals and not to an area—the latter being the far more common unit of intervention for situational measures. Furthermore, it is not clear that the sexual assault interventions—which were the least effective—could be classed as SCP schemes as they aimed to change the behavior of individuals through education, rather than the manipulation of situational factors that might influence opportunities for crime.

A second consideration is the unit of analysis itself. As discussed, for most SCP interventions, the treatment is implemented at the area level and hence the effect sizes calculated reflect changes at this level of aggregation. Relative to other types of interventions (e.g., offender rehabilitation) this makes SCP interventions distinctive in terms of the method by which effect sizes are calculated (which nearly always involves calculation of the relative risk ratio as described in, e.g., Welsh & Farrington, 2008a, b). It also opens up both methodological and philosophical debates. Methodological issues include those concerning statistical assumptions, such as the extent to which it is reasonable to assume that the data-generating process can be described by a Poisson process (Farrington & Welsh, 2004). Philosophical issues include the degree to which such interventions can be dealt with in similar ways to (for example) medical ones, where the administration of treatment is far more direct. We return to some of these issues later on.

A third consideration is the degree to which effectiveness is mediated or moderated by different conditions or contexts. In most of the cases described earlier there were several conditions under which increased or decreased levels of effectiveness might be anticipated. For example, particular types of area, types of crime targeted, geographical locations, or times of the day saw differential effects. This speaks to the benefit of taking an approach to evaluation that more deeply considers circumstance, context, and mechanism as highlighted by Pawson and Tilley (1997). The degree to which mediators and moderators affect the likely outcome of SCP interventions is a subject to which we turn in the next section.

General Patterns for SCP Interventions

In this section, we use the data collected as part of the systematic reviews discussed earlier to draw more general conclusions. To do this, we compiled a database of the 110 different effect sizes calculated across the 63 different studies described in 5 of the systematic reviews. In all cases the effect size measure used was the (odds or) relative risk ratio. Besides collecting information on effect sizes, we also systematically coded information on a number of other factors including the year of publication of the evaluation, the country in which the intervention was implemented, the outcome measured (in terms of crime type), and the physical context of the intervention (e.g., was it implemented in a residential area, a town center, and so on).

Before discussing these effect sizes collectively, it is important to consider the issue of potential overlap between the studies from the five reviews. The concern here is that there may be some double counting of studies; that is, some evaluations

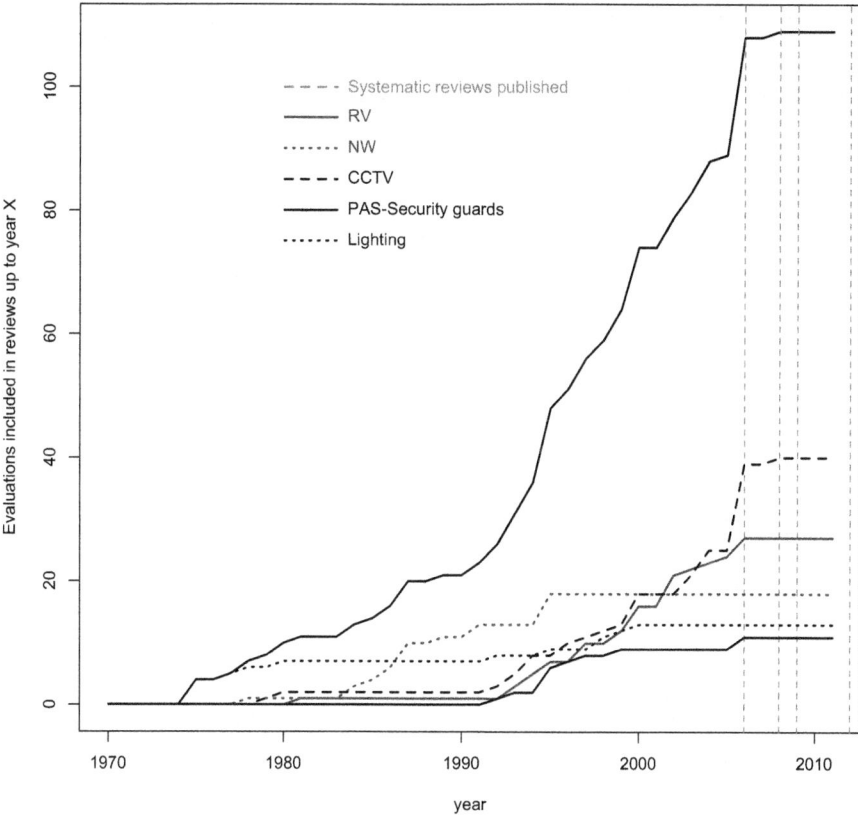

Fig. 4.2 Cumulative number of studies included in the reviews, by year of publication. *RV* repeat victimization strategies, *NW* neighborhood watch, *PAS-Security Guards* public area surveillance and security guards

could be included in more than one systematic review. This could be an issue because area-based interventions rarely comprise a single strategy. When we assessed overlap, we in fact found only one case of repetition. Both the NW and RV systematic reviews included the evaluation of the Kirkholt project (which had one of the largest effect sizes for the NW interventions). The Kirkholt project did include an element of NW but it should be noted that it was predominantly an RV strategy. Further, the two reviews used different evaluation reports (that used slightly different data) of the same project. The lack of overlap for SCP reviews could well be because the interventions are well defined and often involve different hardware, different allocation strategies, and different outcomes. Whatever the reason for the lack of overlap, it means that double counting should not be an issue in terms of the analysis that follows.

Considering the popularity of evaluations of this kind, Fig. 4.2 shows the cumulative number of evaluation studies[4] that were of sufficient methodological adequacy

---

[4] To be entirely accurate, it is in fact the cumulative number of effect size observations within the studies.

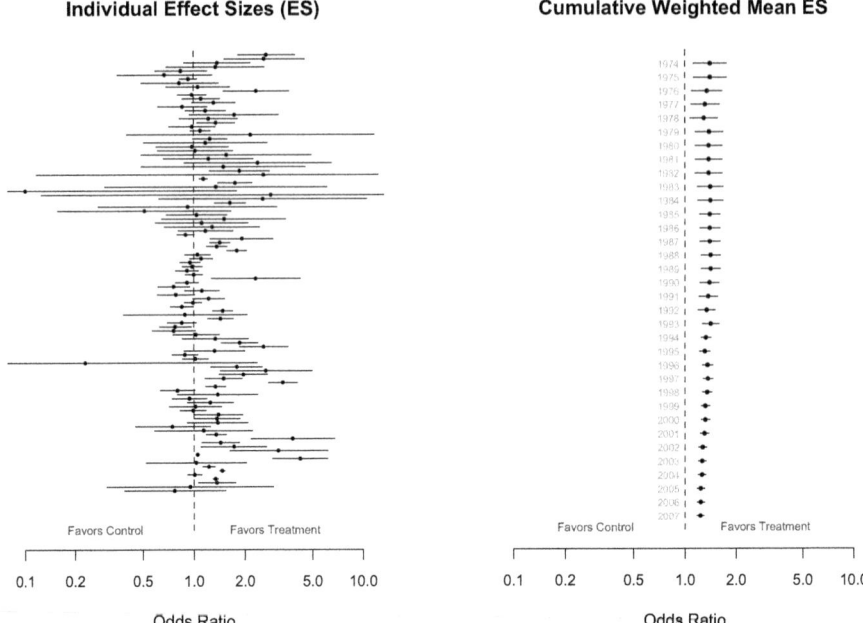

Fig. 4.3 Individual effect sizes for each observation and the cumulative weighted mean effect size, by year of publication

to be included in one of the systematic reviews considered earlier. It is evident that the number of evaluation studies of SCP interventions has been increasing steadily since the mid-1970s, and that there was a notable increase in the number of studies published from the early 1990s onwards. There appear to be few studies published around the start of the most recent decade (2010). However, this most likely reflects the fact that the reviews themselves were published around this time.

Considering trends in the estimates of the effect sizes over time, the left panel of Fig. 4.3 shows the effect size and confidence intervals for each of the observations for which data were available ($n=110$). The effect sizes are arranged sequentially in order of recency, with the most recently published studies shown at the bottom of the plot. It is evident that there is considerable variability in the effect size values, particularly given that the plot is on a logarithmic scale. Visual inspection of this figure suggests that the majority of the effect sizes appear to favor treatment and that many do so significantly. The right panel of Fig. 4.3 shows cumulative weighted mean effect sizes and their associated confidence intervals. One thing that this suggests is that from the very beginning and throughout, the cumulative body of evidence suggested a positive and reliable impact of SCP interventions on crime. As an alternative visualization of the data, Fig. 4.4 displays the information in the order of decreasing magnitude of effect size in favor of treatment. Again, the figure suggests a fairly positive picture in terms of the effectiveness of SCP treatments.

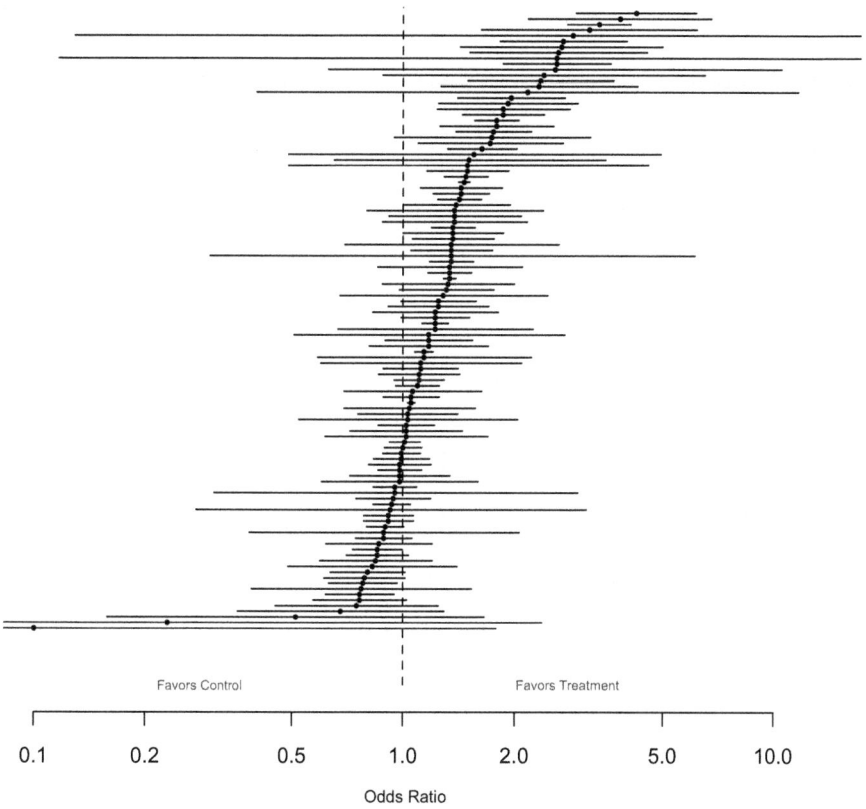

Fig. 4.4 Individual effect sizes for each observation by decreasing magnitude of positive treatment effect

The previous section focused on the individual systematic reviews and hence what the cumulative body of knowledge suggests about the impact of particular *types* of intervention. We next consider what, if anything, might be learned by partitioning the data in different ways. In particular, if we consider the impact of SCP interventions more generally, are particular trends observed for those that are implemented in particular types of areas, in particular countries, in particular decades, or that target particular types of crimes?

To do this, we computed weighted mean effect sizes for studies classified in the ways described. There was considerable heterogeneity in the effect sizes for the different groups and so the weighted mean effect sizes were calculated using random effects models. Moreover, for all studies, when computing the confidence intervals,

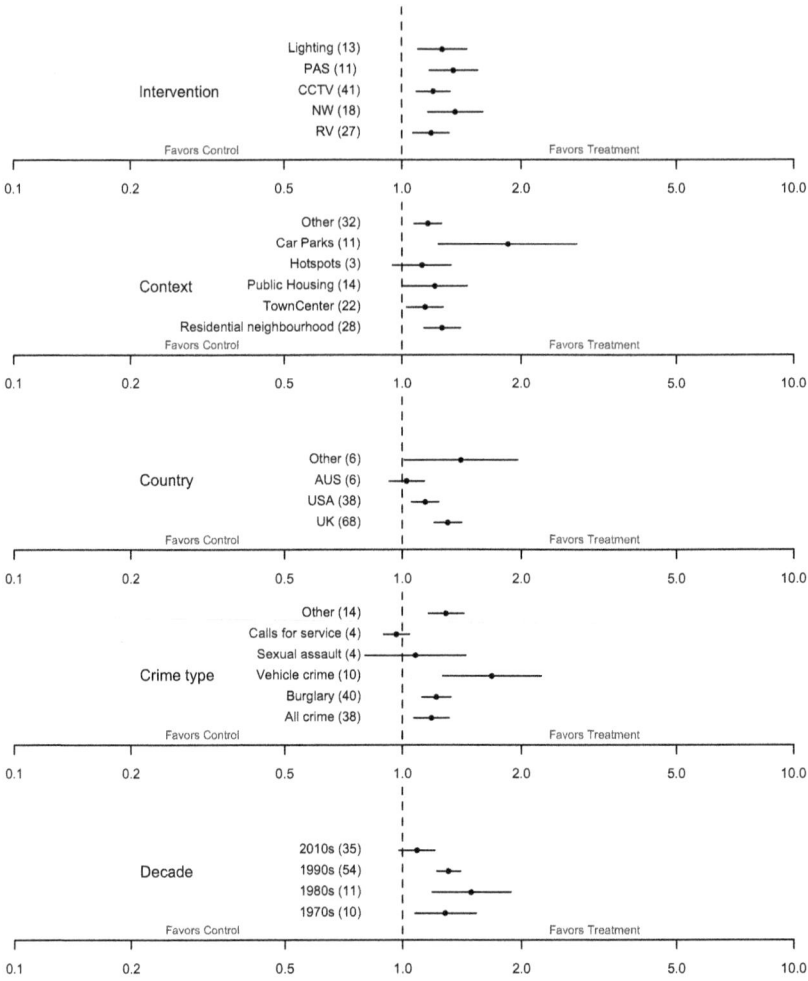

Fig. 4.5 Weighted mean effect sizes by different moderator variables (the number of studies in each group is shown in parentheses)

we multiplied the standard errors by 3.92 (rather than 1.96) to account for potential overdispersion in the data (e.g., Farrington & Welsh, 2004). Figure 4.5 shows the results. In terms of context, we grouped studies according to the general type of environment in which they were implemented. In doing so, five clear categories of land use or area type emerged. For the remainder of studies, the interventions were implemented in one of a range of different types of area, or in more than one type of area. On the basis of this analysis, it would appear to be the case that SCP interventions have positive impacts on crime regardless of the context within which they are implemented (although those implemented in hot spots just fail to demonstrate a significant weighted mean effect). However, those implemented in car parks appear to have the largest (weighted) mean effects by some way, although relative to interventions implemented in other types of area there is more variation in the estimated effects. This is not surprising since this group of effect sizes is made up largely, but not entirely, of the CCTV interventions highlighted earlier as being particularly effective in car parks.

In more general terms, it would appear that SCP interventions implemented in Australia or countries other than the USA or UK tend to have smaller effect sizes associated with them. However, it is also clear that the majority of evaluations are conducted either in the UK ($n=68$) or the USA ($n=38$). Overall, interventions implemented in the UK appear to be slightly more effective than those implemented in the USA. The reasons for variations by country are likely to be contextual in nature; for instance, differences in national policies, infrastructure to encourage partnership working, or funding available for the implementation of SCP interventions.

The effectiveness of SCP measures also appears to vary by crime type. Figure 4.5 suggests that schemes that focus on a single type of property crime such as burglary or vehicle crime, and studies that aim to reduce all recorded crime, tend to have a positive impact on levels of crime, whereas those aimed at reducing calls for service or sexual assault appear less likely to show significant success.

Finally, classifying by decade of study also revealed some differences in the weighted mean effect size. It appears that interventions evaluated in the 1980s tended to demonstrate higher levels of success than preceding or subsequent decades. It is again possible to speculate why this might be the case; SCP was a fresh idea in the 1980s and it was potentially an era where cherished pilot interventions were being placed into more virgin territory by motivated practitioners. Tilley (1993) discusses this and other issues in his assessment of why putative replications of the (very successful) Kirkholt burglary reduction project were less effective at reducing crime than the study they sought to emulate. In that piece, he discusses the issue of implementation intensity and fidelity, which is something to which we will return to later.

Whatever the reason for the variation in weighted effect sizes shown in Fig. 4.5, when classified by different moderating variables, the central point is that variation is apparent. This can also be quantified using Q statistics to partition the variation observed in the effect sizes that may be explained by the categorical (moderator) variable (Q_b), and that which is attributed to the residual pooled within-group portion (Q_w). Q_b and Q_w statistics were calculated for each group of categories shown in Fig. 4.5. The results indicated that in all cases the Q_b values were statistically significant, indicating that there was reliable between-group variability in the individual effect sizes. As this was so for all of the moderator variables, it suggests that factors other than the exact type of intervention may be useful in explaining differences in intervention effectiveness.

However, it is important to add that the Q_w statistics were also highly significant and had larger values than the Q_b statistics. These large Q_w statistics suggest that the variation observed within groups is unlikely to be explained by sampling error, and that the moderator variables selected do not sufficiently identify what those differences might be. This perhaps suggests the importance, of the specific context in which and the precise way in which, interventions are implemented.

Finally, the evaluations considered varied in terms of methodological adequacy. Studies have shown that it is important to consider the mediating effect of study design on outcome of criminal justice initiatives. For example, Weisburd et al. (2001) demonstrate that weaker designs with lower internal validity are more likely to report an outcome in favor of treatment and less likely to find harmful effects. This finding was supported in a more recent replication study by Welsh et al. (2011). In the current study, for 2 of the 110 observations, units were allocated to conditions using a random allocation strategy. For 106 of the observations a quasi-experimental design was used, and for 2 observations it was unclear whether random allocation was employed. Given the small numbers involved, it is not advisable to place too much confidence in any comparison of the effect sizes reported, but it appears that there was a slight trend for larger effect sizes to be reported in the case of the studies that employed a random allocation strategy. Since there is insufficient evidence to systematically test this, no further conclusion can be made here and this factor is not represented in Fig. 4.5.

Discussion

It is clear then that the majority of evaluations of SCP interventions employ a quasi-experimental design, with the majority comparing changes in the rates (be it per unit time or population at risk) of crime in treatment and comparison areas. Such designs rule out some threats to internal validity (e.g., history, maturation)—alternative explanations for observed patterns—that weaker designs invite, but they are still potentially subject to others, including regression to the mean (RTM) and multiple treatment interference (Campbell & Stanley, 1963). RTM can be ruled through the analysis of time-series data for the period prior to intervention and is naturally taken account of in studies that employ an interrupted time-series design. Fewer studies of this kind were identified in the systematic reviews. One reason for this is that such designs are not feasible in cases where the count of crime per unit time is low and so in such cases data are generally aggregated to enable pre- to post-intervention comparisons.

Very few studies employed a random allocation strategy. The advantage of this type of design is that where there are sufficient numbers of units it rules out threats to internal validity, leading to treatment and comparison groups that are matched on those characteristics that are observed and those that are not. The principle of random allocation is simple and it has the advantage of simplifying the statistical analyses that are required to estimate the impact of an intervention.

One reason that RCTs have not been the rule in the evaluation of SCP interventions is that evaluations are often commissioned to examine the effects of an intervention implemented at a particular place. That is, it is often the case that an area is identified as experiencing a crime problem and those responsible for crime and disorder in that area attempt to reduce it. Oftentimes, the actors involved will employ a problem-oriented policing approach (Goldstein, 1979), identifying and then tailoring a potential solution that fits the identified problem. This is quite different to (but not completely incompatible with) the philosophy behind the RCT approach whereby one starts with an intervention of interest and aims to determine the extent to which it reduces crime. In the case of the latter, those involved will be less concerned about the particular places in which the intervention is tested and more about whether a systematic effect is observed, regardless of context. To some extent, in this case, context is more a nuisance factor to be controlled for, although such designs do, through moderator analysis, allow for the examination of the interaction between context and a particular type of intervention.

However, there exist some SCP interventions that are often used in area-based initiatives but that are implemented at the individual level and which those who manufacture them would claim work, presumably regardless of context. This makes them amenable to an RCT and the fact that they are commercial products calls for their systematic study. To take an example, "forensic" or other forms of property marking are used to mark valuable goods so as to either make them less attractive to thieves or aid in their recovery post-theft. Such interventions could easily be evaluated using an RCT design.

For evaluations where the unit of analysis is a place or an area, a further complication relates to implementation intensity. To explain, where interventions are directed at individuals, all of those assigned to the treatment group will usually receive the treatment, and so for each unit of analysis the level of treatment will be all or nothing. In contrast, for place-based interventions, the association between the level of intervention received and the group to which an area is assigned (treatment or control) is rarely so simple. Instead, for the treatment group, the level of intensity will generally vary from (say) 0 to 100 % coverage. To take an example, in the case of CCTV, while an entire area may be designated as a treatment area, it is unlikely that all of it will be covered by cameras. Farrington et al. (2007) usefully examine the relationship between CCTV coverage and effect size. They find a significant correlation of 0.63 ($p=.021$) between a measure of effect size and the CCTV coverage of 13 interventions. This suggests that it is important to consider the extent of treatment, and that measures of outcome are sensitive to changes in the intensity of treatment. In the case of a target hardening initiative, rarely will all homes in the treatment area receive the intervention. In line with this, Grove et al. (2012) find a positive association between RV interventions and levels of intensity. Bowers et al. (2004) report similar findings for area-based interventions more generally.

A further distinction between place-based prevention evaluation and other types of experiment is that the mechanism by which the intervention operates is often less clear. For example, with a clinical drug trial, the drug will be a direct causal agent, and even for other areas within criminology (e.g., drug treatment or correctional interventions) it is easier to trace steps between the treatment and the outcome (Pawson, 2006). For place-based interventions to be reliably tested, care needs to be taken to ensure that implementation went as planned, which in a field with high levels of implementation failure cannot purely be assumed (Knutsson & Tilley, 2009).

As a final point, it is obvious from the results discussed earlier that there are a large number of unmeasured contextual factors that give rise to variation in the effectiveness of SCP interventions. It is far from the case, for example, that the type of measure alone will determine whether a particular scheme will work or not. We have demonstrated via moderator analysis that other factors might in fact be as important in determining effectiveness—for example, the geographical location and context. The more accurate and extensive other information about the intervention context is, the greater our ability to make judgments about its general applicability, and thus the greater the external validity of the evaluation.

Unanticipated Effects

It is difficult to leave a debate on the effectiveness of place-based situational prevention measures without a brief discussion about displacement. One of the most common criticisms of SCP interventions is that crime will simply relocate to other times and places since the "root causes" of crime were not addressed. This phenomenon is known as crime displacement. Spatial displacement (e.g., Hesseling, 1994), which is the movement of crime from an intervention treatment area to an area nearby, is the form most commonly debated and therefore analyzed. On the flip side of the displacement debate is the phenomenon of "diffusion of crime control benefits" (Clarke & Weisburd, 1994). Diffusion occurs when reductions of crime are achieved in areas that are close to crime prevention interventions, even though those areas were not actually targeted by the intervention itself.

There has been no formally conducted Campbell Collaboration systematic review of the degree to which SCP measures displaced crime or lead to diffusion of benefit. However, a review conducted closely in line with procedures recommended by Campbell was conducted by Johnson et al. (2011). This found that for 13 SCP studies in which sufficient quantitative information was available for the calculation of effect sizes, geographic displacement was not an inevitable consequence of this type of intervention. In fact, across the studies examined, it was rarely the case that crime increased in the potential displacement areas following intervention. Furthermore, crime appeared just as likely (or perhaps slightly more so) to decrease in the areas that surround a treatment area following intervention, suggesting a diffusion of benefit. This review was limited in scope by low numbers of suitable studies, and it was noted that there was a tendency for included SCP interventions to be of a certain type (those based on increasing surveillance). However, it is encouraging that displacement is not the inevitable problematic side effect of SCP that some might believe it to be.

Methodological Issues and Future Research

There are a number of issues with the analysis presented in this chapter that require articulation. The first is that we used all 110 effect sizes in the production of the figures presented. This means that it is not possible to assume that the effect sizes are independent of each other. Hence the weighted mean effect sizes calculated are likely to contain multiple observations for the same study. While this would be problematic for a systematic review if it was not addressed in greater depth, we consider it a justifiable position in this situation as we are comparing trends in the weighted mean effect sizes, rather than using the evidence to consider the effectiveness of a particular approach.

A further issue is that the moderator analysis relies on reliable coding in the original studies and consequent categorization of study features. Again, we do not claim that this is absolutely the case here (e.g., we used the systematic reviews rather than the original studies to code the moderator variables) and we ask the reader to consider that we are using the categories selected earlier for illustration purposes. The important point is that various contextual factors can be useful in helping to explain variation in effectiveness.

Finally, we have not considered interactions between the moderator variables. In other words, it might be the case that CCTV schemes had a differential effect in different decades or that SCP schemes that address vehicle crime in Australia are more effective than those in the USA. We suggest that considering these interactions could be a useful avenue for future research.

Conclusion

The general message from this chapter is a positive one; the existing systematic reviews of SCP tend to indicate significant, albeit modest reductions in levels of crime or victimization as a consequence of this type of activity. There are some exceptions; the existing evidence on protecting embassies and diplomats does not indicate reductions in counterterrorist activity and there is insufficient evidence to make conclusions concerning the effectiveness of designated driver interventions. However, the reviews indicate the more "mainstream" situational measures such as CCTV, improved lighting, and public area surveillance appear to be effective, as do some of the situational strategies such as RV schemes and NW.

Of course there are caveats to these conclusions—they are based only upon evidence from systematic reviews, which means the evidence comes from one particular point of view. These findings need to be combined with other evidence about mechanisms to be of more practical use to practitioners. The sort of process undertaken in this chapter can only benefit from more individual-level evaluations and more systematic reviews of situational measures. For example, a review of the effectiveness of blocking or restricting public access to risky places would be particularly beneficial.

References

Bennett, T., Holloway, K., & Farrington, D. (2008). The effectiveness of neighborhood watch. *Campbell Systematic Reviews, 4*(18). http://campbellcollaboration.org/lib/project/50/.

Bowers, K. J., Johnson, S. D., & Hirschfield, A. F. G. (2004). The measurement of crime prevention intensity and its impact on levels of crime. *British Journal of Criminology, 44*(3), 1–22.

Brantingham, P. L., & Brantingham, P. J. (1993). Environment, routine and situation: Toward a pattern theory of crime. *Advances in Criminological Theory, 5,* 259–294.

Campbell, D. T., & Stanley, J. C. (1963). *Experimental and quasi-experimental designs for research.* Dallas: Houghton Mifflin.

Clarke, R. V. (1983). Situational crime prevention: Its theoretical basis and practical scope. *Crime and Justice, 4,* 225–256.

Clarke, R. V. (1995). Situational crime prevention. In M. Tonry & D. P. Farrington (Eds.), *Building a safer society: Strategic approaches to crime prevention. (Crime and justice: A review of research* (Vol. 19). Chicago: University of Chicago Press.

Clarke, R. V., & Cornish, D. B. (1985). Modeling offenders' decisions: A framework for research and policy. *Crime and Justice, 6,* 147–185.

Clarke, R. V., & Newman, G. R. (2006). *Outsmarting the terrorists.* Westport: Praeger. Security International.

Clarke, R. V., & Weisburd, D. (1994). Diffusion of crime control benefits: Observations on the reverse of displacement. In R. V. Clarke (Ed.), *Crime prevention studies* (Vol. 2). Monsey: Criminal Justice Press.

Cornish, D. B., & Clarke. R. V. (2003). Opportunities, precipitators and criminal decisions: A reply to Wortley's critique of situational crime prevention. In M. J. Smith & D. B. Cornish (Eds.), *Theory for practice in situational crime prevention. Crime prevention studies* (Vol. 16). Monsey: Criminal Justice Press.

Cohen, L. E., & Felson, M. (1979). Social change and crime rate trends: A routine activity approach. *American Sociological Review, 44*(4), 588–608.

Ditter, S. M., Elder, R. W., Shults, R. A., Sleet, D. A., Compton, R., & Nichols, J. L. (2005). Effectiveness of designated driver programs for reducing alcohol-impaired driving: A systematic review. *American Journal of Preventative Medicine, 28,* 280–287.

Eck, J. E. (1995). A general model of the geography of illicit retail marketplaces. In D. Weisburd & J. E. Eck (Eds.), *Crime and place. (Crime Prevention Studies* (Vol. 4.) Monsey: Criminal Justice Press.

Eck, J. E. (2006). Preventing crime at places. In L. W. Sherman, D. Farrington, B. Welsh, & D. MacKenzie (Eds.) *Evidence-based crime prevention* (revised ed.). New York: Routledge.

Farrington, D. P., & Welsh, B. C. (2004). Measuring the effects of improved street lighting on crime. *British Journal of Criminology, 44*(3), 448–467.

Farrington, D. P., Gill, M., Waples, S. M., & Argomaniz, J. (2007). The effects of closed-circuit television (CCTV) on crime: Meta-analysis of an English national quasi-experimental multi-site evaluation. *Journal of Experimental Criminology, 3*(1), 21–38.

Goldstein, H. (1979). Improving policing: A problem-oriented approach. *Crime and Delinquency, 24,* 236–258.

Grove, L. E., Farrell, G., Farrington, D. P., & Johnson, S. D. (2012). *Preventing repeat victimization: A systematic review. Report prepared for the Swedish National Council for Crime Prevention.* Stockholm: The Swedish National Council for Crime Prevention.

Guerette, R. T. (2009). The pull, push and expansion of situational crime prevention evaluation: An appraisal of thirty-seven years of research. In N. Tilley & J. Knutsson (Eds.), *Evaluating crime reduction initiatives.* Crime prevention studies (Vol. 24, pp. 29–58). Monsey: Criminal Justice Press.

Hesseling, R. (1994). Displacement: A review of the empirical literature. In R. V. Clarke (Ed.), *Crime prevention studies* (Vol. 3). Monsey: Criminal Justice Press.

Jeffery, C. R. (1971). *Crime prevention through environmental design.* Beverly Hills: Sage.

Johnson, S. D., & Bowers, K. J. (2003). Opportunity is in the eye of the beholder: The role of publicity in crime prevention. *Criminology and Public Policy, 2*, 497–524.

Johnson, S. D., Bowers, K. J., & Guerette, R. (2011). Crime displacement and diffusion of benefit: A review of situational crime prevention measures. In B. Welsh & D. P. Farrington (Eds.), *The Oxford handbook of crime prevention*. Oxford: Oxford University Press.

Johnson, S. D., Bowers, K. J., & Hirschfield. A. (1997). New insights into the spatial and temporal distribution of repeat victimization. *British Journal of Criminology, 37*, 224–241.

Knutsson, J., & Tilley, N. (Eds.). (2009). *Evaluating crime reduction initiatives Crime prevention studies* (Vol. 24). Monsey: Criminal Justice Press.

Lum, C., Kennedy, L. W., & Sherley, A. (2006) The effectiveness of counter-terrorism strategies. *Campbell Systematic Reviews, 2*(2). http://www.campbellcollaboration.org/lib/project/11/.

Merton, R. K. (1938). Social structure and anomie. *American Sociological Review, 3*(5), 672–682.

Newman, O. (1972). *Defensible space: Crime prevention through urban design*. New York: Macmillan.

Pease, K. (1998). *Repeat victimisation: Taking stock. Crime prevention and detection series paper 90*. London: Home Office.

Pawson, R. (2006). *Evidence-based policy: A realist perspective*. London: Sage.

Pawson, R., & Tilley. N. (1997). *Realistic evaluation*. London: Sage.

Rengert, G. F., & Wasilchick, J. (2000). *Suburban burglary: A tale of two suburbs*. Springfield: Charles C. Thomas.

Shaw, C. R., & McKay, H. D. (1942). *Juvenile delinquency in urban areas*. Chicago: University of Chicago Press.

Smith, M. J., Clarke, R. V., & Pease, K. (2002). Anticipatory benefit in crime prevention. In N. Tilley (Ed.), *Crime prevention studies* (Vol. 13). Monsey: Criminal Justice Press.

Tilley, N. (1993). *After Kirkholt: Theory, method and results of replication evaluations*. London: Home Office.

Weisburd, D., Lum, C., & Petrosino, A. (2001). Does research design affect study outcomes in criminal justice? *Annals of American Political and Social Science, 578*, 50–70.

Welsh, B. C., & Farrington, D. P. (2008a). Effects of improved street lighting on crime. *Campbell Systematic Reviews, 4*(13). http://www.campbellcollaboration.org/lib/project/45/.

Welsh, B. C., & Farrington, D. P. (2008b). Effects of closed circuit television surveillance on crime. *Campbell Systematic Reviews, 4*(17). http://www.campbellcollaboration.org/lib/project/49/.

Welsh B.C., Mudge M.E., Farrington D.P. (2010). Reconceptualizing public area surveillance and crime prevention: Security guards, place managers and defensible space. *Security Journal, 23*, 299–319.

Welsh, B., Peel, M., Farrington, D., Elffers, H., & Braga, A. (2011). Research design influence on study outcomes in crime and justice: A partial replication with public area surveillance. *Journal of Experimental Criminology, 7*(2), 183–198.

Yochelson, S., & Samenow, S. E. (1976). *The criminal personality. Vol. 1: A profile for change*. New York: Jason Aronson.

Chapter 5
Policing

Cody W. Telep and David Weisburd

There is a growing evidence base of rigorous studies evaluating policing interventions (see Lum, Koper, & Telep, 2011) and a series of systematic reviews that have synthesized many of these studies. Just a decade ago, there were almost no systematic reviews available about policing, and narrative reviews provided the dominant approach for understanding police practices. We now have 17 completed systematic reviews of police practices. It is, in our view, now useful to conduct a "review of the reviews" to assess what we have learned, questions that remain unanswered, and how we can best move forward with systematic reviews of policing.

Systematic reviews have become an important tool for synthesizing what we know about various topics in criminal justice and have served to help inform researchers, policymakers, and practitioners about what does work and what does not work. Policing reviews appear to have been influential in policymaking and policing circles. The Office of Community Oriented Policing Services (COPS), for example, has a longstanding partnership with the Campbell Collaboration to publish practitioner-friendly guides on systematic reviews relevant to the police. Twelve guides are currently available.[1] The former National Policing Improvement Agency (NPIA) in the UK provided funding for nine systematic reviews and a systematic search (Telep & Weisburd, 2014). A number of policing reviews discussed in this chapter were originally presented at the Jerry Lee Crime Prevention

---

[1] See http://www.cops.usdoj.gov/Default.asp?Item=2614.

C. W. Telep (✉)
Arizona State University, Phoenix, AZ, USA
e-mail: cody.telep@asu.edu

D. Weisburd
Hebrew University of Jerusalem, Jerusalem, Israel
e-mail: david.weisburd@mail.huji.ac.il

George Mason University, Fairfax, VA, USA
e-mail: dweisbur@gmu.edu

Symposium in Washington, DC,[2] which brought together more than 100 academics, policymakers, and police officials annually. The Campbell library of systematic reviews is also listed as a resource on the Department of Justice's CrimeSolutions.gov Website, designed to help inform policymakers and practitioners on what works in policing and criminal justice. The rise in systematic reviews in policing over the past decade represents an important advance in policing research and taking stock of what has been learned is important at this juncture.

In this chapter, we first provide an overview of our search strategy for identifying relevant systematic reviews. We then provide brief summaries of our included reviews. We next turn to lessons learned from the findings of these reviews, focusing our attention on what works, what seems not to be effective, and what seems promising for both crime control effectiveness and increasing fairness and legitimacy in policing. We then discuss what important questions remain unanswered with these reviews, focusing on both the need for more rigorous research and areas of policing where a review might be useful. We next turn to problems encountered with the existing reviews. Finally, we conclude with some thoughts on lessons the police can learn from systematic reviews and our recommendations for the future of systematic reviews on policing.

Search Strategy

We sought to identify any systematic reviews on policing topics that used inclusion criteria ensuring that only more rigorous studies (i.e., randomized experiments and quasi-experiments, preferably with a comparison group) were eligible. While we suspected most of the reviews would focus on crime-related outcomes, we did not limit our search to any particular outcome measure. We did require, however, that reviews feature some sort of intervention or police action that would be associated with an outcome measure. In other words, we were interested in the impact of police programs, training, interventions, or activities on outcome measures. We also included only those reviews that featured exclusively or primarily studies where the police played a significant role in the intervention under review.

We began by examining the Campbell Collaboration Crime and Justice library, which provided us with 11 published and 3 forthcoming reviews related to policing.[3] We do not include reviews here that have some relevance to policing (e.g., Bennett, Holloway, & Farrington, 2008; Farrington & Ttofi, 2010; Lum, Kennedy, & Sherley, 2006; Strang et al., 2013; Welsh & Farrington, 2008), but are not

---

[2] See, for example, http://cebcp.org/jerry-lee-crime-prevention-symposium/ for more on the 2012 Jerry Lee Symposium.

[3] Reviews on community policing, macro displacement, and disorder policing were not yet available in the Campbell library at the time this chapter was published, but results were available in peer-reviewed journal articles that we cite here.

primarily focused on police practices.[4] We next searched the Cochrane Collaboration library for any reviews related to policing. We found one relevant review (Goss et al., 2008) that we included. We considered including the school-based drug prevention review by Faggiano et al. (2008), but because only two of the eligible studies included police and these were part of another review that we identified, we excluded this review.

We then searched online databases to identify additional relevant reviews.[5] We identified several articles described as "systematic reviews" but only two met our inclusion criteria:[6] a systematic review of Drug Abuse Resistance Education (D.A.R.E.) by West and O'Neal (2004) and a systematic review of police efforts to reduce traffic accidents by Blais and Dupont (2005). This left us with a total of 17 systematic reviews for analysis. We summarize these reviews in the next section.

Data Sources

We begin with a discussion of existing systematic reviews on policing. While available space limits our ability to describe each of these reviews in detail, we provide brief information on the purpose and findings of each of these reviews. More information on each completed review is available in Tables 5.1, 5.2, and 5.3.

In the past 5 years or so, there has been a massive increase in the number of systematic reviews related to policing. None of these 17 policing reviews were completed before 2004,[7] and 11 were proposed or completed after 2010. This expansion in the number of policing-related reviews is due in part to funding from the NPIA. As noted earlier, the NPIA provided financial support to a number of Campbell Collaboration reviews on policing or policing-related topics, eight of which we included in this chapter (see Telep & Weisburd, 2014). We begin by discussing the reviews that showed positive results and then discuss those where the programs studied showed little evidence of effectiveness.

---

[4] These reviews are also covered in other chapters in this volume.

[5] We searched Criminal Justice Abstracts, Criminal Justice Periodical Index, Sociological Abstracts, and Google Scholar for "systematic review" AND police OR policing. Because Google Scholar produced over 16,000 hits, we only examined the first 500.

[6] Excluded reviews included a systematic review of the criminal profiling literature that only summarized the state of the literature but did not include interventions (Dowden, Bennell, & Bloomfield, 2007), systematic reviews of weak studies methodologically on police use of improper force (Harris, 2009) and the effects of drug law enforcement on violence (Werb et al., 2011), a systematic review of factors related to police suicide that again did not include any sort of intervention (Hem, Berg, & Ekeberg, 2011), and a systematic review of interventions to reduce problems around bars that included mostly nonpolice interventions (Brennan et al., 2011).

[7] While Campbell did not publish Anthony Braga's hot spots review until 2007, the initial narrative findings were published in a 2001 article and the initial meta-analysis in a 2005 article (see Braga, 2001, 2005, 2007).

Table 5.1 Intervention, outcome measures, study designs, and search characteristics in published and forthcoming policing reviews

Researchers (Date)	Intervention	Comparison group	Outcome	Design	Searches	Time period
West & O'Neal (2004)	Drug Abuse Resistance Education (D.A.R.E.)	Students not receiving D.A.R.E.	Alcohol use, drug use, tobacco use	Randomized experiment or quasi-experiment with comparison group	Online databases, references of acquired studies	1991–2002
Blais & Dupont (2005)	Intensive police programs to prevent traffic accidents	Generally geographic areas not receiving the police program; some before/after studies	Accident with injuries, proxy measures of DWI or speeding	Randomized experiment, quasi-experiment with comparison group, or interrupted time series	Not described	1990–2004
Mazerolle et al. (2007)	Drug law enforcement	Geographic areas receiving "standard model" of policing	Drug offenses, drug calls for service (CFS), property offenses, violent offenses, overall CFS, social disorder	Randomized experiment or quasi-experiment with comparison group	Online databases, hand searches of journals, review of bibliographies, search of agency websites	1990–2001
Weisburd et al. (2008)	Problem-oriented policing	Comparison group of probationers in 2 studies, in all others geographic area not receiving police treatment	Crime (type varied by study) or recidivism	Randomized experiment or quasi-experiment with comparison group	Online databases, agency publication searches, hand searches of journals, forward searches, review of bibliographies, contacted experts	1993–2006
Davis et al. (2008)	Second responder programs for domestic violence	Domestic/family abuse victims not receiving second responder team	Reported abuse to police, reported abuse in survey	Randomized experiment or quasi-experiment with comparison group	Online databases, review of bibliographies, hand searches of journals, review of Violence Against Women Website, contacted experts	1992–2007
Goss et al. (2008)	Police patrols for drunken driving	Geographic areas not receiving increased police presence	Automobile accidents and injuries from accidents	Randomized experiment or quasi-experiment with comparison group, interrupted time series	Online databases, review of bibliographies, hand searches of conference abstracts, contacted experts	1976–2003

5 Policing   141

Table 5.1 (continued)

Researchers (Date)	Intervention	Comparison group	Outcome	Design	Searches	Time period
Bowers et al. (2011)	Micro displacement in focused police interventions	Geographic areas not receiving focused policing strategy; sometimes have catchment areas surrounding comparison site(s) for assessing displacement	Main crime control effect, displacement of crime, diffusion of crime control benefits	Randomized experiment, quasi-experiment with comparison group, or quasi-experiment with catchment area	Online databases, review of bibliographies, forward searches, search of professional agencies, hand searches of journals, contacted experts	1971–2010
Wilson et al. (2011)	DNA for police investigations	Generally cases in which DNA evidence was not used	Variation across studies, generally clearing cases or identifying suspects	Randomized experiment or quasi-experiment with comparison group	Online databases, Home Office, contacted experts	1998–2008
Braga & Weisburd (2012)	Focused deterrence strategies (pulling levers)	Generally geographic areas not receiving police attention (other neighborhoods or similar cities)	Crime (typically gun homicides or assaults)	Randomized experiment or quasi-experiment with comparison group	Online databases, review of bibliographies, forward searches, hand searches of journals, contacted experts	2001–2010
Braga et al. (2012)	Hot spots policing	Hot spots not receiving extra police attention	Crime, displacement and diffusion effects	Randomized experiment or quasi-experiment with comparison group	Online databases, review of bibliographies, forward searches, hand searches of journals, contacted experts	1989–2011
Koper & Mayo-Wilson (2012)	Interventions to reduce gun carrying	Geographic areas not receiving police attention or days intervention not operating	Gun crime	Randomized experiment or quasi-experiment with comparison group	Online databases, agency publication searches, review of bibliographies	1995–2003
Patterson et al. (2012)	Stress management programs (wide variation in interventions)	Police officers (and sometimes civilians) not receiving stress management program	Psychological outcomes, physiological outcomes, behavioral outcomes	Randomized experiment or quasi-experiment with comparison group	Online databases, hand searches of journals, websites searches, review of bibliographies, forward searches, contacted experts	1986–2008

Table 5.1 (continued)

Researchers (Date)	Intervention	Comparison group	Outcome	Design	Searches	Time period
Meissner et al. (2012)	Police interrogation techniques (coded as information gathering or accusatorial or general techniques common to both)	Criminal suspects (or mock suspects in laboratory experiments) receiving accusatorial techniques	Confessions elicited, true confessions elicited	Field study: quasi-experiment (assignment of technique to use) or systematic observation/coding of interview; Laboratory: randomized experiment	Online databases, review of bibliographies, review of abstracts from recent conferences, contacted experts	1996–2011
Mazerolle et al. (2013)	Programs and practices to increase procedural justice and citizen perceptions of legitimacy	Individuals not receiving police program or practice designed to increase legitimacy	Perceived legitimacy, procedural fairness (or perceived procedural fairness), willingness to cooperate with police, trust/confidence in police, social ties, compliance, satisfaction, reduction in reoffending or crime (indirect outcome)	Randomized experiment, quasi-experiment with comparison group, or quasi-experimental times series analysis	Online databases, review of bibliographies, review of references of influential authors	1987–2009
Gill et al. (2014)	Community-oriented policing	Geographic areas not receiving police attention	Property crime, violent crime, fear of crime, perceived disorder, citizen satisfaction, police legitimacy	Randomized experiment, quasi-experiment with comparison group, or quasi-experimental times series analysis	Online databases, review of bibliographies, forward searches, search of professional agencies, review of journal abstracts	1986–2010

Table 5.1 (continued)

Researchers (Date)	Intervention	Comparison group	Outcome	Design	Searches	Time period
Telep et al. (2014)	Displacement in interventions in medium sized or large geographic areas	Geographic areas not receiving social control intervention	Main crime control effect, displacement of crime, diffusion of crime control benefits	Randomized experiment, quasi-experiment with comparison group, or quasi-experimental times series analysis	Online databases, review of bibliographies, forward searches, search of professional agencies, review of journal abstracts, contacted experts	1971–2013
Braga et al. (2015)	Policing disorder	Geographic areas not receiving policing disorder intervention	Total crime, violent crime, property crime, disorder/drug crime	Randomized experiment, quasi-experiment with comparison group	Online databases, search of professional agencies, review of bibliographies, forward searches, hand searches, contacted experts	1985–2013

*$p < 0.05$

Table 5.2 Participants, number of studies, and results in published and forthcoming policing reviews

Researchers (Date)	Participants	Number of studies	Number of experiments	Effect size/significance (CI = Confidence Interval) (SD = Standard Deviation)	Moderators
West & O'Neal (2004)	Middle and high school students	11	1	Cohen's d 0.023; CI = −0.04, 0.08	None
Blais & Dupont (2005)	Geographic areas receiving intensive police response	33	0	Average % reduction in injuries with accident = 24.42 (SD = 10.00)	Type of intervention (results fairly consistent across intervention type)
Mazerolle et al. (2007)	Geographic areas receiving police response (hot spots, problem-oriented policing, or community-wide policing) to address drugs	14 (15 comparisons in meta-analysis)	3	Odds ratio (large number of meta-analyses, see full report for additional effect sizes) Drug CFS = 1.330 CI = 1.071, 1.642* Drug offenses = 1.530 CI = 0.749, 3.126 Total calls for service = 1.180 CI = 1.075, 1.296* Total offenses = 1.090 CI = 0.968, 1.227	Type of intervention (hot spots, POP, community-wide), implementation year, publication year, study design, length of follow-up period, methodological rigor
Weisburd et al. (2008)	Probationers in 2 studies; in all others geographic areas receiving POP response	10 in main analysis; 45 in separate pre/post analysis	4	Cohen's d (SD) Mean = 0.126 (0.047)* Largest = 0.296 (0.142)* Mean for experiments = 0.147 (0.011)* Mean for quasi-experiments = 0.158 (0.098)	None
Davis et al. (2008)	Domestic/family abuse victims	10	5	Cohen's d (SD) Overall mean reports to police = 0.082 (0.088) Mean reports to police in experiments = 0.117 (0.055)* Mean reports on survey = 0.021 (0.072)	None
Goss et al. (2008)	Geographic areas receiving increased police presence to address drunk driving	32	1	No mean effect sizes reported, only individual results from studies	None

Table 5.2 (continued)

Researchers (Date)	Participants	Number of studies	Number of experiments	Effect size/significance (CI=Confidence Interval) (SD=Standard Deviation)	Moderators
Bowers et al. (2011)	Geographic area receiving focused policing strategy; catchment areas surrounding target site(s) for assessing displacement	44 (16 studies in meta-analysis)	5	Odds ratio Best case treatment effect=1.39 CI=1.22–1.59* Best case displacement=1.14 CI=1.03–1.14* (significant diffusion) Worst case treatment effect=1.15 CI=1.05, 1.27* Worst case displacement=1.04 CI=0.95–1.13	Study design, intervention type, size of intervention
Wilson et al. (2011)	Cases in which DNA evidence was used	5	1	No mean effect size	None
Braga & Weisburd (2012)	Generally high rate offenders/gang members living in specified geographic areas	10	0	Cohen's d (SD) Overall mean = DMI=0.661 (0.213)* Gang/group=0.770 (0.127)* Individual=0.186 (0.057)* Near-equivalent quasi-experiments=0.196 (0.057)* Nonequivalent quasi-experiments=0.766 (0.112)*	Program type (high-risk individuals, gang group, Drug Market Initiative [DMI]), Research design (non-equivalent quasi-experiment, near equivalent quasi-experiment)
Braga et al. (2012)	High crime micro geographic units that typically receive extra police attention	19 (25 tests)	10	Cohen's d (SD) Mean=0.185 (0.035)* POP studies=0.232 (0.049)* Presence studies=0.113 (0.034)* Experiments=0.116 (0.026)* Quasi-experiments=0.325 (0.012)* Displacement/diffusion=0.104 (0.016)* - supports diffusion	Type of intervention (increasing presence vs. POP); Methodological quality (experiment vs. quasi-experiment)

Table 5.2 (continued)

Researchers (Date)	Participants	Number of studies	Number of experiments	Effect size/significance (CI=Confidence Interval) (SD=Standard Deviation)	Moderators
Koper & Mayo-Wilson (2012)	Geographic areas where crime reduction areas were implemented (e.g., beats, neighborhoods, or citywide)	4 (7 tests)	0	No mean effect size	None
Patterson et al. (2012)	Police officers (and sometimes civilians) receiving stress management program; 906 total included across 12 studies	12	9	Hedge's g (SD) Psychological outcomes=0.038 (0.098) Behavioral outcomes=−0.176 (0.277) Physiological outcomes=0.196 (0.196)	For psychological outcomes (length of stress management intervention, type of stress management intervention, population, gender, years of police experience, random assignment to conditions, attrition)
Meissner et al. (2012)	Criminal suspects (or mock suspects in laboratory experiments) receiving information-gathering techniques; Total of 608 interrogations coded in field studies; 1,814 participants in laboratory studies	17	12 (laboratory experiments)	Logged odds ratio transformed into Cox index *Field-studies* (eliciting confessions) Accusatorial=0.90, CI=0.38, 1.41* Information gathering=0.86 CI=0.04, 1.69* General=0.19 CI=−0.69, 1.06 *Laboratory* (eliciting true and false confession) Accusatorial vs. Control: True=0.46 CI=0.06, 0.86* False=0.74 CI=35, 1.12* Information-gathering vs. Control: True=0.67 CI=0.02, 1.32* False=−0.23 CI=−0.98, 0.52 Accusatorial vs. Information-gathering: True=0.64 CI=0.01, 1.28* False=−0.77 CI=−1.46,…,−0.08*	Different experimental paradigms in laboratory studies ("ALT key" paradigm, "cheating" paradigm)

Table 5.2 (continued)

Researchers (Date)	Participants	Number of studies	Number of experiments	Effect size/significance (CI = Confidence Interval) (SD = Standard Deviation)	Moderators
Mazerolle et al. (2013)	Varied, but all focused on individuals interacting with police in the context of police efforts to enhance legitimacy perceptions	30 (41 comparisons in meta-analysis)	4	Odds ratio: Legitimacy = 1.58 CI = 0.85, 2.95 Procedural justice = 1.47 CI = 1.16, 1.86* Compliance/cooperation = 1.62 CI = 1.13, 2.32* Satisfaction/confidence = 1.75 CI = 1.54, 1.99* Cohen's d: Reoffending = −0.07 CI = −0.14, 0.00	Intervention type, research design, respondent type, crime type, year of publication, country of publication
Gill et al. (2014)	Geographic areas (often neighborhoods) receiving community policing program	25 (covering 65 tests)	1	Odds ratio: Property crime = 1.05 CI = 0.98, 1.13 Violent crime = 1.10 CI = 1.02, 1.19* Perceived disorder = 1.24 CI = 0.92, 1.66 Fear of crime = 1.17 CI = 0.93, 1.46 Citizen satisfaction = 1.37 CI = 1.10, 1.72* Police legitimacy = 1.28 CI = 0.97, 1.67	Problem-solving as component of treatment
Telep et al. (2014)	Geographic area receiving social control intervention (typically a policing treatment); catchment areas surrounding target site(s) for assessing displacement	33 (covering 43 tests; 20 included in meta-analysis)	0	Odds ratio: Treatment effect mean = 1.46 CI = 1.25, 1.69* Displacement mean = 1.069 CI = 0.95, 1.20 Best case displacement = 1.11 CI = 0.99, 1.25 Worst case displacement = 1.02 CI = 0.92, 1.15 Police-led displacement = 1.01 CI = 0.87, 1.18	Whether the intervention was primarily police-led

Table 5.2 (continued)

Researchers (Date)	Participants	Number of studies	Number of experiments	Effect size/significance (CI = Confidence Interval) (SD = Standard Deviation)	Moderators
Braga et al. (2015)	Geographic areas (range of sizes) receiving policing disorder intervention	28 (covering 30 tests)	9	Cohen's d (SD): All crime = 0.21 (0.04)* Violent crime = 0.23 (0.07)* Property crime = 0.19 (0.05)* Disorder/drug crime = 0.27 (0.05)* Problem-solving = 0.27 (0.05)* Order maintenance = 0.06 (0.05)	Research design, whether the intervention used community problem solving or aggressive order maintenance

*$p < 0.05$

Table 5.3 Authors' summary of findings in published policing reviews

Researchers (Date)	Authors' summary of findings
West & O'Neal (2004)	"Given the tremendous expenditures in time and money involved with D.A.R.E., it would appear that continued efforts should focus on other techniques and programs that might produce more substantial effects" (p. 1028)
Blais & Dupont (2005)	"…different intervention types bring similar results. No particular intervention seems more effective than the others in improving road safety. In our study the implementation of intensive police programmes was associated with average reductions varying between 23 and 31 per cent of accidents with injuries" (p. 932)
Mazerolle et al. (2007)	"…rather than simply increasing police presence or intervention (e.g. arrests) at drug hotspots, street-level drug law enforcement should (1) focus on forging productive partnerships with third parties, (2) target drug hotspots rather than spreading intervention efforts across neighborhoods, and (3) make efforts to alter the underlying criminogenic conditions that exist in places with street-level drug market problems" (p. 3)
Weisburd et al. (2008)	"Despite a small number of eligible studies, we find an overall positive impact of POP across different units of analysis, different types of problems, and different types of outcome measures" (p. 34)
Davis et al. (2008)	"While second responder programs may slightly increase victims' confidence in the police to report abuse, they do not reduce the likelihood of repeat violence" (p. 18)
Goss et al. (2008)	"Studies examining increased police patrol programs were generally consistent in reporting beneficial effects on traffic crashes and fatalities, but study quality and reporting were often poor" (p. 2)
Bowers et al. (2011)	"…message from this review is a positive one to those involved in the sort of operational policing initiatives considered, the main point being that displacement is far from inevitable as a result of such endeavor, and, in fact that the opposite, a diffusion of crime control benefits appears to be the more likely consequence" (p. 4)
Wilson et al. (2011)	"The evidence suggests that DNA testing has value when used to investigate a broad range of crime types. There are caveats to this conclusion, and additional high quality evaluations are needed to establish the robustness and generalizability of these findings" (p. 5)
Braga & Weisburd (2012)	"While the evaluation evidence needs to be strengthened and the theoretical underpinnings of the approach needs further refinement, we believe that jurisdictions suffering from gang violence, overt drug markets, and repeat offender problems should add focused deterrence strategies to their existing portfolio of prevention and control interventions" (p. 28)

Table 5.3 (continued)

Researchers (Date)	Authors' summary of findings
Braga et al. (2012)	"The results of our updated systematic review and meta-analysis provide strong support for the basic conclusions of the original Campbell review: hot spots policing programs generate modest crime control gains and are likely to produce a diffusion of crime control benefits into areas immediately surrounding targeted high-activity crime places" (p. 19)
Koper & Mayo-Wilson (2012)	"With one exception, the included studies suggest that directed patrols focused on illegal gun carrying reduce gun violence at high-risk places and times. Inferences are limited, however, by the small number of available trials, variability in study design and analytical strategy, and the absence of randomized trials" (p. 33)
Patterson et al. (2012)	"These results do not provide evidence to support the efficacy of stress management interventions for police officers or recruits. Given the weakness of the research designs, we can neither claim that these programs are effective or ineffective" (p. 4)
Meissner et al. (2012)	"The available data support the effectiveness of an information-gathering style of interviewing suspects. Caution is warranted, however, due to the small number of independent samples available for the analysis of both field and experimental studies" (p. 7)
Mazerolle et al. (2013)	"Our review finds that police can use a variety of police-led interventions (including conferencing, community policing, problem-oriented policing, reassurance policing, informal police contact, and neighborhood watch) as vehicles for promoting and enhancing citizen satisfaction with and confidence in police, compliance and cooperation, and perceptions of procedural justice" (pp. 75–76)
Gill et al. (2014)	"The results of this systematic review of community-oriented policing (COP) strategies provide robust evidence that community policing increases satisfaction with police, elements of police legitimacy, and citizen perceptions of disorder…We do not find evidence that COP reduces fear of crime or officially recorded crime" (p. 423)
Telep et al. (2014)	"Both our narrative results and meta-analysis suggest that the most likely outcome from meso and macro-level studies is neither displacement nor a diffusion of benefits, although there is some suggestive evidence that diffusion may be somewhat more likely than displacement" (p. 544)
Braga et al. (2015)	"The results of our systematic review and meta-analysis suggest that disorder policing strategies generate noteworthy crime control gains…Aggressive order maintenance strategies that target individual disorderly behaviors do not generate significant crime reductions. In contrast, community problem-solving approaches that seem to change social and physical disorder conditions at particular places produce significant crime reductions" (pp. 580–581)

Reviews with Positive Results

Hot Spots Policing Braga, Papachristos, and Hureau (2012; see also Braga, 2007) examined the effectiveness of police efforts to target small geographic units with high rates of crime. The updated hot spots review found a number of additional studies not included in Braga's (2007) original review. Their meta-analysis of experimental studies found an overall mean Cohen's *d* of 0.184 (equivalent to an odds ratio of 1.396), suggesting a significant benefit of the hot spots approach in treatment compared to control areas. Of the 25 comparisons from 19 eligible studies, 20 showed notable crime declines as a result of the hot spots intervention. Braga et al. (2012) also compared the findings from studies that used increased police presence as a hot spots strategy with those using a problem-oriented intervention. They found that problem-oriented hot spots policing overall tends to lead to greater crime control benefits, although the authors caution that these comparisons are based on a smaller number of studies and that both types of strategies can lead to decrease in crime. Braga's (2007, p. 18) conclusion that "extant evaluation research seems to provide fairly robust evidence that hot spots policing is an effective crime prevention strategy" remains true in the updated review (see Braga et al., 2012).

Focused Deterrence Strategies Braga and Weisburd (2012) reviewed the impact of focused deterrence strategies. Many of these strategies employed the "pulling levers" framework popularized in Boston with Operation Ceasefire (Braga et al., 2001), in which gangs were notified that violence would no longer be tolerated and if violence did occur, every available legal lever would be pulled to bring an immediate and certain response. They found that such approaches had significant beneficial impacts on crime, particularly violent crime. Nine of the ten eligible studies showed significant positive impacts on crime. One concern is that there were no randomized trials included in the review, in part because of the difficulty in evaluating focused deterrence strategies in a randomized experimental framework (i.e., many of the interventions were implemented either citywide or in areas that were so unique in the jurisdiction that there was no reasonable comparison group).

Problem-Oriented Policing (POP) Weisburd, Telep, Hinkle, and Eck (2008) examined the effectiveness of interventions that used the scanning, analysis, response, assessment (SARA) model (see Eck & Spelman, 1987) for a problem-oriented policing intervention. Based on their meta-analysis of ten eligible studies, problem-oriented policing has a modest but statistically significant impact on reducing crime and disorder. The authors also collected more numerous but less rigorous pre/post studies without a comparison group. The results of these studies indicated an overwhelmingly positive impact of POP.

Policing Disorder Braga, Welsh, and Schnell (2015) identified 30 experimental and quasi-experimental studies in their review of policing disorder strategies, which included a range of interventions. These strategies typically draw on the "broken windows" argument from Wilson and Kelling (1982), which posits that addressing social and physical disorder can contribute to reductions in more serious crime.

Braga et al. (2015) found an overall positive and statistically significant impact of policing disorder strategies on crime. Program type was important; the average effect for community problem-solving programs was significant and much larger than the nonsignificant overall mean effect for aggressive order maintenance programs.

Strategies to Reduce Illegal Possession and Carrying of Firearms Koper and Mayo-Wilson (2012) reviewed the impact of police strategies to reduce the illegal possession and carrying of firearms on gun crime. They found a small number of eligible studies (and no randomized experiments), but their overall results suggest directed patrol in high gun crime areas can have a significant impact on reducing gun-related crime. These directed patrol strategies involved increasing officer enforcement and proactivity at these high crime areas. Koper and Mayo-Wilson (2012), however, cautioned that these results were based only on a small number of comparisons, and because of the heterogeneity across studies, they did not undertake a meta-analysis.

DNA Testing in Investigative Work Wilson, Weisburd, and McClure (2011) looked at the use of DNA testing in police investigations in order to increase the identification of offenders, as well as arrests, convictions, and case clearances. They found only a small number of eligible studies, but generally the use of DNA evidence was beneficial in investigations across multiple categories of crime. The evidence base for more serious crimes was particularly weak though, while the strongest evidence came from a multisite study on the use of DNA testing in property crime cases (see Roman et al., 2009). Across the five sites in that study, the use of DNA evidence as opposed to traditional investigatory techniques was associated with large increases in the number of suspects identified, arrested, and prosecuted.

Drug Law Enforcement Mazerolle, Soole, and Rombouts (2007) evaluated police-led drug enforcement programs, focusing in particular on whether more innovative approaches were more effective than traditional policing strategies (such as random preventive patrol). They found overall evidence of effectiveness in terms of reducing drug calls for service and incidents for problem-oriented approaches and "community-wide" approaches compared to intensive police efforts at drug hot spots. Community-wide efforts refer to interventions encouraging police/community collaboration as a means to address drug problems in neighborhoods. For nondrug calls and incidents, community-wide interventions were particularly effective in reducing disorder, and intensive hot spots approaches were most effective for addressing serious property and violent crime. The authors concluded that multiagency and multipartner interventions that do not make use of exclusively intensive law enforcement are most likely to be successful in addressing drug markets (see similar conclusions in an earlier review by Mason & Bucke, 2002).

Micro Displacement in Police Interventions Bowers, Johnson, Guerette, Summers, and Poynton (2011) did not focus on a single policing intervention, but instead examined the extent to which displacement is likely as a result of geographically focused police interventions. They found that, overall, geographically focused police interventions tended to show a main effect in favor of treatment, and in areas surrounding the treatment area, there tended to be no significant evidence of crime displacement. The data were more supportive of a diffusion of crime control benefits (Clarke & Weisburd, 1994) to areas nearby than displacement. Overall, they concluded that displacement is not an inevitable outcome of focused policing interventions.

Police Patrols to Prevent Drunk Driving Goss et al. (2008) examined the effects of increased police patrols to prevent drunk driving in a Cochrane Collaboration review. The authors concluded that increased patrols generally reduced the number of traffic accidents and fatalities resulting from drunk driving, but noted that the poor methodological quality of most studies made drawing strong conclusions very difficult. The authors lamented the fact that although millions are spent annually on police efforts to target drunk drivers, so little high-quality research on the topic has been undertaken.

Intensive Police Programs to Reduce Traffic Accidents Blais and Dupont (2005) examined a number of different police interventions to address traffic accidents, as well as driving while intoxicated (DWI) and speeding. These included random breath testing, sobriety checkpoints, random road watch, red-light cameras, speed cameras, and multicomponent programs. While this review included some quasi-experiments without a comparison group, the overall results were very positive. Thirty of the thirty-three included studies showed reductions in traffic accidents with injuries. In a related systematic review, Elder et al. (2002) found that sobriety checkpoints for drunk driving were associated with reductions in traffic accidents and traffic deaths.[8] This was true whether officers used random breath testing checkpoints (officers give breath tests to all drivers) or selective breath testing checkpoints (officers only test drivers they believe have been drinking).

Reviews with Promising Results

Community Policing Gill, Weisburd, Telep, Vitter, and Bennett (2014) examined the impact of community policing on crime and disorder, fear of crime, legitimacy, and citizen satisfaction. Their results suggest community policing has a moderate positive effect on citizen satisfaction and perceived levels of police legitimacy. Community policing had an overall very small impact on violent crime and a non-significant impact on fear of crime and citizen perceptions of disorder. These results suggest that while community policing may have little or no impact on crime in the short-term, there could be a more substantial long-term positive relationship through increased levels of legitimacy and satisfaction.

---

[8] We did not include this review because all but one of the most rigorous studies captured in this review were also included in the Blais and Dupont (2005) review.

Interview and Interrogation Techniques Meissner, Redlich, Bhatt, and Brandon (2012) assessed police interview and interrogation techniques to determine which method of interrogation is more successful in maximizing valid confessions and minimizing false confessions from suspects. They compared the accusatorial method common in the USA to the less confrontational information-gathering method common in the UK. Field studies suggested that both methods increased the likelihood of confessions compared to general questioning methods. Laboratory experiments, however, revealed that information-gathering methods reduced false confessions and in certain instances increased the likelihood of true confessions, while accusatorial methods made false confessions more likely.

Interventions to Increase Legitimacy Mazerolle, Bennett, Davis, Sargeant, and Manning (2013) examined police interventions designed to enhance procedural justice and/or increase citizen perceptions of police legitimacy. They focused on interventions that either explicitly concentrated on increasing legitimacy or incorporated at least one component of procedural justice (participation, neutrality, dignity/respect, and trustworthy motives). Their findings suggest the promise of police efforts to enhance legitimacy. There was strong evidence that such interventions increased citizen satisfaction, compliance and cooperation, and levels of procedural justice. The overall effect of these programs on perceptions of legitimacy was large, but not statistically significant, indicating variability across studies. The impact of these interventions on reducing reoffending was also mixed.

Macro Displacement Telep, Weisburd, Gill, Vitter, and Teichman (2014), like Bowers et al. (2011), examined the likelihood of displacement in policing and other criminal justice interventions.[9] Their focus, however, was on units of geography larger than crime hot spots, what might be called macro- or meso-level displacement. Their findings suggest a limited number of studies at very large units of geography (e.g., jurisdictions), but at more medium-sized units (e.g., neighborhoods, police beats), displacement is not very likely and a diffusion of crime control benefits is just as likely to occur. One concern is that none of the eligible studies in this review was a randomized experiment.

Reviews with Limited Evidence of Effectiveness

Drug Abuse Resistance Education (D.A.R.E.) West and O'Neal (2004) examined 11 published studies of Drug Abuse Resistance Education (D.A.R.E.), a school-based drug education program delivered by police officers. Their overall results suggested D.A.R.E. has little or no impact on drug use, alcohol use, or tobacco use. These results are in line with an earlier meta-analysis by Ennett et al. (1994), which found that D.A.R.E. showed little evidence of effectiveness in reducing drug use, particularly in the long term.

---

[9] While the Telep et al. (2014) review included non-policing studies, the vast majority of eligible studies focused on interventions with at least some level of police involvement.

Second Responder Programs for Domestic Violence Davis, Weisburd, and Taylor (2008) assessed the impact of second responder programs for victims of domestic and family violence. These programs involve follow-up services for domestic violence victims usually from a team consisting of a police officer and a victim advocate. Davis et al. (2008) found that such programs do not reduce the likelihood of future violence reported either to police or on victimization surveys. There was some evidence that those receiving second responder services reported slightly more violence to police. It is not entirely clear if this represents a backfire effect or victims having greater confidence in the police.

Stress Management Training for Police Patterson, Chung, and Swan (2012) examined the effects of stress management and development programs on stress-related outcomes for police officers. They found that overall stress management interventions did not have a significant impact on psychological, behavioral, or physiological outcomes. The authors cautioned that the low methodological rigor of the studies limited the conclusions they could reach, and there was considerable heterogeneity across the studies in the particular components that made up each stress management program. The lack of positive findings are a concern, as Patterson et al. (2012) note, because it is clear that stress has negative consequences for officers.

Lessons Learned

Collectively, these systematic reviews can help us identify both effective and ineffective strategies and tactics. While the systematic reviews do not focus exclusively on crime control outcomes, we have the most data on outcomes related to crime control, and so that will be the primary focus of the section below. We also examine, to the extent possible, the impact of interventions on perceptions of police legitimacy. Enhancing police legitimacy and ensuring fairness are also primary goals of the police (NRC, 2004) and have become especially important in light of recent events concerning police/community relationships (see President's Task Force, 2015). While we think it is important to also develop the evidence base on additional outcomes (e.g., fear of crime, cost-effectiveness), the available data limit our discussion to crime and disorder and legitimacy.

What Works?

In Fig. 5.1, we present a forest plot with mean effect sizes for all of the systematic reviews where a meta-analysis on a crime-related outcome was available. All of these effects have been converted to odds ratios, where an odds ratio of greater than 1 indicates a crime decline. This is not a meta-analysis of meta-analyses, because we are not interested in a mean effect size, but we do think it is useful to display graphically what we see overall about different policing strategies that have been

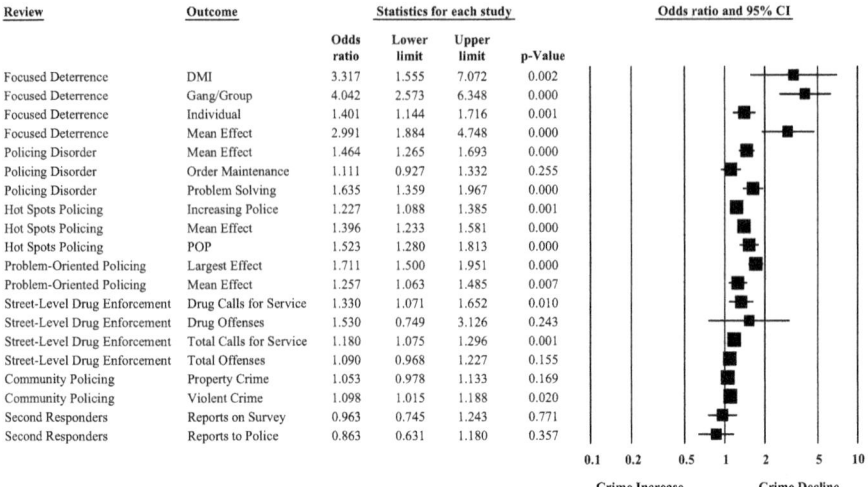

Fig. 5.1 Forest plot of mean effect sizes for reviews examining crime-related outcomes

the subject of a systematic review. Not all of the reviews we described above are included, largely because some of these reviewers chose not to use meta-analysis because of limited eligible studies and/or the heterogeneity of these studies.

Figure 5.1 reveals the largest overall mean effects come from the focused deterrence review (Braga & Weisburd, 2012). The largest effect in the plot is for the gang/group studies (e.g., Braga et al., 2001), which have a large odds ratio of 4.042. While the effect is large and highly significant, we urge some caution because, as noted earlier, none of the studies in this review is a randomized experiment.

The policing disorder review (Braga et al., 2015) shows the second largest mean effect size, with an odds ratio of 1.464. As noted above, this mean effect is largely driven by the success of community problem-solving projects, which have a mean effect of 1.635. Conversely, aggressive order maintenance disorder policing projects have a nonsignificant mean effect of just 1.111. Hot spots policing (Braga et al., 2012) also shows significant positive effects (odds ratio 1.396), particularly studies that use problem-oriented policing in crime hot spots. The mean odds ratio for problem-oriented hot spots studies was 1.523. The significant crime control benefits of hot spots policing found in meta-analyses are in line with the narrative review by the National Research Council (2004) that argued that existing research evidence most strongly supported the effectiveness of hot spots policing. Although not included in Fig. 5.1 because Koper and Mayo-Wilson (2012) did not conduct a meta-analysis, directed patrol strategies to reduce gun violence, which in some sense are a hot spots strategy in somewhat larger areas, also show evidence of effectiveness.

Problem-oriented policing (Weisburd et al., 2008) overall shows a modest but significant mean odds ratio of 1.257. As noted earlier, the less rigorous studies collected in the review showed more strongly positive results. It appears that combining problem solving with hot spots policing or disorder policing (or sometimes both) is a particularly effective approach. Additionally, the Mazerolle et al. (2007) drug enforcement review found POP strategies in drug markets to be an effective strategy. The Mazerolle et al. (2007) review reports a large number of mean effect sizes based on type of intervention, but based on Fig. 5.1, it appears such efforts are most successful at reducing drug calls for service (and to a lesser extent drug offenses, where the effect is not statistically significant). The evidence also suggests the effectiveness of DNA in police investigations, particularly in property crime cases where DNA tends to be used less frequently. The findings of the Roman et al. (2009) multisite experiment and the Wilson et al. (2011) review suggest using DNA evidence can be a cost-effective means to identify, arrest, and convict more offenders.

These results overall suggest a very different portrait of the effectiveness of policing than even as recently as the early 1990s, when it was widely believed that the police were ineffective crime fighters. David Bayley (1994, p. 3), for example, began his book *Police for the Future* with a chapter on "The Myth of Police" and a powerful first sentence: "The police do not prevent crime." But over the last two decades there has been a dramatic change in the underlying conclusions that scholars have reached regarding the effectiveness of the police in reducing crime. Our results suggest a number of effective policing programs focused on reducing crime and disorder.

What Seems to Have Little or No Effect?

Figure 5.1 also suggests the overall less-supportive evidence for second responder programs. For second responder programs (Davis et al., 2008), neither of the mean effects are statistically significant, but both suggest that victims receiving second responder services reported more subsequent abuse than comparison victims. The crime-related effects for community policing are very small in magnitude and statistically nonsignificant for property crime (Gill et al., 2014). Additionally, stress management programs for police do not have strong evidence of effectiveness, based on the Patterson et al. (2012) review. Because of variation across programs and the multifaceted nature of most of the interventions, it is difficult to determine what exactly is causing these programs to show limited evidence of effectiveness, but greater efforts are needed to better address the very important problem of police stress. Finally, D.A.R.E. programs also show little effect in reducing adolescent alcohol, cigarette, and drug use (West & O'Neal, 2004).

What's Promising?

The review by Meissner et al. (2012) suggests the potential benefits of a shift in interrogation techniques in investigations. While the accusatorial model dominates US detective work, the findings of the Meissner et al. (2012) review suggest the potential negative consequences of this approach in terms of increased false confessions, which raises important concerns about both fairness and efficiency. The information-gathering method, more common in the UK, relies on establishing rapport with the suspect, obtaining the suspect's side of the story, and using honesty and clarity to carefully gather information during the interrogation. This approach is promising for both increasing true confessions and reducing false ones.

Police programs designed to help increase procedural justice and citizen perceptions of legitimacy also seem promising. Although the Mazerolle et al. (2013) review had a small number of rigorous studies, a number of different strategies including training, directives, and a range of interventions appear promising for enhancing legitimacy. When police incorporate at least one component of procedural justice into daily routines or as part of a special program, they tend to see benefits in terms of citizen satisfaction, cooperation, and perceived fairness. Research suggests that when citizens perceive the police as more legitimate, they are more likely to cooperate with police and comply with the law (see Tyler, 2004). Indeed, the information-gathering method of interrogation described above is grounded in the importance of using procedural justice as a means to ensure suspect cooperation with the investigation (see Meissner et al., 2012).

Finally, as noted above, the results in Fig. 5.1 from the community policing review suggest a very limited impact on crime (Gill et al., 2014). Community policing had a more substantial impact on some noncrime-related outcomes with meta-analyses showing a positive effect on citizen satisfaction and citizen perceptions of legitimacy. This suggests that community policing programs may be one way for the police to incorporate principles of procedural justice into their interactions with citizens and as a result improve police/community relations. Based on Tyler's (2004) process-based model, it could be the case that community policing is a more effective crime control program in the long-term, as enhanced citizen perceptions of police legitimacy may contribute to increased compliance with the law and reduced crime.

What Do the Reviews Cover and What Areas Are Absent?

Our assessment of systematic reviews in policing suggests we have reviews on quite an array of issues of concern to policing. In Tables 5.1, 5.2, and 5.3 we provide a summary of the previous sections, with additional information on all of the reviews. We also note here the number of eligible studies, and how many of these studies were randomized experiments. We are particularly interested in the methodological quality of the included studies in each review. While high-quality systematic reviews typically have strict inclusion criteria with minimum standards for methodological rigor, most quasi-experimental designs do not have the same level of internal validity as randomized experiments, which are typically recognized as the strongest research design in evaluation research (see Boruch, Snyder, & DeMoya, 2000; Cook & Campbell, 1979; Weisburd, 2003).

Some of the systematic reviews are drawing upon a large base of highly rigorous studies. The hot spots review (Braga et al., 2012), for example, includes ten randomized experiments and nine quasi-experiments with a comparison group. In other areas though, the evidence points to the effectiveness of particular interventions, but the rigor of this evidence could be stronger. In the focused deterrence review (Braga & Weisburd, 2012), for example, there are no randomized experiments. The same is true for the review of directed patrol to reduce gun violence (Koper & Mayo-Wilson, 2012). While the quasi-experimental evidence in both of these reviews is consistent with a treatment effect, the lack of experimental trials limits our ability somewhat to reach strong conclusions regarding effectiveness.[10] In the problem-oriented policing review (Weisburd et al., 2008), the problem is not a lack of randomized experiments (four of the ten eligible studies were randomized trials). However, because of the range of different problems police address using problem-oriented approaches and the multitude of different possible responses, the available evidence made it difficult to reach strong conclusions about the relative effectiveness of different approaches. It is no surprise then that almost all of the systematic reviews on policing conclude by noting the need for additional rigorous research.

Overall, there are 337 publications (some of which include information on multiple studies) across the 17 reviews in Tables 5.1, 5.2, and 5.3. Some of these publications are repeats, as a single paper may appear in multiple reviews (e.g., Weisburd & Green, 1995 appears in the hot spots review, the problem-oriented policing review, the drug law enforcement review, the policing disorder review and the micro displacement review). Removing overlapping publications, there are 285 total papers covered in the completed reviews. This overlap raises important questions of what aspects of particular interventions are driving their success (or lack of success). Ignoring the overlap for a moment, 65 of these papers are randomized experiments and 272 are quasi-experiments (typically, although not always, quasi-experiments with a comparison group). Thus, fewer than 20% of the publications included in systematic reviews on policing are randomized experiments. When we focus on the nonrepeats, 49 of the 285 total papers (17.2%) report on randomized experiments. While we think it is noteworthy that these reviews are drawing from more than 280 rigorous primary studies in policing, and that there are a large number of randomized experiments in policing evaluations, it is still the case that randomized experiments are much outnumbered by other evaluation methods.

---

[10] We recognize that some nonexperimental studies can provide very credible results. For example, regression discontinuity designs (e.g., see Cook, Shadish, & Wong, 2008), or propensity score matching with very systematic knowledge of underlying causal structures and rich data to account for them (e.g., see Shadish, Clark, & Steiner, 2008) have been found to provide outcomes similar to randomized designs. Nonetheless, the bulk of the nonexperimental designs in these policing reviews were much weaker quasi-experimental comparisons.

What Do the Reviews Cover?

In a 2006 book, Weisburd and Braga identify a number of police innovations that have been developed in recent decades (Weisburd & Braga, 2006). Most of the topics in that book are now covered by completed or in progress systematic reviews. These include community policing (Gill et al., 2014), hot spots policing (Braga et al., 2012), broken windows policing (Braga et al., 2015), problem-oriented policing (Weisburd et al., 2008), pulling levers policing (also known as focused deterrence strategies; Braga & Weisburd, 2012), and third party policing (Mazerolle, Higgins, and Eggans, in progress).[11] At this point, most of the key areas of policing, particularly related to innovations in policing, have been covered.

Are there other areas where a review might be useful? The Weisburd and Braga (2006) book also devotes chapters to Compstat (Weisburd et al., 2006) and evidence-based policing (Welsh, 2006). As Weisburd et al. (2004) note, Compstat has become an incredibly popular police innovation since its inception in New York City in the 1990s, but there remains only limited evidence on the contribution of Compstat to crime reduction. A systematic review in this area may be useful, but it is not clear that there would be a sufficient body of rigorous evidence to draw upon. It is often the case, as it was in New York City, that overlapping and simultaneous interventions make it difficult to assess the effectiveness of Compstat on its own. Evidence-based policing is an overarching category relevant to all of these reviews. Systematic reviews are designed, in part, to provide clearer answers to practitioners on what strategies do or do not have a strong evidence base. It seems unnecessary to devote a review to evidence-based policing, and it is unclear what such a review would entail.

Moving beyond police innovations, a larger concern may be the more traditional tactics in policing where there are not currently reviews. These more traditional approaches make up what Weisburd and Eck (2004) refer to as the "standard model" of policing. While such strategies are generally seen as outdated and ineffective, they continue to occupy a substantial portion of police time and resources and so more systematic inquiry into their effects may be warranted. For example, random preventive patrol is routinely dismissed as an ineffective strategy that police should not be using (see Telep & Weisburd, 2012) based largely on the results of a single study, the Kansas City preventive patrol experiment (Kelling et al., 1974). As Sherman and Weisburd (1995) note, the small sample of beats in the study created low statistical power, which made it difficult for the evaluation to discern a significant difference between the study groups even if one had existed. We are not suggesting that random preventive patrol is likely to be an effective approach. The data on the clustering of crime in small geographic areas (e.g., see Sherman, Gartin, & Buerger, 1989; Weisburd et al., 2004) and the strong evidence of effectiveness for hot spots policing (Braga et al., 2012) suggest the greater effectiveness of focused police efforts compared to beat-based random patrol. Nonetheless, a more systematic ex-

---

[11] The review by Mazerolle et al. was in progress when this chapter was completed, and so was not included in the previous section.

amination of the impact of increasing patrol in beats or large geographic areas may provide a stronger answer to the question of "does random preventive patrol work?" than simply citing the Kansas City study as the final answer (see Sherman, 2013).[12]

Similarly, other parts of the "standard model" of policing may be worthy of systematic review, such as the broad question of the impact of the number of police officers on crime. While others have reviewed prior studies on this issue (e.g., see Marvell & Moody, 1996; Eck & Maguire, 2000), there is not a consensus on the impact more police officers have on crime (see Telep & Weisburd, 2012). While it may be difficult to examine this question with highly rigorous studies (i.e., a researcher would have to be creative to use a randomized design in a study of adding police officers), this is an important question for agencies and local government, particularly in the current era of reduced budgets for public safety.

Problems Encountered

While the systematic reviews described in this chapter have provided a wealth of information for researchers, policymakers, and practitioners, some issues and problems have also arisen. Not all of these are unique to policing reviews; they help to highlight the problems more generally in conducting systematic reviews in crime and justice. A first problem was cited above. In some areas we do not yet have systematic reviews and in others our conclusions are limited somewhat by the available studies.

A second major problem is the difficulties researchers sometimes face in calculating effect sizes for meta-analyses. Sometimes the difficulty is a result of limited studies and in those cases, a meta-analysis may not be appropriate because of the small number of eligible cases. In other cases though, the problem is more of descriptive validity (see Gill, 2011; Perry, Weisburd, & Hewitt, 2010). The authors of included studies often do not provide sufficient data on outcomes to make consistent effect size calculation possible. As a result, review authors are often forced to be rather creative in generating effect sizes that can be compared across studies. Weisburd et al. (2008), for example, used six different methods to generate Cohen's *d* effect sizes for the ten eligible studies in the POP review.

While there is nothing inherently wrong with using different methods for calculating effects across studies, the more manipulations made to the original data, the greater potential for inconsistencies across reviews and problems with correctly calculating overall effects. For example, the Weisburd et al. (2008) review used an odds ratio method described by Farrington et al. (2007) to calculate effect sizes for four of the studies. Because this calculation is "a nonstandard use of the term 'odds ratio'" (Farrington et al., 2007, p. 35), it is not clear that the standard error estimates

---

[12] Weisburd, Telep, Wire, and Farrington (in progress) have begun a systematic review to look at the impact of increasing police presence (in both random patrol and hot spots interventions) on crime.

for this odds ratio are correct (see also Bowers et al., 2011). Of course any errors in individual study effect size standard errors will carry over to mean effect size calculations. A related problem is the reporting of different effect sizes for the same study across different reviews. The Weisburd et al. (2008) review, for example, reported much smaller effects for the Braga et al. (1999) study than the Braga (2007) hot spots review. The updated Braga et al. (2012) review, however, has adjusted these effect sizes to more closely reflect those in the Weisburd et al. (2008) review. As systematic reviews continue to be updated and refined, it is important that authors report consistent effect sizes for the same study (assuming they are examining the same outcome measures) and explain any discrepancies.

Third, in policing, as in crime and justice more generally, treatments tend to not be entirely consistent across studies and the outcome measures often vary due to data availability or author choices. This tends to be less of a problem in medical trials, for example, where a series of experiments may examine the exact same treatment and the exact same outcome measures. This variation creates additional heterogeneity that can affect mean effect size calculations. This heterogeneity typically makes it important to use random effects models as opposed to fixed effects models, but even with this adjustment, a high degree of heterogeneity across studies could raise concerns about the use of meta-analysis in the first place. For example, in the area of hot spots, nearly all of the hot spots experiments and quasi-experiments did not follow the original Minneapolis model (Sherman & Weisburd, 1995) of simply increasing police presence on street segments. Instead, these later studies tended to use particular strategies in combination with increased presence, such as problem-oriented policing (e.g., Braga et al., 1999). Additionally, some studies focus on calls for service while others examine crime incidents. Since all of the studies in the Braga et al. (2012) review are focused on the overall approach of concentrating police resources at small geographic areas, a meta-analysis still seems warranted, but the heterogeneity across studies cannot be ignored.

Overall, we think it is important that the effect size calculations in systematic reviews be interpreted with caution. As with any quantitative approach, meta-analysis only provides a best guess at the true effect for each study and for the studies overall based on a number of statistical assumptions. As we noted above, the heterogeneity across studies in many of the reviews and the difficulties in generating effect size estimates should make one hesitant to oversell the findings from any review. It is important for authors to be as comprehensive and transparent as possible in discussions of effect size calculations. Systematic reviews on policing have been an important tool in evaluating what does and does not work in policing, but the limitations, particularly in reviews with a small number of eligible studies, should not be overlooked.

We also think it is important to consider unit of analysis when interpreting effect size magnitude. For Cohen's d, the convention is to view effect sizes of 0.2 as small, 0.5 as medium, and 0.8 as large (see Borenstein, Rothstein, & Cohen, 2001). In terms of crime declines, a small effect is equivalent to about a 20% proportional decline in the treatment relative to the control group, a medium effect is associated with about a 38.5% proportional decline, and a large effect represents a 48.7%

proportional decline. These effects, however, may represent quite different overall outcomes when considering people versus places. For a person, for example, reducing recidivism risk from 50 to 40% (a small effect) is noteworthy, but still a fairly small change. However, when thinking about the same effect in a crime hot spot, a 20% reduction in crime in the treatment group relative to the control could be quite meaningful. Indeed, even smaller effect sizes may suggest significant crime declines in places. This is particularly important to consider in policing, where many of the interventions in the reviews considered here are place-based rather than person-based.

Finally, multifaceted interventions create a challenge for determining the effectiveness of particular policing strategies. Policing interventions often combine multiple innovations simultaneously, which makes it difficult to discern what particular aspect of the program is driving the results. A number of studies in the problem-oriented policing review (Weisburd et al., 2008), for example, also appear in the hot spots policing review (Braga et al., 2012). Is problem-oriented policing driving the effectiveness of the Jersey City POP at violent places study (Braga et al., 1999) or is it the focus on high violent crime hot spots? Or is it that hot spots policing and problem-oriented policing work particularly well in concert? Such multifaceted interventions are common in policing, and it can be difficult to disentangle these different components using systematic reviews. This, of course, is not a problem limited to systematic reviews. It can be difficult or even impossible to isolate these components in primary evaluation studies as well.

Discussion and Conclusions

In recent years, systematic reviews have been an important means of synthesizing existing rigorous research on important practices and approaches in policing. We have summarized these reviews and focused on the lessons we have learned from systematic reviews in policing, what might be missing with existing reviews, and problems encountered in current reviews. Overall, systematic reviews have proven to be an essential resource for academics, criminal justice policymakers, and police practitioners interested in knowing with greater confidence whether particular programs, strategies, or tactics are effective. As we complete our review of what we have learned about systematic reviews in policing, we think it is useful to discuss collective lessons the police can draw from these reviews and also briefly look into what the future might hold.

What Can Police Learn from These Reviews Overall?

The evidence we have reviewed from systematic reviews on policing suggests certain generalizations the police can draw from these reviews. First, the police are most effective when they focus on high-activity people and places (see also Telep & Weisburd, 2012; Weisburd & Eck, 2004). When police narrow in on specific high-crime places or high-offending individuals, they can more efficiently use their resources to address crime problems. Many of the most effective policing strategies in terms of crime control focus on small geographic areas (e.g., hot spots policing) or a small group of high rate offenders (e.g., focused deterrence strategies). The police can also draw important lessons from the fact that interventions at micro or meso scales will not simply lead to displacement and push crime to areas nearby. Focusing on a high crime street segment will not just push that hot spot to the next street block. A more likely occurrence than displacement is a diffusion of crime control benefits to nearby areas.

Second, police should focus in particular on proactive problem-solving (Lum et al., 2011; Weisburd & Eck, 2004). The police should view themselves not just as a crime response agency that waits for 911 calls before springing into action, but instead as a crime prevention agency that can address underlying conditions that allow crime to develop in certain areas. Proactivity is a key component of most of the successful strategies described above, and in particular, the benefits of problem-solving are clear in the POP review and the drug law enforcement review.

Third, police should, when possible, not rely exclusively on law enforcement and arrest to address crime and disorder (Weisburd & Eck, 2004). While arrest is an important tool of the police, as Goldstein (1990) argues, police can be more effective when they expand the toolbox to include other efforts to address crime such as partnerships with other agencies. This was a clear conclusion of the reviews by Mazerolle et al. (2007) and Braga et al. (2015), and Weisburd et al. (2008) also note the benefits of multiagency POP efforts. Focused deterrence projects typically require a multiagency working group to be successful (e.g., see Braga et al., 2001). These partnerships do not need to just be with other law enforcement agencies either. The work of Mazerolle et al. (2007) and Gill et al. (2014) suggest that police efforts to collaborate with the community can have significant benefits. As noted above, even if these benefits are not crime-related in the short-term, increases in satisfaction and legitimacy may lead to long-term increases in compliance with the law.

The Future of Systematic Reviews in Policing

As we noted earlier, there are some areas in policing where a new systematic review may be useful. Moving forward, it is important though to balance research generation and research synthesis. Perhaps we have reached a saturation point when it comes to systematic reviews in policing, and there is a need for additional rigorous studies to build the evidence base which these systematic reviews draw upon. Nearly every systematic review reaches the conclusion that more primary research is needed to reach stronger conclusions. Many of these reviews are targeted at interventions where researchers were aware of significant research efforts already undertaken, suggesting that other areas may not have enough research output for a strong review. Of course, without a systematic search one cannot be certain of this.

The good news is that primary research appears to be growing at a rapid rate. In the updated hot spots review (Braga et al., 2012), for example, there were 19 eligible studies, up from nine in Braga's (2007) original review. The problem-oriented policing review is currently being updated, and there will similarly be an increase in eligible studies, as multiple experiments examining POP have been published since the initial review by Weisburd et al. (2008). The key for the future of systematic reviews may be to ensure that the pace of primary research keeps up with review completion to ensure that systematic reviews continue to provide useful information for researchers, policymakers, and practitioners.

References

Bayley, D. (1994). *Police for the future*. New York: Oxford University Press.
Bennett, T., Holloway, K., & Farrington, D. (2008). The effectiveness of neighborhood watch. *Campbell Systematic Reviews, 4*(18).
Blais, E., & Dupont, B. (2005). Assessing the capability of intensive police programmes to prevent severe road accidents. *British Journal of Criminology, 45*, 914–937.
Borenstein, M., Rothstein, H., & Cohen, J. (2001). *Power and precision*. ™ Englewood: Biostat, Inc.
Boruch, R., Snyder, B., & DeMoya, D. (2000). The importance of randomized field trials. *Crime & Delinquency, 46*, 156–180.
Bowers, K., Johnson, S., Guerette, R. T., Summers, L., & Poynton, S. (2011). Spatial displacement and diffusion of benefits among geographically focused policing interventions. *Campbell Systematic Reviews, 7*(3).
Braga, A. A. (2001). The effects of hot spots policing on crime. *Annals of the American Academy of Political and Social Science, 578*, 104–125.
Braga, A. A. (2005). Hot spots policing and crime prevention: A systematic review of randomized controlled trials. *Journal of Experimental Criminology, 1*, 317–342.
Braga, A. A. (2007). The effects of hot spots policing on crime. *Campbell Systematic Reviews, 3*(1).
Braga, A. A., & Weisburd, D. (2012). The effects of "pulling levers" focused deterrence strategies on crime. *Campbell Systematic Reviews, 8*(6).
Braga, A. A., Weisburd, D. L., Waring, E. J., Mazerolle, L. G., Spelman, W., & Gajewski, F. (1999). Problem-oriented policing in violent crime places: A randomized controlled experiment. *Criminology, 37*, 541–580.
Braga, A. A., Kennedy, D. M., Waring, E. J., & Piehl, A. M. (2001). Problem-oriented policing, deterrence, and youth violence: An evaluation of Boston's Operation Ceasefire. *Journal of Research in Crime and Delinquency, 38*, 195–225.
Braga, A. A., Papachristos, A. V., & Hureau, D. M. (2012). Hot spots policing effects on crime. *Campbell Systematic Reviews, 8*(8).
Braga, A. A., Welsh, B. C., & Schnell, C. (2015). Can policing disorder reduce crime? A systematic review and meta-analysis. *Journal of Research in Crime and Delinquency, 52*, 567–588.
Brennan, I., Moore, S. C., Byrne, E., & Murphy, S. (2011). Interventions for disorder and severe intoxication in and around licensed premises, 1989–2009. *Addiction, 106*, 706–713.
Clarke, R. V., & Weisburd, D. (1994). Diffusion of crime control benefits: Observations on the reverse of displacement. In R. V. Clarke (Ed.), *Crime prevention studies* (Vol. 2, pp. 165–184). Monsey: Criminal Justice Press.
Cook, T. D., & Campbell, D. (1979). *Quasi-experimentation: Design and analysis issues for field settings*. Chicago: Rand McNally.

Cook, T. D., Shadish, W. R., & Wong, V. C. (2008). Three conditions under which experiments and observational studies produce comparable causal estimates: New findings from within-study comparisons. *Journal of Policy Analysis and Management, 27,* 724–750.

Davis, R. C., Weisburd, D., & Taylor, B. (2008). Effects of second responder programs on repeat incidents of family abuse. *Campbell Systematic Reviews, 4*(15).

Dowden, C., Bennell, C., & Bloomfield, S. (2007). Advances in offender profiling: A systematic review of the profiling literature published over the past three decades. *Journal of Criminal Psychology, 22,* 44–56.

Eck, J. E., & Maguire, E. (2000). Have changes in policing reduced violent crime? In A. Blumstein & J. Wallman (Eds.), *The crime drop in America* (pp. 207–265). New York: Cambridge University Press.

Eck, J. E., & Spelman, W. (1987). *Problem solving: Problem-oriented policing in Newport News.* Washington, DC: Police Executive Research Forum.

Elder, R. W., Shults, R. A., Sleet, D. A., Nichols, J. L., Zaza, S., & Thompson, R. S. (2002). Effectiveness of sobriety checkpoints for reducing alcohol-involved crashes. *Traffic Injury Prevention, 3,* 266–274.

Ennett, S. T., Tobler, N. S., Ringwalt, C. L., & Flewelling, R. L. (1994). How effective is drug abuse resistance education? A meta-analysis of project DARE outcome evaluations. *American Journal of Public Health, 84,* 1394–1401.

Faggiano, F., Vigna-Taglianti, F. D., Versino, E., Zambon, A., Borraccino, A., & Lemma, P. (2008). School-based prevention for illicit drugs use: A systematic review. *Preventive Medicine, 46,* 385–396.

Farrington, D. P., & Ttofi, M. M. (2010). School-based programs to reduce bullying and victimization. *Campbell Systematic Reviews, 6*(6).

Farrington, D. P., Gill, M., Waples, S. J., & Argomaniz, J. (2007). The effects of closed-circuit television on crime: Meta-analysis of an English national quasi-experimental multi-site evaluation. *Journal of Experimental Criminology, 3,* 21–38.

Gill, C. E. (2011). Missing links: How descriptive validity impacts the policy relevance of randomized controlled trials in criminology. *Journal of Experimental Criminology, 7,* 201–224.

Gill, C. E., Weisburd, D., Telep, C. W., Bennett, T., & Vitter, Z. (2014). Community-oriented policing to reduce crime, disorder, and fear and increase legitimacy and citizen satisfaction in neighborhoods. *Journal of Experimental Criminology, 10,* 399–428.

Goldstein, H. (1990). *Problem-oriented policing.* New York: McGraw-Hill.

Goss, C. W., Van Bramer, L. D., Gliner, J. A., Porter, T., R., Roberts, I. G., et al. (2008). Increased police patrols for preventing alcohol-impaired driving. *Cochrane Database of Systematic Review, 4.*

Harris, C. J. (2009). Police use of improper force: A systematic review of the evidence. *Victims and Offenders, 4,* 25–41.

Hem, E., Berg, A. M., & Ekeberg, O. (2001). Suicide in police-a critical review. *Suicide and Life Threatening Behavior, 31,* 224–233.

Kelling, G. L., Pate, A. M., Dieckman, D., & Brown, C. (1974). *The Kansas City preventive patrol experiment: Technical report.* Washington, DC: Police Foundation.

Koper, C. S., & Mayo-Wilson, E. (2012). Police strategies to reduce illegal possession and carrying of firearms: Effects on gun crime. *Campbell Systematic Reviews, 8*(11).

Lum, C., Kennedy, L. W., & Sherley, A. J. (2006). The effectiveness of counter-terrorism strategies. *Campbell Systematic Reviews, 2*(2).

Lum, C., Koper, C., & Telep, C. W. (2011). The evidence-based policing matrix. *Journal of Experimental Criminology, 7,* 3–26.

Marvell, T. B., & Moody, C. E. (1996). Specification problems, police levels, and crime rates. *Criminology, 34,* 609–646.

Mason, M., & Bucke, T. (2002). Evaluating actions against local drug markets: A 'systematic' review of research. *The Police Journal, 75,* 15–30.

Mazerolle, L., Soole, D. W., & Rombouts, S. (2007). Street-level drug law enforcement: A meta-analytic review. *Campbell Systematic Reviews, 3*(2).

Mazerolle, L., Bennett, S., Davis, J., Sargeant, E., & Manning, M. (2013). Legitimacy in policing. *Campbell Systematic Reviews, 9*(1).

Mazerolle, L., Higginson, A., & Eggins, E. (in progress). Third party policing for reducing crime and disorder: A systematic review. *Campbell Systematic Reviews*.

Meissner, C. A., Redlich, A. D., Bhatt, S., & Brandon, S. (2012). Interview and interrogation methods and their effects on true and false confessions. *Campbell Systematic Reviews, 8*(13).

National Research Council. (2004). *Fairness and effectiveness in policing: The evidence*. Committee to Review Research on Police Policy and Practices. In W. Skogan & K. Frydl (Eds.), *Committee on Law and Justice, Division of Behavioral and Social Sciences and Education*. Washington, DC: National Academies Press.

Patterson, G. T., Chung, I. W., & Swan, P. G. (2012). The effects of stress management interventions among police officers and recruits. *Campbell Systematic Reviews, 8*(7).

Perry, A. E., Weisburd, D., & Hewitt, C. (2010). Are criminologists describing randomized controlled trials in ways that allow us to assess them? Findings from a sample of crime and justice trials. *Journal of Experimental Criminology, 6*, 245–262.

President's Task Force on 21st Century Policing. (2015). *Final report of the President's task force on 21st century policing*. Washington, DC: Office of Community Oriented Policing Services, U.S. Department of Justice.

Roman, J. K., Reid, S. E., Chalfin, A. J., & Knight, C. R. (2009). The DNA field experiment: A randomized trial of the cost-effectiveness of using DNA to solve property crimes. *Journal of Experimental Criminology, 5*, 345–369.

Shadish, W. R., Clark, M. H., & Steiner, P. M. (2008). Can nonrandomized experiments yield accurate answers? A randomized experiment comparing random and nonrandom assignments. *Journal of the American Statistical Association, 103*, 1334–1343.

Sherman, L. W. (2013). The rise of evidence-based policing: Targeting, testing, and tracking. In M. Tonry (Ed.), *Crime and justice: A review of research* (vol. 42, pp. 377–451). Chicago: University of Chicago Press.

Sherman, L. W., & Weisburd, D. (1995). General deterrent effects of police patrol in crime hot spots: A randomized controlled trial. *Justice Quarterly, 12*, 625–648.

Sherman, L. W., Gartin, P. R., & Buerger, M. E. (1989). Hot spots of predatory crime: Routine activities and the criminology of place. *Criminology, 27*, 27–56.

Strang, H., Sherman, L. W., Mayo-Wilson, E., Woods, D., & Ariel, B. (2013). Restorative justice conferencing (RJC) using face-to-face meetings of offenders and victims: Effects on offender recidivism and victim satisfaction. A systematic review. *Campbell Systematic Reviews, 9*(12).

Telep, C. W., & Weisburd, D. (2012). What is known about the effectiveness of police practices in reducing crime and disorder? *Police Quarterly, 15*, 331–357.

Telep, C. W., & Weisburd, D. (2014). Generating knowledge: A case study of the National Policing Improvement Agency program on systematic reviews in policing. *Journal of Experimental Criminology, 10*, 371–398.

Telep, C. W., Weisburd, D., Gill, C. E., Teichman, D., & Vitter, Z. (2014). Displacement of crime and diffusion of crime control benefits in large-scale geographic areas: A systematic review. *Journal of Experimental Criminology, 10*, 515–548.

Tyler, T. R. (2004). Enhancing police legitimacy. *The Annals of the American Academy of Political and Social Science, 593*, 84–99.

Weisburd, D. (2003). Ethical practice and evaluation of interventions in crime and justice: The moral imperative for randomized trials. *Evaluation Review, 27*, 336–354.

Weisburd, D., & Braga, A. A. (2006). Introduction: Understanding police innovation. In D. Weisburd & A. A. Braga (Eds.), *Police innovation: Contrasting perspectives* (pp. 1–23). New York: Cambridge University Press.

Weisburd, D., & Eck, J. E. (2004). What can the police do to reduce crime, disorder, and fear? *Annals of the American Academy of Political and Social Science, 593*, 42–65.

Weisburd, D., & Green, L. (1995). Policing drug hot spots: The Jersey City drug market analysis experiment. *Justice Quarterly, 12,* 711–736.

Weisburd, D., Bushway, S., Lum, C., & Yang, S.-M. (2004). Trajectories of crime at places: A longitudinal study of street segments in the city of Seattle. *Criminology, 42,* 283–321.

Weisburd, D., Mastrofski, S. D., Willis, J. J., & Greenspan, R. (2006). Changing everything so that everything can remain the same: Compstat and American policing. In D. Weisburd & A. A. Braga (Eds.), *Police innovation: Contrasting perspectives* (pp. 284–301). New York: Cambridge University Press.

Weisburd, D., Telep, C. W., Hinkle, J. C., & Eck, J. E. (2008). Effects of problem-oriented policing on crime and disorder. *Campbell Systematic Reviews, 4*(14).

Weisburd, D., Telep, C. W., Wire, S., & Farrington, D. (In progress). The effects of increased police patrol on crime and disorder. *Campbell Systematic Reviews.*

Welsh, B. C. (2006). Evidence-based policing for crime prevention. In D. Weisburd & A. A. Braga (Eds.), *Police innovation: Contrasting perspectives* (pp. 305–321). New York: Cambridge University Press.

Welsh, B. C., & Farrington, D. P. (2008). Effects of closed circuit television surveillance on crime. *Campbell Systematic Reviews, 4*(17).

Werb, D., Rowell, G., Guyatt, G., Kerr, T., Montaner, J., & Wood, E. (2011). Effect of drug law enforcement on drug market violence: A systematic review. *International Journal of Drug Policy, 22,* 87–94.

West, S. L., & O'Neal, K. K. (2004). Project D.A.R.E. outcome effectiveness revisited. *American Journal of Public Health, 94,* 1027–1029.

Wilson, J. Q., & Kelling, G. L. (1982). Broken windows: The police and neighborhood safety. *Atlantic Monthly, 211,* 29–38.

Wilson, D. B., Weisburd, D., & McClure, D. (2011). Use of DNA testing in police investigative work for increasing offender identification, arrest, conviction and case clearance. *Campbell Systematic Reviews, 7*(7).

Chapter 6
Sentencing and Deterrence

Amanda E. Perry

Since the inception of the International Campbell and Cochrane Collaborations (www.campbellcollaboration.org; www.cochrane.org), interest in systematic reviews and meta-analytical techniques to identify "what works" in research has expanded rapidly. Over the past three decades, many systematic reviews and meta-analytical studies of experimental and quasi-experimental studies have been published. It is highly important to consolidate and take stock of the evidence on sentencing and deterrence strategies given their impact on the public, offenders, and victims of crime.

Resources linked to sentencing options and the role these play in deterring individuals away from crime are stretched to capacity with evermore incarcerated individuals. As the population of incarcerated offenders rises there is renewed interest in the relative effectiveness of different sentences, and in particular the effectiveness of custodial versus alternative community-based sentences (Marsh, Fox, & Sarmah, 2009).

In the past decade, changes to the Criminal Justice Act in the UK and similar shifts in the USA demonstrate a transition from the traditional use of custodial sentencing to an alternative approach encompassing the needs of the individual offender. Such examples include the introduction of community orders and drug and MHC initiatives, which have been established in New Zealand, Australia, and North America and more recently in the UK (see www.gov.uk/community-sentences/overview). These alternatives often use a therapeutic provision providing an element of individualization for each offender.

Evaluations of interventions devised to focus on deterring individuals from crime are sparsely reported in the literature (Shepherd, 2001). Although deterrence is an established theme in the Criminal Justice System (CJS), the role of deterrence, and the extent to which people can be deterred from causing criminal activity, focuses on the theoretical implications around the rational choice (Coben & Larkin, 1999; Petrosino, Turpin-Petrosino, & Buehler, 2003). Deterrence within the

---

A. E. Perry (✉)
Department of Health Sciences, University of York, Heslington, UK
e-mail: amanda.perry@york.ac.uk

© Springer Science+Business Media New York 2016
D. Weisburd et al. (eds.), *What Works in Crime Prevention and Rehabilitation*,
Springer Series on Evidence-Based Crime Policy, DOI 10.1007/978-1-4939-3477-5_6

literature concerns itself with the issue of desistance from crime through the fear of punishment. Sentencing policies focusing on the deterrent effect have included "getting tough on crime" and the "three strikes and you're out" (www.threestrikes.org/). Such initiatives are designed to deter with the threat of imposing substantial terms of imprisonment. The concept of deterrence is therefore subjective and relies upon an individual having the correct knowledge about the sentencing policy and its proposed deterrent effect. If the sentence severity and deterrence effect is not known, it is unlikely to have an impact on subsequent criminal behavior. In this regard, research illustrates that the general public tend to underestimate the severity of sanctions generally imposed (Von Hirsch, Bottoms, Burney, & Wikstrom, 1999; Williams, 1980). Furthermore, evidence tells us that an increase in the *certainty* of punishment as opposed to the *severity* of punishment is more likely to produce a deterrence effect (Nagin & Pogarsky, 2001; Von Hirsch et al., 1999; Williams, 1980). With such a broad range of different sentencing alternatives, the debate that surrounds appropriate deterrence strategies and public opinion is recognized as a central issue within the CJS.

Systematic reviews and meta-analyses provide a mechanism to collate different primary research studies to form an independent summary of the research evidence. The purpose of this chapter is to review the evidence on sentencing and deterrence strategies and to assess what we know about the effectiveness of different sentencing options and how deterrence strategies can impact an individual's involvement in the CJS.

Methodology

The main aim of this review was to evaluate systematic reviews and meta-analytical studies of sentencing and deterrence in the CJS. For this purpose, we used the Cochrane Collaboration definition of a systematic review to identify whether studies were eligible for inclusion. The definition states:

> A systematic review is a review using a clearly formulated question that employs systematic and explicit methods to identify, select, and critically appraise relevant research, from studies that are included in the review.

In addition, we were interested in including studies using meta-analytical approaches that combine individual studies to produce an overall effect. Meta-analyses within the context of systematic reviews are often limited by the number of available studies and their heterogeneity, but are also published as a study in their own right (Gould & Clum, 1993). We therefore included any review using systematic principles and/or meta-analytical techniques. Reviews were not required to employ both methodologies to be included in the review.

Defining Sentencing and Deterrence

For the purpose of this review, the term sentencing was defined as "any sanction imposed by a judge via legal proceedings." This definition incorporates a variety of different mandated custodial and non-custodial sentences at different stages within the CJS. Examples, though not exhaustive, include electronic monitoring, drug courts, MHCs, financial or suspended sanctions, and post-diversion schemes. For reviews of deterrence, we included interventions that were primarily aimed at deterring individuals from either committing a crime or repeating some form of criminal activity. These included programs where (i) the underlying theory was based on a deterrence theory such as rational choice and /or (ii) the primary aim of the intervention or sentencing option was to deter an individual from a criminal activity (Petrosino et al., 2003). We specifically excluded interventions of CCTV and hot spots policing as these are covered elsewhere in this book (Chap. 4 and 5, respectively).

Database Searches

A total of five databases[1] and two websites[2] were searched between the date of database inception and week 3 in February 2012. The databases were chosen specifically to identify systematic reviews and meta-analyses of evidence in the social science and criminal justice arena (e.g., The Campbell Collaboration). A specific search strategy was devised by a specialist information officer, and a search filter was used to identify relevant publications. The example below shows the combination of search terms used to identify systematic reviews and meta-analyses in the Applied Social Sciences Index and Abstracts (ASSIA) database:

> KW = (sentencing OR sentences OR court* OR corrections OR offending OR custodial sentenc* OR custodial sanction* OR custodial penalt* OR custodial punish* OR prison sentenc* OR penal sanction* OR custodial disposal* OR prison disposal* OR community sanction* OR community sentenc* OR community penalt* OR community disposal* OR community punish* OR crime reduction OR crime prevent* OR reparation OR probation OR diversion OR alternative sanction* OR public safety OR community service* OR recidiv* OR deterrence OR deter OR deterring)
> And

---

[1] PsychINFO (OVID), Social Policy and Practice, Applied Social Sciences Index and Abstracts (ASSIA), Social Science Citation Index and Public Affairs Information Service (PAIS).

[2] Campbell Collaboration (see www.campbellcollaboration.org) and the The Evidence for Policy and Practice Information and Co-ordinating Centre (EPPI Centre).

> TI = (metaanaly* OR meta-analy*) OR AB = (metaanaly* OR meta-analy*) OR KW = (meta study OR meta synthes* OR meta evaluat*) OR DE = (literature reviews) OR KW = (synthes* WITHIN 3 literature*) OR KW = (synthes* WITHIN 3 research*) OR KW = (synthes* WITHIN 3 studies) OR KW = (synthes* WITHIN 3 data) OR KW = (synthes* WITHIN 3 trials) OR KW = (synthes* WITHIN 3 findings) OR KW = (synthes* WITHIN 3 evidence) OR KW = (quantitative synthes*) OR KW = (pooled analys*) OR KW = ((data WITHIN 3 pool*) AND studies) OR KW = (pooling studies) OR KW = (medline OR medlars OR embase OR cinahl OR cochrane OR scisearch OR psychinfo OR psycinfo OR psychlit OR psyclit) OR KW = ((hand OR manual* OR database* OR computer* OR electronic*) WITHIN 3 search*) OR KW = ((electronic* OR bibliographic*) WITHIN 3 database*) OR KW = (review* WITHIN 3 (systematic* OR methodologic* OR quantitative* OR research* OR literature* OR studies OR trial* OR effective*)) OR KW = (overview* WITHIN 3 (systematic* OR methodologic* OR quantitative* OR research* OR literature* OR studies OR trial* OR effective*)) OR KW = (evaluation synthes*) OR KW = (evaluation review*) OR KW = (what works)

Further search combinations can be obtained from the author. Once identified, the records were uploaded into a bibliographic database. Because a number of different databases were searched, duplicated references were removed prior to screening the title and abstracts.

Inclusion and Exclusion Criteria

The review included the following types of studies:

1. Reviews that either defined themselves as "systematic" or used "meta-analytical techniques."
2. Reviews that reported clearly defined searches, search strategies, listed databases and search terms, and reported systematic principles.
3. Reviews where sentencing options and/or deterrence were the main focus of the review.
4. Reviews of quantitative and qualitative analyses.
5. Reviews including outcomes of recidivism and/or criminal activity measures such as arrest.

Reviews incorporating sentencing options within the scope of a larger review (e.g., the overall effectiveness of the CJS) were not included. In addition, reviews focusing on the psychological attributes of jury decision making (although part of the sentencing process) were excluded because such reviews did not consider the effectiveness a sentencing option per se (Cross, Walsh, Simone, & Jones, 2003; Schutte & Hosch, 1997). Other exclusions included systematic reviews of pre-trial and pre-booking systems where offenders are diverted away from the CJS prior to formal charges being laid. The majority of persons served by these types of programs often suffer from a mental illness, and diversion is therefore the preferred option.

Data Extraction and Synthesis

A standardized data extraction sheet was used to collect information from each review. The elements included author details, year, focus of the review (intervention and comparison), number and type of studies identified, outcome measures, and number of databases searched (see Table 6.1). Details of the participant level of risk, number of studies, effect sizes, and significant moderators were also extracted (see Table 6.2). Finally, the studies were grouped into five categories based on the "what works" principles (see Table 6.3). Following extraction by a single reviewer, a narrative synthesis of the results was conducted and papers were themed into two domains (sentencing options and deterrence strategies). A number of successive reviews were identified representing cumulative evidence on the effectiveness of drug courts. For these reviews a narrative of the findings is described to demonstrate the progression and growth of literature. However, only the latest review is reported as part of the data extraction tables as this review subsumes all previous findings (Mitchell, Wilson, Eggers, & MacKenzie, 2012). Where outcome measures of effectiveness were reported we converted standardized mean differences (Cohen's *d* and Hedges' *g*) and relative risk outcomes into odds ratios (ORs) to allow us to compare across reviews (see Fig. 6.3). An OR greater than 1 indicates a desirable effect (e.g., a decrease in offending behavior).

Results

The PRISMA flowchart in Fig. 6.1 shows the publication findings at each stage of the review (Moher, Liberati, Tetzlaff, Altman and the PRISMA Group, 2009). A total of 3906 citations were identified. After the application of the inclusion criteria these were reduced to a possible 73 studies. Papers were excluded in the later stage of the review due to (i) not complying with the Cochrane definition of systematic review criteria, (ii) reviews not focusing solely on the elements of sentencing options and/or deterrence (contact the author for a list of excluded studies), and/or (iii) reviews appearing elsewhere in this book (e.g., McDougall, Cohen, Swaray, & Perry, 2003; see Chap. 11). This process left 25 full papers for further examination. Of this selection, three papers could not be easily accessed via electronic journals or via the Internet and contact with the authors was sought without response. The final selection resulted in 22 publications reporting on 16 reviews.

Table 6.1 Systematic reviews of sentencing and deterrence: summary of evidence

Author, year	Intervention(s)	Comparison(s)	Study design	Outcome measure(s)	Number of databases
Reviews of sentencing					
Feder & Wilson (2005)	Court-mandated interventions for offenders with domestic violence	Alternative sentencing options	RCTs	Re-offending, criminal behavior	18
Finfgeld-Connett & Johnson (2011)	Drug court treatment gender-specific correctional programs community-based drug program outpatient day treatment program	Not an intervention design, comparison group not applicable	Qualitative	No reported outcomes at the start of the review	8 databases
Lange et al. (2011)	A range of different diversion schemes relating to mental health	A range of different schemes including diversion schemes and prison alternatives	Meta-analyses RCTs quasi-experimental retrospective cohort pre-post test descriptive cost-effectiveness	Recidivism days incarcerated mental health service utilization substance use quality of life	5 databases websites of relevant literature
Wilson et al. (2005)	Correctional boot camps	Alternative sentencing option	RCT quasi experimental	Recidivism	9 databases 1 internet site
Mitchell et al. (2012)	Drug courts effects on juveniles and adults	Alternative sentencing options including prison	154 evaluations 34 juvenile drug courts 92 adult drug courts 28 DWI courts	Recidivism	11 Google internet search Research organizations
Sarteschi et al. (2011)	Assessing the effectiveness of mental health courts	Control, comparison, or waiting list group. No further details reported	RCTs quasi-experimental pre- and post-test (but analyzed separately)	Recidivism mental and or clinical health	12 journal hand-search mental health governmental websites email survey

Table 6.1 (continued)

Author, year	Intervention(s)	Comparison (s)	Study design	Outcome measure(s)	Number of databases
Reviews of deterrence					
Coben & Larkin (1999)	Ignition interlock devices in reducing drunk driving recidivism	Offences relating to drunk driving	RCT quasi-experimental studies retrospective cohort	Re-arrest rate, recidivism impaired driving during recidivism	9
Petrosino et al. (2003)	Studies including a component whereby program participants visit a prison facility	Juveniles receiving treatment as usual	RCT	Criminal activity	19 an extensive mail campaign
Von Hirsch et al. (1999)	Deterrence and sentencing severity	Sentencing alternatives	Cohort longitudinal correlational time series	Recidivism	Not stated
Yang & Lester (2008)	Deterrence effects of executions	Geographical areas with and without the death penalty	Time-series studies cross-sectional studies panel data studies single execution studies studies on publicity	Number of executions	4

Table 6.2 Systematic reviews of sentencing and deterrence: summary of evidence

Author, year	Time period	Participants and (level of risk)	Studies (N)	Odds ratio (95% CI)	Moderators
Reviews of sentencing					
Feder & Wilson (2005)	1986 Jan to 2003	3614 adult men, sentenced for violence against the partner	10	Victim report measures: experiments—1.02 (0.82-1.27) quasi-experiments—0.82 (0.40-1.63) Official report measures: experiments—1.60 (1.06-2.48) quasi-experiments—0.78 (0.45-1.75) for no treatment comparison group quasi-experiments—5.80 (1.24-27.14) for treatment drop-outs as comparison	Different study design official and self-report victim outcomes
Finfgeld-Connett & Johnson (2011)	Up to March 2011	$N=70$ Mean age 34–44 women attending substance abuse programs referred through CJS to participate outside of high security jails	5	Meta-analysis not completed	Not applicable
Lange et al. (2011)	Jan 1995 to Jan 2011	Adults with mental illness and co-occurring substance abuse disorders	43	Meta-analysis not completed	Not applicable
Wilson et al. (2005)	1986 to Dec 2003	120,000 adults and juvenile male and females under the supervision of the CJS	32	Any recidivism Experiments only—0.92 (0.61–1.38) All studies—1.02 (0.90–1.14)	Moderators focused on method characteristics, offender characteristics, and boot program characteristics

Table 6.2 (continued)

Author, year	Time period	Participants and (level of risk)	Studies (N)	Odds ratio (95% CI)	Moderators
Mitchell et al. (2012)	Final search August 2011	Male, female, adult and juvenile offenders (level of risk not reported)	154	Overall mean reduction in recidivism Experiments – DWI Drug Courts 1.15 (0.79–1.67) Adult Drug Courts 1.45 (0.80–2.62) Juvenile Drug Courts 1.39 (0.50–3.85) All studies – DWI Drug Courts 1.65 (1.35-2.02) Adult Drug Courts 1.66 (1.50–1.84) Juvenile Drug Courts 1.37 (1.15-1.63)	Numerous moderators investigated including study quality, publication bias, and outcome measures by court type
Sarteschi et al. (2011)[a]	Through July 2009	Individuals aged 17 years and older with a mental illness	18	Overall mean recidivism 2.66 (1.92–3.69)	Study design/recidivism/publication type/study quality
Reviews of deterrence					
Coben & Larkin (1999)[b]	Database inception (from 1964) to 1997	$N = 88$ Included drivers who had at least one prior conviction for driving while intoxicated (level of risk not reported)	6	Re-arrest Experiment: 2.74 (1.56–4.83)	None reported
Petrosino et al. (2003)	1945 and 1993	946 juveniles aged 15–17 years	9	Experiments: 0.76 (0.61–0.95)	Sensitivity analysis conducted
Von Hirsch et al. (1999)	1980 onwards	Not reported	8	Meta-analysis not completed	Not applicable
Yang & Lester (2008)	1975 onwards	Not reported	95	Meta-analysis not completed	Not applicable

[a] This conversion from a Hedges' g is for recidivism using quasi-experimental studies, using $g*1.8414$. Two trials were reported but no data were presented in the paper to enable the calculation of an effect size.

[b] This odds ratio is based on only one reported RCT study in the review (Beck, 1997) and has been re-calculated from the raw data in the paper.

Table 6.3 The taxonomy of what works evidence presented in systematic reviews of sentencing and deterrence

Conclusion	Mental health courts	Jail-based courts	FACT	Court based	Mental health and parole	Adult Drug courts	Juvenile drug courts	Court-mandated interventions for domestic violence	Ignition interlocking devices for drunk driving	Scared Straight program	Sentence and deterrence	Deterrence effects linked to executions	Boot camps
What works	•												
What is promising		•	•	•	•								
No evidence of any effect						•			•		•		•
What is harmful							•	•		•			
What is uncertain												•	

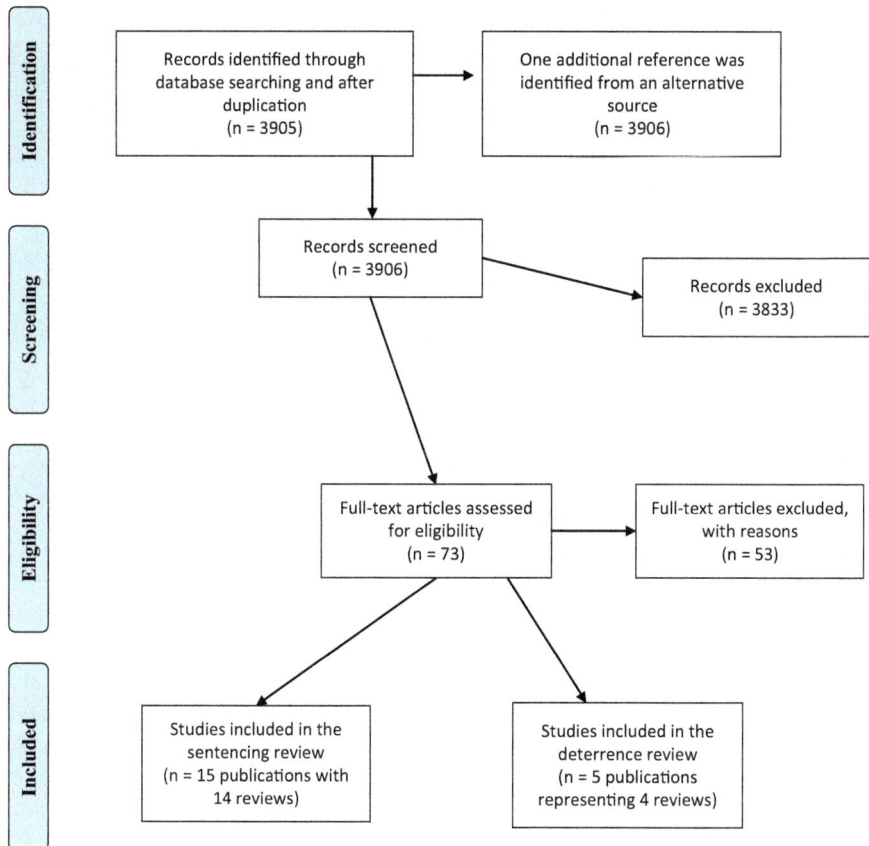

Fig. 6.1 The process of publication selection

The included publications were divided into two domains: sentencing options or deterrence strategies. This resulted in 14 sentencing papers describing 12 reviews of sentencing and 5 deterrence papers describing 4 systematic reviews.

Overall Study Details

The 16 reviews were conducted between 1999 and 2012 and were mainly published in the USA (see Tables 6.1 and 6.2). The studies included all sectors of the CJS including males and females, juvenile and adults, and offenders suffering from mental illness. We were particularly interested to record the level of risk or offence type for each population; however, we found in many cases that this information was not reported, or it was used as a generic term to describe the study populations (Feder & Wilson, 2005; Mitchell et al., 2012).

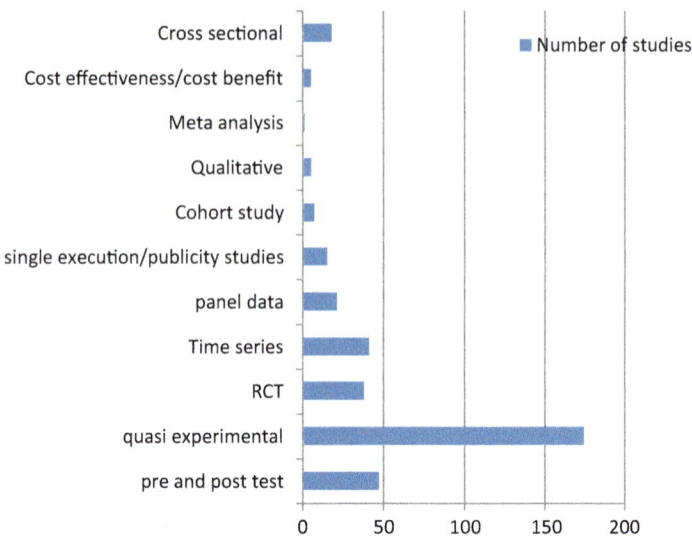

Fig. 6.2 Type of study included in systematic reviews of sentencing and deterrence

The extent of searching varied across the studies and the number of databases searched ranged from 5 (Lange, Rehm, & Popova, 2011) to 19 (Petrosino et al., 2003). Many authors also included searches of the Internet, specific journal hand searches, and email surveys. Six publications included a meta-analysis and considered a variety of different moderators. The most commonly investigated moderator included an examination of study quality, official and self-report measurement differences, and study type.

The majority of reviews included studies using a quasi-experimental design[3] and trial data (see Fig. 6.2), although many also reported on the use of pre- and post-test studies. We identified one qualitative review. This study reported on women's engagement with enforced substance abuse treatment in the community (Finfgeld-Connett & Johnson, 2011; see also Chap. 9).

A range of different interventions and comparison sentencing options were included in the review. These included Mental Health Courts (MHCs) (Sarteschi, Vaughn, & Kim, 2011) and different diversion schemes where conviction for a sentence had been granted (Feder & Wilson, 2005; Lange et al., 2011). The largest body of evidence related to the emergence and evaluation of drug courts. This accounted for seven of the 12 sentencing reviews (Belenko, 2001; Jenson & Mosher, 2006; Lowenkamp, Holsinger, & Latessa, 2005; Lowenkamp, Latessa, & Holsinger, 2006; Mitchell et al., 2012; US Government Accountability Office (GAO), 2005; Wilson, Mitchell, & Mackenzie, 2006). Many outcomes were reported across the reviews, most cited was recidivism and criminal behavior, although diversion schemes (in

---

[3] Quasi-experimental studies also included those studies using a prospective design.

particular) also considered other measures such as the provision of mental health services and quality-of-life measures.

Two reviews reported on court-mandated interventions (Feder & Wilson, 2005) and correctional boot camps (Wilson, MacKenzie, & Mitchell, 2005), respectively. These were assessed individually and the results reported separately.

The deterrence reviews reported on singular topics including deterrence and sentence length (Von Hirsch et al., 1999), interventions aimed at reducing drunken driving (Coben & Larkin, 1999), the deterrence effect of executions (Yang & Lester, 2008), and the impact of Scared Straight programs for at risk youths (Petrosino et al., 2003).

Overall Measures of Effectiveness

Of the 16 reviews only 6 reported on outcomes of effectiveness using meta-analytical techniques (Coben & Larkin, 1999; Feder & Wilson, 2005; Mitchell et al., 2012; Petrosino et al., 2003; Sarteschi et al., 2011; Wilson et al., 2005). These systematic reviews not reporting outcomes of effect were either qualitative in nature (Finfgeld-Connett & Johnson, 2011) or focused on the presence of deterrence (Von Hirsch et al., 1999; Yang & Lester, 2008). Figure 6.3 shows a summary of each review reported by outcome and confidence interval. Many studies reported on multiple outcomes at different time points. For example, the Wilson review produced 199 ORs with most studies reporting multiple outcomes (Wilson et al., 2005). In such instances, we took the overall mean effect reported for the primary outcome by the authors of each review. Where possible, we reported effect sizes on trial data and quasi-experimental studies separately.

Boot Camps To our knowledge, only one systematic review considered the effect of boot camp programs on the criminal behavior of convicted adult and juvenile offenders (Wilson et al., 2005). The review included 32 studies producing 43 independent comparisons. The results of a random effects model produced a mean OR of 1.02 (95% CI 0.90–1.14) for all studies and a mean OR of 0.92 (95% CI 0.61–1.38) for experiments, indicating very little benefit to boot camp participants in relation to comparison participants and potentially even a harmful effect. The authors report that the current evidence suggests that boot camps are not effective in reducing post-boot camp offending (Wilson et al., 2005).

Drug Courts Five systematic reviews and one meta-analytical study were found to assess the drug court literature (Belenko, 2001; Jenson & Mosher, 2006; Lowenkamp et al., 2005, 2006; Mitchell et al., 2012; US Government Accountability Office (GAO), 2005; Wilson et al., 2006). Each of these reviews used different criteria to review the effectiveness of drug courts on two main outcome measures; recidivism and substance use or relapse. The latest review by Mitchell subsumes previous results, but a brief description of the earlier literature is described below.

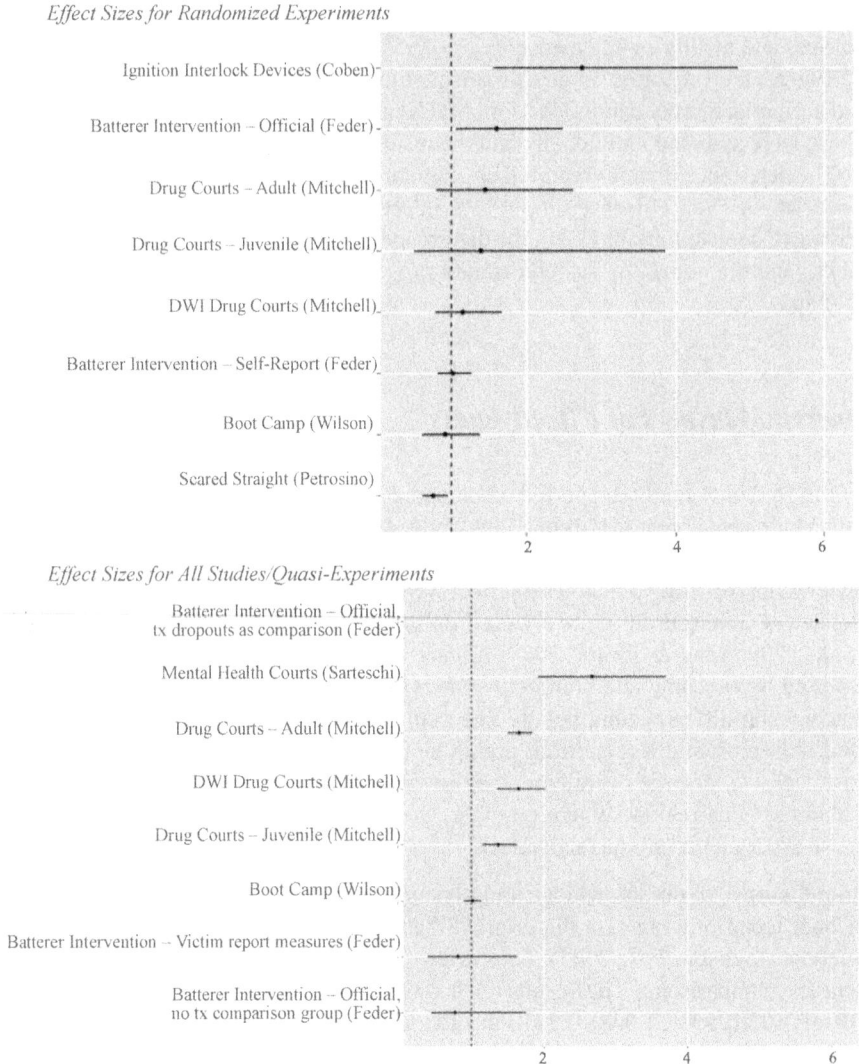

Fig. 6.3 Forest plot of recidivism outcomes for sentencing and deterrence alternatives

Belenko (2001) was one of the first to evaluate the effectiveness of drug courts and identified 37 published and unpublished studies between 1999 and April 2001. His findings indicated that drug use and criminal activity were "relatively reduced" but the longer term impacts were less clear. In an attempt to update the Belenko review, Jensen & Mosher (2006) searched published evaluations from 2001 to June 2005, this added a further 11 studies. Despite this additional literature, a number of methodological limitations were identified, (i) including the ways in which recidivism was measured, (ii) the length and scope of the study, and (iii) the use of nonequivalent comparison groups (Jensen & Mosher, 2006, p. 464). Finally, an external critique of the review also identified the failure to include the unpublished or gray literature (Stern & Simes, 1997).

In 2005, the review conducted by the US Government Accountability Office found a further 27 evaluations. Of these, five studies employed random assignment. The review focused on "within-program" evaluations, thus limiting the conclusions to evaluations where post-program recidivism was measured up to 1 year post completion. The authors argued that participants were found to have fewer incidents of re-arrest or reconvictions following the drug court. Inconsistent findings were shown between official drug test results and self-report testing mechanisms.

The systematic review conducted by Wilson and colleagues differed from the previous reviews in that it included both published and unpublished reports and used a statistical meta-analysis to produce an estimate of overall effect across studies. This review identified a substantial amount of unpublished literature (62%), helping to refute earlier criticisms concerning a possible bias linked to peer-reviewed publications. The conclusions led the reviewers to establish that drug offenders participating in drug courts were less likely to reoffend than similar offenders when sentenced to traditional correctional options.

One further meta-analytical study conducted by Lowenkamp et al. (2005) reported on similar findings identifying 22 outcome evaluations which utilized some measure of criminal activity. The authors assessed the long term results using follow-up periods of more than 2 years which demonstrated a larger reduction in recidivism. This review also included an evaluation of offender risk level. The results showed a big effect linked to those participants who had previously been involved with the CJS. This notion supports other research which suggests that treatment programs should be reserved for offenders at high risk of future offending behavior (Lowenkamp et al., 2005).

The most recent review conducted by Mitchell et al. (2012) found 154 evaluations of drug courts including 92 adult drug courts, 34 juvenile drug courts and 28 courts investigating driving while intoxicated (DWI). Despite the large number of research studies, most of these studies were found to employ quasi-experimental designs. Only eight randomized controlled trials (RCTs) of adult drug courts, one RCT of a juvenile court and four RCTs were identified evaluating DWI courts were identified. Overall, the findings support the effectiveness of drug courts in reducing recidivism but the strength of this evidence was found to vary by court type. Consistently strong evidence was shown in adult courts in the reduction of recidivism with a much smaller effect on recidivism for the juvenile drug courts. DWI courts found less consistent results especially in those studies which employed an experimental design (Mitchell et al., 2012).

In summary, despite the large amount of research and investment in drug court evaluations over the last three decades only a handful of RCTs has been conducted. The findings of these vary and provide tentative evidence to support the use of adult drug courts; however, the effectiveness of juvenile and DWI courts still remains undecided.

Mental health diversion schemes The impact of MHCs has recently been examined using a meta-analytical study focusing on health and criminological outcomes (Sarteschi et al., 2011). The study included both published and unpublished literature as well as an email survey of MHC program directors. In all, they identified 18 studies and synthesized the data by outcome measure, study design and publication type. The results indicated that MHCs have the greatest impact on reduction in recidivism with white males in their mid-30s. The authors raise concerns about such results given that women offenders are more likely to suffer from a diagnosed mental illness than their male counterparts. This suggests one of two ideas: either females are not accessing such services and/or research is not being conducted with females (Fazel & Danesh, 2002).

The authors also noted that many of the MHCs did not provide adequate information about the individuals who did not complete the MHC program. This lack of detail makes the detail of the intervention and suitability for clients different to ascertain. Compliance with the program was clearly identified as a factor for success. Participants receiving the "full dose" did significantly better than those who did not. Different judges and court personnel were found to have their own individual preferences for the referral procedures and poor program descriptions leave us with gaps in our knowledge about why such schemes may work better than others.

Although the authors felt that MHCs showed some positive effects, these conclusions were based on the findings of quasi-experimental studies. High-quality research using RCT designs are required. As a consequence, the extent to which we can rely upon the findings about the effectiveness of MHCs is limited.

The second review in this domain evaluated the effectiveness of post-booking and post-incarceration diversion programs in North America (Lange et al., 2011). Forty-three articles, 41 in America and 2 in Canada, described post-booking diversion schemes designed to identify individuals in court or jail for diversion at some point after arrest and booking. Schemes included jail-based diversion programs, court-based diversion programs, and MHCs. Post-incarceration diversion is intended to guide the transition of an offender following release into the community. Such schemes are mainly reserved for people suffering from mental illness. The review evaluated mental health probation and parole and Forensic Assertiveness Community Treatment (FACT).

The evidence of effectiveness was measured using (i) reduced recidivism, (ii) fewer days incarcerated, (iii) improved mental health status, (iv) reduced substance, and (v) increased quality of life. Overall, the authors report that post-booking diversion schemes show a moderate to high degree of success in reducing recidivism. The biggest impact was shown in schemes using jail-based diversion and MHCs as opposed to court-based diversion which only found moderate effects. Only five studies of post-incarceration diversion programs were identified. Mental health probation and parole showed evidence of moderate effectiveness and were found to increase service utilization but showed less success in the reduction of time spent in prison and recidivism rates.

FACT was found to reduce recidivism, had limited to moderate effects on the number of days incarcerated, and showed a reduction in substance use. Limitations are noted on a number of different aspects based on the quality of the research. In particular, the authors note problems with failure to include control groups, relatively small sample sizes, poor external generalizability, and an absence of longitudinal designs to assess long-term outcomes. This means that without further high-quality research we are unable to draw firm conclusions about the effectiveness of sentencing diversionary schemes. No meta-analysis has been completed in this area and the evidence relies upon mainly descriptive information.

Non-mental Health Diversion Programs We identified one qualitative systematic review which was employed to understand more about the supervision of women in court-mandated substance abuse treatment programs (Finfgeld-Connett & Johnson, 2011). The systematic review contained five US papers published between 2006 and 2009 and included programs of supervision and monitoring through law enforcement correctional system as well as a variety of therapeutic services.

The overall findings showed that women were generally reluctant to participate into referred court sanctioned substance abuse treatment programs, but once engaged they often complied well with treatment, with many completing the full complimentary service. The results identified the need for gender-specific programs which use the general themes of hope to provide individualized care for women. One of the challenges facing those devising treatment attributes considered how such schemes can be implemented and sustained in a highly demanding and complex clinical setting. Contrary to other research the authors found that although the length of time varied greatly (3–24 months), time enrolled was not identified as a relevant factor in terms of treatment success.

Court-mandated Interventions This review assessed the effects of post-arrest court-mandated interventions for perpetrators of domestic violence. The review included experimental and quasi-experimental studies measuring official or victim reports of further domestic violent behavior. Such interventions used two different theoretical approaches: (i) a psychosocial educational type intervention or (ii) an intervention based on cognitive behavioral therapy. The results showed modest benefit for official reports of domestic violence from experimental studies (OR = 1.60; CI = 1.06–2.48), but not for victim-reported violence (OR = 1.02; CI = 0.82–1.27). The findings raise doubts about the effectiveness of court-mandated batterer intervention programs in reducing re-assault among men convicted of misdemeanor domestic violence (Feder & Wilson, 2005).

Systematic Reviews and Meta-Analytical Studies of Deterrence

Four reviews were identified on deterrence, these included the literature between 1967 and 2001. A wide range of different populations including juveniles at risk of offending behavior and adults in prison were covered across the four reviews with the majority of the literature published in the USA. The reviews included different types of study designs including ten RCTs and four quasi-experimental designs.

The research evidence focused on interventions aimed at reducing drunk driving using interlock devices (Coben & Larkin, 1999), deterrence and sentencing length (Von Hirsch et al., 1999), the deterrence of executions (Yang & Lester, 2008), and deterring young people from crime (Petrosino et al., 2003). Two of the four reviews included a meta-analytical approach, but overall the evidence on the application of deterrence theory using experimental studies in the CJS is lacking.

Ignition Interlock Devices in Reducing Drunk Driving Coben and Larkin (1999) identified six studies investigating the use of ignition interlocks as deterrence for offenders with drink driving offences. Five experimental studies found that programs utilizing ignition interlocks were effective in reducing DWI recidivism. These five studies showed a significant effect where participants were between 15 and 69 % less likely to be re-arrested for DWI than those in the control group. The study results should be interpreted with caution and are limited by the nature of their quasi-experimental design. The single RCT demonstrated a 65 % reduction in DWI, which is encouraging, but replication of this study in different settings and countries is required before firm conclusions can be made (Coben & Larkin, 1999).

Sentencing Length and the Impact of Deterrence The review conducted by Von Hirsch et al. (1999) explored the certainty of severity and punishment and the likelihood of being convicted. The authors noted that the review findings did not provide a basis for inferring that increasing the severity of sentences generally enhanced any deterrent effect. Despite this, they concluded that deterrence does work in certain circumstances. In particular; they found that the impact of social ties played an important role in deterring offenders from crime. The results showed that those with strong family and community links were found to be much more likely to be deterred by the prospect of being caught than the lone, persistent burglar, who often acts impulsively (Von Hirsch et al., 1999). With regards to the certainty of being caught and punished, or the prospect of a really severe punishment, they concluded the evidence showed that passing ever harsher sentences did not "enhance the deterrent effect."

Deterrence and the Effect of Executions Yang and Lester (2008) undertook a meta-analysis of studies investigating the deterrent effect of executions on murder. This review contained one of the largest meta-analyses across all the systematic review studies, combining 95 studies by study type. Overall, the findings showed that the deterrent impact of executions on murder was affected by the type of study design (e.g., time series and panel data vs. cross sectional data) and the effects of publicity. In addition, other researchers have specified the main problems with such research designs are their inability to specify the non-capital sanction components of the sanction regime for the punishment of homicide, and that such studies do not take into consideration the perceptions of potential murderers and their response to the capital punishment component of a sanction regime (Nagin & Pepper, 2012).

Scared Straight The "Scared Straight" program is aimed at deterring young people from criminal activity. The program comprised organized visits to prisons by juvenile delinquents adjudicated by a juvenile court or children in trouble (who were not officially adjudicated as delinquents). The findings of the review showed the intervention to do more harm than good, with a mean OR of 0.76 (CI = 0.61–0.95). As a result, the authors concluded that program such as Scared Straight are likely to have a harmful effect and increase delinquency relative to doing nothing at all (Petrosino et al., 2005).

Discussion

This chapter provides an overview of systematic reviews and meta-analytical studies of sentencing and deterrence in crime and justice. Overall, 16 reviews were identified with the majority of evidence focusing on alternative sentencing options. Table 6.3 shows the summary of evidence by intervention type described in this review. Fifteen different intervention categories were used to describe the findings. Those that were classified as "what works" included adult drug courts, where the majority ($n=8$) RCTs have been conducted, which show generally consistent results in reducing subsequent recidivism. The largest body of evidence showed some promising findings but requires additional research to ascertain firm conclusions. The interventions that were classified as promising included: MHCs, post-booking schemes, FACT, jail-based courts, mental health and probation and parole schemes, and DWI initiatives. We remain "uncertain" about the findings about juvenile drug courts and courts assessing DWI offenders, the use of court-mandated domestic violence schemes, and use of the death penalty. The broad category of sentencing and deterrence, specifically in relation to sentence severity and boot camps, was found to have "no evidence of any effect." We excluded one intervention of women mandated to substance abuse treatment from this taxonomy because the systematic review of qualitative studies was not identified to assess the effectiveness of the program but the *process* by which women engaged in such services. More recent requirements by funding bodies to encompass the use of traditional qualitative research alongside large RCTs with economic analyses generate a rich data source not only about what works, but also *how* does it work, *why* does it work, and *how much* does it cost (See also Chap. 9).

As with all judgments of effectiveness, the extent to which we can conclusively say a program works is limited by the quality of available evidence. In terms of research design, the quality of evidence is usually based upon the extent to which we can ascertain the causal relationship about the effectiveness of a particular intervention or sentencing option; ideally through a RCT design. For this reason, we were particularly interested in investigating the distribution of RCTs within the classification system of "what works." Figure 6.4 shows the majority of trials are classified under "what works," with a smaller number identified under the "what is harmful" and the "what is uncertain" categories. These findings suggest that trials have been repeatedly conducted in an area of research where (1) the results of the study have been harmful and (2) the differing trial outcomes under the "what is uncertain" category relate to a lack of process evaluation detail, which describes why something does or does not work.

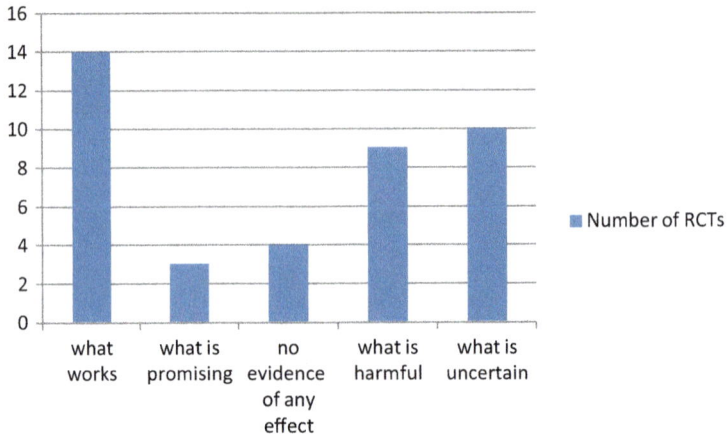

Fig. 6.4 The number of RCTs categorized by the 'What Works' taxonomy

However, these conclusions warrant a number of caveats. First, most of the research evidence comes from the USA; this highlights the issue of limited external generalizability and the paucity of evidence from judicial systems outside of the USA. In many of these examples, the results are based upon one or two single studies that have been combined using meta-analytical techniques. Although useful, the conclusions drawn from such limited evidence must be caged with caution as replicability of the results plays an important role in generating a body of evidence which produces consistent results.

Most of the reviews identified differing levels of success on the same outcome measure. Different reporting mechanisms of recidivism (e.g., official and self-report information) generated different outcomes of success. Such differences may be linked to measurement problems, including error caused by social desirability in responses and recall bias, missing attributes on large databases, and limitations of standardized data entry procedures.

Drug court evaluations comprised the biggest body of literature identified. Tentative conclusions about their relative effectiveness reveal some illustrative criticisms (Fischer, 2003). These involve the general lack of program retention; what Fischer referred to as "skimming practices," where the most treatable or lowest risk offenders are put forward for programs, leading to the possibility of selection bias; and a lack of long-term post-intervention follow-up, meaning that any measures of effect are limited to 1 or 2 years of follow-up. At the other end of the spectrum, the element of coercion has a powerful effect on the impact of successful completion using drug courts as an alternative to traditional sentencing. Success within drug courts has also varied, with more success for adult as opposed to juvenile drug courts. In the Mitchell et al. (2012) review, only one study in a juvenile court was classified as an RCT. Until a substantial body of good-quality evidence is developed, the implementation and variation within drug court programs will remain difficult to untangle.

Although many questions still remain over the effectiveness of MHCs and diversion schemes for the mentally ill, they provide a service which has important clinical implications. Within this context, offenders are not treated as criminals but as individuals with an illness that impairs their psychological ability to refrain from behavior which ultimately leads to crime. The demand for clinical services highlights a need for more research of high methodological quality that includes descriptions of program implementation. Information about the program content and individuals who do not complete such initiatives will help us to explore what exactly seems to work and for whom. Lange et al. (2011) propose that a holistic approach is required whereby the criminal justice and health care systems work together to prevent the criminalization of persons suffering from mental illness (Lange et al., 2011).

Being able to provide information to policy makers based on not only evidence of effectiveness but also cost effectiveness is of great importance. Four studies included cost-benefit information showing, that drug court treatment was likely to yield a net benefit (US Government Accountability Office [GAO], 2005). Basic policy decisions must rely upon who benefits most from a particular intervention and at what cost. Clearly, such information is not being included as part of RCTs in the criminal justice setting. Where public expenditure on such initiatives involves a dependence upon taxpayers' money, cost-benefit information should become standard for conducting RCTs. Only when this becomes a recognized requirement will such evidence eventually filter into systematic reviews and meta-analyses, whereupon such information will become a powerful tool upon which policy makers can base policy formulation decisions (see also Chap. 11 of this volume).

Aside from the sentencing reviews identified within this paper, the most striking lack of evidence comes from those focusing on deterrence. As a result, philosophers, criminologists, judges, lawyers, and others have debated whether and to what extent the CJS serves as a deterrent. Deterrence requires the would-be criminal to possess some degree of reflective capacity before the crime is committed, at least enough reflection to consider the possible consequences of violating the law if caught. Since many crimes are committed during "the heat of the moment" when an individual's reflective capacities are severely compromised, most observers agree that some crimes simply cannot be deterred. Individuals who commit crimes for the thrill of "getting away with it" and outwitting law enforcement officials probably cannot be deterred either. The biggest missing area of research in this area includes the absence of a systematic inquiry into the extent of that awareness. The importance of this comes into play when sentence severity is changed. General deterrence is directed at both potential and convicted offenders, and the issue of dissemination of sentencing policy is a critical and unexplored area of research. Without such information it is difficult to draw valid inferences concerning the marginal deterrent effects of changes in sanction levels. In addition, recent findings of a review of the deterrence literature in relation to the death penalty on behalf of the National Research Committee on Law Enforcement and Criminal Justice concluded that the current research does not explore the issue of the deterrent effects of capital punishment relative to other penalties such as life without parole (Blumstein, Cohen, & Nagin, 2012). As a result, simple questions about whether the legal status of the death penalty does indeed affect the homicide rate and whether the intensity of the death penalty affects its use are as yet unknown despite this form of sentencing being used for numerous decades. The death penalty, which is frequently used as sentencing option and a measure of deterrence in the USA, is poorly understood, and the research evidence is not adequate to support the notion that the death penalty acts as deterrence for potential murderers.

Conclusions

The evidence summarized in this review identifies what we know about what works in relation to sentencing and deterrence. Currently, cautionary judgments about what works can be deduced from the literature but they are limited by the large amount of gaps in our knowledge about many of the basic questions surrounding sentencing and deterrence. The paucity of evidence relating to the impact of deterrence provides us with little scope to draw conclusions about the elements of effectiveness or whether a particular sentencing option works. Large investments of money are needed to develop and encourage high-quality, focused, and detailed research on the effectiveness of sentencing and deterrence, as this will remain a topic of importance throughout the CJS.

Acknowledgment The author thanks Kate Light, Information Specialist, Centre for Reviews and Dissemination, University of York, for her assistance with developing the search strategies and conducting the searches. The author also thanks Catherine Hewitt, The Trials Unit, University of York, UK and Alese Wooditch, Center for Evidence-Based Crime Policy, University of George Mason, USA, for their help in converting effect sizes into ORs.

References

Beck, K. H., Rauch, W. J., & Baker, E. A. (1997). *The effects of alcohol ignition interlock license restrictions on multiple alcohol offenders: A randomized trial in Maryland.* College Park, MD: Department of Psychology: University of Maryland.

Belenko, S. (2001). *Research on drugs courts: A critical review, 2001 update.* New York: National Center on Addiction and Substance Abuse: Columbia University.

Coben, J. H., & Larkin, G. L. (1999). Effectiveness of ignition interlock devices in reducing drunk driving recidivism. *American Journal of Preventive Medicine, 16*(1 Suppl), 81–87.

Cross, T. P., Walsh, W. A., Simone, M., & Jones, L. M. (2003). Prosecution of child abuse: A meta-analysis of rates of criminal justice decisions. *Trauma, Violence, & Abuse, 4*(4), 323–340.

Fazel, S., & Danesh, J. (2002). Serious mental disorder in 23 000 prisoners: A systematic review of 62 surveys. *Lancet, 359,* 545–550.

Feder, L., & Wilson, D. B. (2005). A meta-analytic review of court-mandated batterer intervention programs: Can courts affect abusers' behavior? *Journal of Experimental Criminology, 1*(2), 239–262.

Finfgeld-Connett, D., & Johnson, E. (2011). Substance abuse treatment for women who are under correctional supervision in the community: A systematic review of qualitative findings. *Issues in Mental Health Nursing, 32*(10), 640–648.

Fischer, B. (2003). Doing good with venegeance: A critical assessment of the practices, effects and implications of drug treatment courts in North America. *Criminology & Criminal Justice, 3*(3), 227–248.

Gould, R. A., & Clum, G. A. (1993). A meta-analysis of self-help treatment approaches. *Clinical Psychology Review, 13*(2), 169–186. doi:10.1016/0272-7358(93)90039-o.

Jenson, E., & Mosher, C. (2006). Adult drug courts: Emergence, growth, outcome evaluations and the need for a continuum of care. *Idaho Law Review, 42*(2), 443–470.

Lange, S., Rehm, J., & Popova, S. (2011). The effectiveness of criminal justice diversion initiatives in North America: A systematic literature review. *The International Journal of Forensic Mental Health, 10*(3), 200–214.

Lowenkamp, C. T., Holsinger, A. M., & Latessa, E. J. (2005). Are drug courts effective: A meta analytic review. *Journal of Community Corrections, Fall, 5–10,* 28.

Lowenkamp, C. T., Latessa, E. J., & Holsinger, A. M. (2006). The risk principle in action: What have we learned from 13,676 offenders and 97 correctional programs? *Crime & Delinquency, 52*(1), 77–93.

Marsh, K., Fox, C., & Sarmah, R. (2009). Is custody an effective sentencing option for the UK? Evidence from a meta-analysis of existing studies. *Probation Journal, 56*(2), 129–151.

McDougall, C., Cohen, M. A., Swaray, R., & Perry, A. (2003). The costs and benefits of sentencing: A systematic review. *Annals of the American Academy of Political and Social Science, 587,* 160–177.

Mitchell, O., Wilson, D. B., Eggers, A., & MacKenzie, D. L. (2012). Drug courts' effects on criminal offending for juveniles and adults. *Campbell Systematic Reviews, 8*(4). doi:10.4073.

Moher, D., Liberati, A., Tetzlaff, J., Altman, D. G., & PRISMA Group. (2009). Preferred reporting items for systematic reviews and meta-analyses: the PRISMA statement. *PLoS Medicine, 6*(7), e1000097. doi:10.1371/journal.pmed.1000097.

Nagin, D., & Pepper, D. S. (2012). *Deterrence and the death penalty.* Washington, DC: National Academies Press.

Nagin, D., & Pogarsky, G. (2001). Integrating celerity, impulsivity and extralegal sanction threats into a model of general deterrence: Theory and evidence. *Criminology, 39*(4), 865–892.

Petrosino, A., Turpin-Petrosino, C., & Buehler, J. (2003). Scared Straight and other juvenile awareness programs for preventing juvenile delinquency: A systematic review of the randomized experimental evidence. *Annals of the American Academy of Political and Social Science, 589,* 41–62.

Petrosino , A., Turpin-Petrosino, C., & Buehler, J. (2005). Brief report: The effects of scared straight and similar programs on delinquency: A systematic review. *Scientific Review of Mental Health Practice, 4*(1).

Sarteschi, C. M., Vaughn, M. G., & Kim, K. (2011). Assessing the effectiveness of mental health courts: A quantitative review. *Journal of Criminal Justice, 39*(1), 12–20.

Schutte, J. W., & Hosch, H. M. (1997). Gender differences in sexual assault verdicts: A meta-analysis. *Journal of Social Behavior & Personality, 12*(3), 759–772.

Shepherd, J. P. (2001). Criminal deterrence as a public health strategy. *The Lancet, 358*(9294), 1717–1722.

Stern, J., & Simes, J. (1997). Publication bias: Evidence of delayed publication in a cohort study of clinical research projects. *British Medical Journal, 315,* 640–645.

US Government Accountability Office (GAO). (2005). Adult drug courts: Evidence indicates recidivism reductions and mixed results for other outcomes. GAO-05-219, February 2005.

Von Hirsch, A., Bottoms, A. E., Burney, E., & Wikstrom, P. O. (1999). *Criminal deterrence and sentence severity: An analysis of recent research.* Oxford: Hart Publishing.

Williams, K. R., Gibbs, J. P., Erickson, M. L. (1980). Public knowledge of statutory penalities: The extent and basis of accurate perception. *Pacific Sociological Review, 23*(1). 105–128.

Wilson, D. B., MacKenzie, D. L., & Mitchell, F. N. (2005). Effects of correctional boot camps on offending. *Campbell Systematic Reviews, 1*(6), 1–45.

Wilson, D. B., Mitchell, O., & Mackenzie, D. L. (2006). A systematic review of drug court effects on recidivism. *Journal of Experimental Criminology, 2*(4), 459–487.

Yang, B., & Lester, D. (2008). The deterrent effect of executions: A meta-analysis thirty years after Ehrlich. *Journal of Criminal Justice, 36*(5), 453–460.

Chapter 7
Correctional Programs

David B. Wilson

Throughout most of human history, punishment for wrongdoing was physical and often brutal. The idea of punishing someone by simply locking them up for a period of time is a relatively recent approach and represented an important paradigmatic shift in penal philosophy. This shift found expression in the penitentiary system that developed in the early 1800s, such as Eastern State Penitentiary in Philadelphia. The very name *penitentiary* reflects that these institutions were to be a place of penance or repentance of sins. The early penitentiaries in the USA incorporated religious education and work as key rehabilitative elements. Thus, the development of the penitentiary system represented a movement toward the rehabilitative ideal and away from the corporal punishments and public shaming that dominated prior centuries, at least within Western societies, although the implementation fell far short of the ideal and was often brutal in its own right (Rothman, 2002).

The rehabilitative ideal is the notion that criminal justice sanctions should be designed to change individual offenders such that they are "cured" of crime (Cullen, Fisher, & Applegate, 2000). This utilitarian goal is clearly seen in the use of the word *correctional* in the name for most systems for handling the sentences imposed on convicted offenders. We can quibble over the implementation of the rehabilitative ideal throughout recent history (see Rothman, 2002 for a critique), but providing offenders with opportunities for personal improvement in some form has been a cornerstone of modern correctional practice.

Public support for the rehabilitation of offenders is high, despite calls for more punitive sentences. In summarizing public opinion surveys, Cullen et al. (2000) showed that while support for rehabilitation declined from the 1960s through the mid-1990s, "rehabilitation remains widely endorsed by citizens as an important function of the correctional system" (p. 47). This support is even greater with respect to juveniles. These surveys were conducted during the "nothing works" era following the Martinson and Lipton (e.g., Lipton, Martinson, & Wilks, 1975) treaty against the effectiveness of rehabilitative programs. Thus, support has remained

D. B. Wilson (✉)
George Mason University, Fairfax, VA, USA
e-mail: dwilsonb@gmu.edu

high for the goal of rehabilitation even during a period of general pessimism regarding the ability of the correctional system to "cure" offenders of their criminal ways.

Rehabilitative programs locate the causes of crime within the individual or at least presume that by bringing about change within an individual he or she will be less likely to continue to commit crime. A popular framework for thinking about rehabilitation is the risk-need-responsivity (RNR) model (Andrews & Bonta, 2010). Within this model, criminogenic factors are those things that support or lead to criminal behavior, such as substance abuse, and low educational attainment. Correctional programming should, according to this model, address these criminogenic factors. The RNR model has received empirical support and is widely used throughout the US criminal justice system (Smith, Gendreau, & Swartz, 2009).

The range of rehabilitative programs developed for offenders is extensive and it would be difficult, if not impossible, to catalog all of them. There are the standard programs, such as remedial education, and the just plain wacky, such as a program to build self-esteem in female prisoners by teaching them how to apply makeup. Despite this diversity, the majority of programs for general offenders provided within an adult correctional setting can be categorized into one of the following four groups: (1) educational, vocational, or work related; (2) religious; (3) substance abuse; and (4) psychosocial or behavioral (e.g., cognitive-behavioral). There are also specialty programs and services for (5) sex offenders and those with (6) mental illness.

The objective of this chapter is to summarize the findings from meta-analyses of correctional programs suitable for incarcerated adult offenders. This summary will organize the meta-analyses around the six categories identified above. Although not all correctional programs have been subjected to meta-analysis, these reviews provide evidence on the effectiveness (or ineffectiveness) of the more typical programs found within Western correctional systems.

Method of Reviewing Reviews

Numerous meta-analyses have been conducted on the effectiveness of correctional programs (e.g., Lipsey & Cullen, 2007). The focus of this chapter is the subset of reviews that examined programs suitable for incarcerated adult offenders, even if some of the reviewed studies were of community-based programs. Toward this aim, the following criteria were used to determine eligibility for this chapter. First, the review must have used meta-analytic methods to summarize the results across studies. The minimum criteria were the calculation of effect sizes reflecting the effectiveness of the correctional program and statistical analysis of those effect sizes, such as the computing of a mean effect. No quality standards were imposed on the methods of meta-analysis, although the quality of the meta-analytic methods are summarized in Table 7.1 and commented on in the text when necessary. An exception was made to these criteria for religious programs where no meta-analyses were found but one review using systematic review methods was identified. This review was included because it was the only one to address this program category.

Table 7.1 Characteristics of the reviewed meta-analyses by treatment category

Treatment category, study author, publication date	Designs[a]	No. of RCTs	Searches	Time period	Participants	Meta-analysis	No. of studies
Educational, vocational, & work							
Chappell (2004)	QEs, One-group designs	0	Includes gray literature	1990–1999	Incarcerated adults	Sample size weighted (Hunter and Schmidt method)	15
Wilson et al. (2000)	RCTs, QEs	3	Includes gray literature	1975–1997	Incarcerated adults	Random-effects inverse-variance weighted	33
Religious programs							
Dodson et al. (2011)	QEs, One-group designs	0	Includes gray literature	1976–2002	Adult and juvenile offenders	No meta-analysis	7
Substance abuse treatment							
Mitchell et al. (2007)	RCTs, QEs	4	Multiple sources, gray literature included	1980–2004	Incarcerated offenders	Random-effects inverse-variance weighted	53
Pearson & Lipton (1999)	RCTs, QEs	2	Based on CDATS, includes gray literature	1968–1996	Incarcerated offenders	Random-effects inverse-variance weighted	26
Tong & Farrington (2008)	RCTs,[c] QEs	9	Multiple sources, gray literature	1988–2006	Adult and juvenile; incarcerated and in community	Fixed/Random-effects inverse-variance weighted	19
Landenberger & Lipsey (2005)	RCTs, QEs	19	Multiple sources, gray literature	1980–2004	Adult and juvenile; incarcerated and in community	Random-effects inverse-variance weighted	58
Wilson et al. (2005)	RCTs, QEs	4	Multiple sources, gray literature	1985–1999	Adult and juvenile; incarcerated and in community	Random-effects inverse-variance weighted	20

Table 7.1 (continued)

Treatment category, study author, publication date	Designs[a]	No. of RCTs	Searches	Time period	Participants	Meta-analysis	No. of studies
Cognitive-behavioral programs							
Dowden et al. (2003)	RCTs, QEs	[b]	Multiple sources, gray literature	1983–1999	Mostly adult offenders	Unknown, violated independence	24
Pearson et al. (2002)	RCTs, QEs	7	Based on CDATS, includes gray literature	1968–1996	Adult and juvenile; incarcerated and in community	Random-effects inverse-variance weighted	69
Sex offender programs							
Hanson et al. (2009)	RCTs, QEs[d]	4	Multiple sources; gray literature	1980–2009	Adult and juvenile sex offenders; incarcerated or in community	Random-effects inverse-variance weighted	23
Lösel & Schmucker (2005)	RCTs, QEs	7	Multiple sources, gray literature	1968–2003	Adult and juvenile sex offenders; incarcerated or in community	Random-effects inverse-variance weighted	69
Gallagher et al. (1999)	RCTs, QEs	2	Multiple sources; gray literature	1975–1999	Adult and juvenile sex offenders; incarcerated or in community	Random-effects inverse-variance weighted	25
Hall (1995)	RCTs, QEs	3	Published studies only	1988–1994	Adult and juvenile sex offenders; incarcerated or in community	Fixed effects, Rosenthal method	12
Mental health services							
Morgan et al. (2012)	RCTs, QEs, One-group	Unknown	Multiple sources, gray literature	1973–2004	Adult offenders with mental illness; incarcerated or in community	Random-effects inverse-variance weighted	26

[a] RCTs = true experiments or randomized controlled trials; QEs = nonequivalent comparison group quasi-experimental designs
[b] Cannot determine directly. Twenty-four studies produced forty effect sizes, ten of which came RCT designs
[c] RCTs include sequential assignment
[d] Author applied a structured data quality instrument and excluded studies that failed to meet a minimum quality standard

Second, the review must have examined the effectiveness of a correctional program on future criminal behavior. Reviews may have examined other outcomes as well but the focus here is on the effectiveness of these interventions to rehabilitate offenders in the classic sense. Most reviews and primary evaluations of correctional programs rely on official measures of recidivism, such as arrest. Reviews that used alternative measures, such as self-report or other-report, were also eligible.

Third, reviews must have evaluated a program provided to adult offenders in an institutional setting, such as a prison or jail. Reviews did not, however, need to be restricted to incarcerated adult samples. The important demarcation was that the intervention being assessed be appropriate for an adult prison population and that some portion of the primary studies included in the review used a sample of adults in prison or jail. Thus, many of the reviews of cognitive-behavioral programs and sex offender programs included both adult and juvenile samples, and incarcerated and community-based samples. Substance abuse treatment reviews, however, were restricted to prison-based studies in part because of the availability of reviews focused specifically on such programs and also because community-based substance abuse programs are reviewed in Chap. 8. Educational, vocational, and work-related programs were also similarly restricted. Such programs in a prison context are likely to be quite different than their community counterpart.

The following databases were searched to identify relevant meta-analyses: Criminal Justice Abstracts, Google Scholar, National Criminal Justice Reference Service (NCJRS), PsychNET, Sociological Abstracts, and Social Science Citation Index. The reference list of the systematic review of reviews in corrections by Lipsey and Cullen (2007) was examined as well as two bibliographies of systematic reviews related to criminal justice, one compiled by Amanda Perry that included 253 systematic reviews (personal communication) and the other by Wells (2009) that included 179 publications. The search strategy was tailored to each database, taking advantage of unique features, such as the ability to restrict a search to meta-analyses or systematic reviews (PsychNET) or literature reviews (NCJRS). The keywords that served as the basis for the search including the Boolean logic were offender or criminal or prisoner or inmate or jail or correctional; program or rehabilitation or treatment or cognitive or education or religious or service or work or industries; and meta-analysis or review). This produced 638 hits across the databases. From all of these sources, 45 titles were identified as representing a potentially eligible meta-analysis of a correctional rehabilitation program for adults. This was reduced to 15 meta-analyses after closer inspection and removal of duplicate reviews as discussed below.

Duplicate reviews of the same literature present a complication. These reviews generally contain overlapping collections of studies and as such do not provide separate evidence of the effectiveness or ineffectiveness of an intervention or program area. However, these overlapping reviews, when conducted by different scholars, do provide an independent assessment of the literature, often based on somewhat different inclusion/exclusion criteria and other decisions regarding the review methods. Thus, related reviews by different review groups were retained. The newest and most complete review was generally given the primary focus in the narrative section unless it was viewed as methodologically flawed. When an older review was completely redundant with a newer review, it is only mentioned briefly in the text to indicate whether the findings were consistent with a more recent meta-analysis. Two or more reviews by the same author(s) were handled differently: only the newer review was retained unless the reviews differed in important ways, thus making independent contributions to the discussion.

Each relevant meta-analysis was carefully read and the information needed for Tables 7.1 and 7.2 was extracted. The result from a meta-analysis that used either the standardized mean difference or correlation coefficient as the effect size were converted to an odds ratio, with values greater than 1 indicating less recidivism for the rehabilitative program.[1] A few of the meta-analyses did not provide confidence intervals. If possible, these were estimated using the provided p-values by solving for the standard error that would produce the z value associated with the reported p-value.

Summary of Findings By Program Category

Educational, Vocational, and Work Programs

Educational and vocational programs have been a mainstay of correctional rehabilitation. Inmates enter prison undereducated and with poor work histories relative to the general population. For example, the 2003 *National Assessment of Adult Literacy Prison Survey* showed that 57% of US inmates entered prison without a high school diploma or general equivalence certificate compared with 19% in the general population (Greenberg, Dunleavy, & Kutner, 2007). Similarly, inmates have fewer job-related skills and a more impoverished work history than the general population (Holzer, Raphael, & Stoll, 2003).

Common sense suggests that addressing the educational and vocational deficits of an offender will reduce future recidivism through enhancing his/her prospects for meaningful employment upon release. Thus, the presumed effect of prison-based educational and vocational programs is indirect and works through its impact on postrelease employment. Empirically, the connection between work and crime is well established, although the strength of the relationship tends to be weak (e.g., Bushway, 2011).

Two systematic reviews were found that addressed prison-based educational, vocational, and work-related programs(Chappell, 2004; Wilson, Gallagher, &

---

[1] A standardized mean difference was converted to a logged odds ratio using $\ln(\text{OR}) = d\left(\dfrac{\pi}{\sqrt{3}}\right)$, and then converted to an odds ratio (OR) using $\text{OR} = e^{\ln(\text{OR})}$. A correlation coefficient was first converted to standardized mean difference and then converted to an odds ratio using the above formulas. The equation used to convert from a correlation to a standardized mean difference was $d = \dfrac{2r}{\sqrt{1-r^2}}$.

Table 7.2 Mean odds-ratio and 95% confidence interval by program type for the reviewed meta-analyses

Treatment category, study author, publication date	Intervention(s)	Comparison	Outcomes	No. of studies	Mean odds ratio	95% CI
Educational, vocational, & work						
Chappell (2004)	Postsecondary education	Treatment as usual	Criminal recidivism	15	3.26	[3.00–3.55]
Wilson et al. (2000)	Adults basic/GED	Treatment as usual	Criminal recidivism	14	1.44	[1.15–1.82]
	Postsecondary education	Treatment as usual	Criminal recidivism	13	1.74	[1.36–2.22]
	Vocational training	Treatment as usual	Criminal recidivism	17	1.55	[1.18–1.86]
	Work program	Treatment as usual	Criminal recidivism	4	1.48	[0.92–2.17]
	Multicomponent	Treatment as usual	Criminal recidivism	5	1.33	[0.89–1.98]
Religious						
Dodson et al. (2011)	Prison Fellowship Ministries	Matched controls	Criminal recidivism	2	a, b	
	Faith-based prison	Vocational prison	Criminal recidivism	1	a, c	
Substance abuse treatment						
Mitchell et al. (2007)	Therapeutic communities	Treatment as usual	Criminal & drug recidivism	30	1.38	[1.17–1.62]
	Counseling (group)	Treatment as usual	Criminal & drug recidivism	25	1.50	[1.25–1.79]
	Boot camps	Treatment as usual	Criminal & drug recidivism	2	1.10	[0.62–1.96]
	Narcotic maintenance	Treatment as usual	Criminal & drug recidivism	5	0.84	[0.54–1.29]
Pearson & Lipton (1999)	Therapeutic communities	Treatment as usual	Criminal recidivism	7	1.61	[1.00–2.66]
	Group counseling	Treatment as usual	Criminal recidivism	7	1.16	[0.97–1.38]
	Boot camps	Treatment as usual	Criminal recidivism	6	1.20	[0.83–1.73]
	Methadone maintenance	Treatment as usual	Criminal recidivism	4	a	a
	Education	Treatment as usual	Criminal recidivism	2	a	a

Table 7.2 (continued)

Treatment category, study author, publication date	Intervention(s)	Comparison	Outcomes	No. of studies	Mean odds ratio	95 % CI
Cognitive behavioral programs						
Tong & Farrington (2008)	Reasoning & Rehabilitation	Treatment as usual	Criminal recidivism	32	1.16	[1.04–1.31]
Landenberger & Lipsey (2005)	Cognitive-behavioral (mixed)	Treatment as usual	Criminal recidivism	58	1.53	[1.19–1.97]
Wilson et al. (2005)	Reasoning & Rehabilitation	Treatment as usual	Criminal recidivism	7	1.36	[0.95–1.99]
	Moral Reconation	Treatment as usual	Criminal recidivism	6	1.92	[1.60–2.30]
	Other group-based	Treatment as usual	Criminal recidivism	7	2.52	[2.03–3.19]
Dowden et al. (2003)	Relapse prevention	Unspecified	Criminal recidivism	24	1.73	[1.49–2.02]
Pearson et al. (2002)	Cognitive-behavioral (mixed)	Treatment as usual	Criminal recidivism	44	1.70	[1.38–2.09]
	Behavioral	Treatment as usual	Criminal recidivism	23	1.27	[0.93–1.75]
Sex offender programs						
Hanson et al. (2009)	Psychological (any)	No/alternative treatment	Recidivism (sexual)	22	1.52	[1.12–2.04]
		No/alternative treatment	Recidivism (violent)	10	1.23	[0.88–1.72]
		No/alternative treatment	Recidivism (general)	13	1.64	[1.25–2.13]
Lösel & Schmucker (2005)	Cognitive-behavioral	No/alternative treatment	Recidivism	35	1.45	[1.12–1.86]
	Classic behavioral	No/alternative treatment	Recidivism	7	2.19	[1.22–3.92]
	Insight oriented	No/alternative treatment	Recidivism	5	0.98	[0.51–1.89]
	Therapeutic community	No/alternative treatment	Recidivism	8	0.86	[0.54–1.35]
	Other psychosocial, unclear	No/alternative treatment	Recidivism	5	0.94	[0.53–1.65]
	Hormonal medication	No/alternative treatment	Recidivism	6	3.08	[1.40–6.79]
	Surgical castration	No/alternative treatment	Recidivism	8	15.34	[7.34–32.1]
Gallagher et al. (1999)[d]	Behavioral	No/alternative treatment	Recidivism	4	1.36	[0.83–2.18]
	Cognitive-behavioral	No/alternative treatment	Recidivism	13	2.26	[1.66–3.08]
	General psychosocial	No/alternative treatment	Recidivism	3	1.36	[0.73–2.57]
	Hormonal medication	No/alternative treatment	Recidivism	14	3.50	[1.57–7.76]
	Surgical castration	No/alternative treatment	Recidivism	1	27.14	[6.48–111.71]

Table 7.2 (continued)

Treatment category, study author, publication date	Intervention(s)	Comparison	Outcomes	No. of studies	Mean odds ratio	95 % CI
Hall (1995)	Psychological and medical	Unspecified	Recidivism	12	1.55	[a]
Hanson et al. (2009)	Psychological (any)	No/alternative treatment	Recidivism (sexual)	38	1.23	[1.08–1.43]
		No/alternative treatment	Recidivism (general)	31	1.79	[1.56–2.00]
Mental health services						
Morgan (2012)	Psychological and psychiatric	Unspecified	Criminal recidivism	4	1.22	[0.43–3.50]

[a] Not computed by study author
[b] One study reported a statistically significant benefit, another did not
[c] Statistically significant difference between the groups
[d] Additional data needed for this table obtained through personal communication with the authors

MacKenzie, 2000). Wilson et al. (2000) examined the effectiveness of basic and postsecondary educational programs, vocational programs, and correctional work programs (e.g., prison industries), whereas Chappell (2004) focused solely on the effectiveness of postsecondary educational programs.

The methodological rigor of this body of literature is generally weak with only three randomized experiments, one of which suffered from high levels of attrition (Wilson et al., 2000, p. 354). Although many of the quasi-experimental designs involved post hoc matching or some form of statistical controls, only one quasi-experimental design in the Wilson et al. (2000) meta-analysis was judged as adequately addressing selection bias. Thus, the findings in this area need to be interpreted cautiously. That said, the evidence is generally positive across program types.

Focusing on educational programs, Wilson et al. (2000) found a small positive effect for adult-basic and general equivalence diploma (GED) type programs (mean odds ratio of 1.44). The effect was somewhat larger for postsecondary educational programs (mean odds ratio 1.74). Postsecondary programs are any educational program beyond high school, such as community college courses, certificate programs, etc. Both of these effects were statistically significant. Given the large confidence intervals, the difference between the two is not. Chappell (2004) also found a positive effect for postsecondary educational programs in a correctional setting. This meta-analysis, however, suffers from numerous weaknesses, including the inclusion of studies using pre-post, one-group designs. As such, this meta-analysis adds little to the evidence on the effectiveness of these programs.

Vocational programs also fair favorable in the Wilson et al. (2000) meta-analysis. Across the 17 available studies, the mean odds ratio was 1.55, with a confidence interval ranging from 1.18 to 1.86. Assuming a 50% recidivism rate in the control condition, this translates into a recidivism rate for the vocational training group of 39%, a meaningful reduction in recidivism.

Correctional work programs produced similar results (mean odds ratio=1.48) although this was based on only four studies and was not statistically significant. Thus, there is currently insufficient evidence to conclude that these programs work, although the pattern of evidence is encouraging. Scholars have noted, however, that prison-based work programs often provide training in jobs that persons with a criminal record are barred from holding outside of prison (Petersilia, 2009, p. 174), potentially undermining any program benefits.

A subset of studies included in the Wilson et al. (2000) meta-analysis also examined employment as an outcome. In a post hoc analysis, Wilson et al. (2000) showed that a program's effectiveness at improving employment was related to its effectiveness in reducing recidivism. That is, there was a correlation between employment and recidivism effects. This is consistent with the presumed causal model: education and vocation programs increase employment which decreases involvement in crime.

The causal connection between work and crime is unlikely to simply reflect an income substitution effect, that is, legitimate work providing the income that would be gain through illegal means. As Bushway (2011) pointed out, legal employment provides a normative social context and it is this context that may have a larger impact on behavior. Thus, it may be that the pressures to conform that exist within an employment setting (i.e., informal social control within the Sampson and Laub theoretical framework) produce the positive behavior changes associated with work and not the income per se (Uggen, 2000).

Furthermore, Uggen (2000) argued that any informal social control effect of employment may not kick in until after an individual has fully transitioned into adulthood. He found empirical support for this claim with a reanalysis of the *National Supported Work Demonstration Project* experimental study. This project from the late 1970s randomly assigned a job or no job to individuals referred to the project by criminal justice, social welfare, and job-training agencies. The reanalysis found positive effects of the program for individuals of 27 years or older but no effects for those younger than 27 years. This raises the possibility that prison-based programs focusing on improving employability may be most effective for those individual who will be in their late 20s or older upon release.

Religious Programs

The history of prisons and of punishment more generally is intertwined with religion. The penitentiary system that developed in the early nineteenth century in the USA was based on the idea that solitude focused on religious penance and physical labor would cure the offender of the moral disease of crime (Clear, Hardyman, Stout, Lucken, & Dammer, 2000). With the recent increase in conservative politics, religiously based interventions within the correctional context have increased over the past two decades (Clear et al., 2000; Sumter, 2006), including the establishment in 2002 of a faith-based residential program within the US Federal Bureau of Prisons (Sumter, 2006). The personal religious transformations that are the goal of these programs, either in the form of conversion or a reaffirmation of faith, are presumed to have a secondary benefit of reducing an individual's involvement in criminal behavior.

One systematic review was identified that examined the effectiveness of religious programming on postrelease recidivism (Dodson, Cabage, & Klenowski, 2011), although this review did not perform a meta-analysis. Dodson et al. (2011) identified seven studies that examined faith-based programs, including both community and prison programs as well as programs for youths and adults. Three of the studies examined prison-based programs for adults and are the focus of what is discussed below and presented in Tables 7.1 and 7.2.

Two of these three studies examined the effectiveness of Prison Fellowship Ministries in reducing recidivism, and both used a matched comparison group design. One found a statistically significant positive effect, whereas the other did not, at least for an intent-to-treat analysis. A third study examined a Brazilian faith-based prison and compared it with a vocational or work-based prison. This study found a substantial relative reduction in recidivism for those released from the faith-based prison despite being at higher risk at baseline, on average, than the vocational prison. The authors interpreted these findings as supporting the conclusion that faith-based programs "work" to reduce recidivism. Given the small number of studies, this conclusion is unwarranted. At best, we can conclude that the evidence is encouraging.

The existing evaluation evidence is clearly Christian-centric. No evaluations were found of the utilitarian benefits of programming based on other religious faiths, such as Islam, Judaism, Buddhism, Native American religions, etc. Furthermore, the very nature of this research presumes a tangible societal benefit from these programs. As Clear et al. (2000) point out, using social science methods to investigate the value of religion is a poor fit. A primary goal of these programs is spiritual and not the utilitarian outcome of reduced criminal behavior. The utilitarian benefits of religious programming for inmates may also be more immediate. Clear et al. (2000) conducted qualitative interviews with inmates who were participating in religious programs in several prisons throughout the USA. They found that participation in these programs helped counteract the dehumanizing aspects of the prison experience and facilitated effective adaptation to prison life. Thus, any value of religious programs may be less tangible than reduced criminal conduct.

Prison-Based Substance Abuse Programs

Drug and alcohol abuse and dependence are common problems among correctional populations and have long been presumed contributors to crime. Karberg & James (2005) estimated that roughly 68% of the jail population in 2002 abused or was dependent on illicit drugs or alcohol. The rate is also high for both US state and federal prison inmates with nearly 70% reporting regular drug use (Mumola & Karberg, 2006). Furthermore, drug use is believed to be intertwined with other criminal behaviors. For example, Mumola & Karberg (2006) found that nearly a third of state and federal prisoners in the USA were under the influence of an illicit drug at the time they committed their offense. Studies have regularly established a correlation between drug use and criminal behavior (e.g., French et al., 2000). The assumption is that by reducing or stopping drug use, individuals will be more successful at transitioning to a crime-free lifestyle.

Any causal pathway between drug use and crime is likely to be indirect. That is, drug dependent individuals are known to engage in property and sexual crimes (e.g., prostitution) to support a drug habit. Crimes also occur as part of the sale and distribution of drugs. Drug use, however, may also simply reflect a criminal lifestyle, and as such may share a common cause (or causes). Whatever the connection between drugs and crime, providing substance abuse treatment services to offenders while they are incarcerated makes intuitive sense and is a commonly available treatment option within many prison systems. Despite this availability, however, Belenko and Peugh (2005) drew attention to the inadequacy of drug treatment services within the US prison system to meet existing needs, particularly the need for intensive drug treatment.

Two meta-analyses of substance abuse treatment programs for incarcerated adult offenders were eligible for this review (Mitchell, Wilson, & MacKenzie, 2007; Pearson & Lipton, 1999). The Mitchell et al. (2007) review subsumes most of the studies included in the earlier Pearson and Lipton (1999) review. As such, the following discussion will focus on the former.

The Mitchell et al. (2007) (see also Mitchell, Wilson, & MacKenzie, 2006) meta-analysis systematically searched for both published and unpublished studies during the time period of 1980 through 2004. Only four eligible studies were true experiments (i.e., randomized controlled trials, RCTs); the vast majority were nonequivalent comparison group designs. The comparison condition was no treatment or minimal treatment. Given the incarceration context, comparison offenders often received other nonsubstance-related rehabilitation programming or less intensive substance abuse-related services. Several types of treatments were examined, including therapeutic communities, group counseling, substance-abuse treatment focused boot camps, and narcotics maintenance.

The strongest positive evidence is for the effectiveness of therapeutic communities. Within a prison setting, a therapeutic community is separated from the general population and represents an intensive form of treatment, often lasting 6–12 months or longer. The treatment model is based on the idea that an individual with a substance abuse problem needs to address broad psychological problems beyond its drug dependence. A therapeutic community is a phased program and participants become increasingly involved in helping run the program as they progress through the phases. The therapeutic approach is confrontational with both staff and clients actively confronting the dysfunctional behaviors and attitudes of others in the program in daily group therapy sessions.

Mitchell et al. (2007) found 30 comparison group studies that evaluated the effectiveness of therapeutic communities. The overall mean odds ratio for general criminal recidivism (i.e., any future criminal behavior upon release) was 1.38 and was statistically significant (this translates into a reduction in recidivism from 50 to 42%); this is arguably small but meaningful. The meta-analysis found similar results for drug-related crimes. Two of these 30 evaluations employed a true experimental design with random assignment to conditions. These two studies demonstrated a positive and statistically significant mean odds ratio of 1.90 (95% confidence interval of 1.22–2.97). Thus, the evidence suggests that prison-based therapeutic communities are effective at reducing recidivism upon release from prison. Furthermore, a study by Prendergast, Farabee, and Cartier (2000) showed that therapeutic communities facilitate prison management by reducing inmate infractions and reducing staff absenteeism.

Another common form of substance abuse treatment within prisons is group counseling. This represents a diverse collection of therapeutic approaches including eclectic approaches with no clear therapeutic orientation or treatment model. The 25 studies identified by Mitchell et al. (2007) generally found positive benefits of group counseling with an overall mean odds ratio of 1.50. This translates into a reduction in recidivism from 50 to 40%. Not surprising given the diversity in programs, the results were highly variable across studies. As with the therapeutic communities, two studies used random assignment to conditions. The mean odds ratio for these two studies was near the null value (1.05) and was not statistically significant. The strongest effects were for the methodologically weakest studies. Thus, the evidence is encouraging for group counseling programs but the effectiveness is in doubt given the near null findings of the highest quality studies. It is likely that some programs are effective and others are ineffective (or even harmful). The moderator analyses did show that larger effects were associated with more mature programs of longer duration and of a voluntary nature. The descriptive information in the studies regarding the therapeutic model used was too limited to gain insights into potentially effective or ineffective approaches.

A subset of correctional boot camps are designed specifically for substance abusing offenders and provide drug treatment as part of the boot camp experience. Both Mitchell et al. (2007) and Pearson and Lipton (1999) examined the few studies that have assessed the effectiveness of these specialty boot camps: The evidence suggests that they are ineffective. Mitchell et al. (2007) found two such evaluations and the overall mean odds ratio was near the null value (1.10) and statistically nonsignificant. The top end of the 95% confidence interval (0.62–1.96) includes values of clear practical and policy significance, so the evidence does not preclude positive (or negative) effects. The meta-analysisby Pearson and Lipton (1999) included six studies of substance abuse boot camps and found a similar, albeit slightly larger, overall mean odds ratio. The additional studies identified by Pearson and Lipton (1999) were deemed ineligible for the Mitchell et al. (2007) review. Combined with the evidence of the ineffectiveness of correctional boot camps more generally (e.g., Mackenzie, Wilson, & Kider, 2001), these reviews suggest that specialized boot camps for substance abusers are unlikely to produce large meaningful benefits.

Narcotics maintenance programs, such as methadone and buprenorphine maintenance, generally are used in prison to sustain treatment continuity for individuals on a substitution maintenance program upon entering prison (Stallwitz & Stöver, 2007). They may also be used for those entering prison with an untreated narcotics addiction to avoid problematic withdrawal. These programs have been shown to be effective in the community at reducing drug dependence and improving treatment participation (Mattick, Breen, Kimber, & Davoli, 2009). Community-based maintenance programs may also reduce criminal behavior, although with the exception of heroin replacement, the evidence is less strong (Egli, Pina, Christensen, Aebi, & Killias, 2009). The evidence on the effectiveness of substitution maintenance in prison with respect to reducing future criminal behavior is disappointing. Mitchell et al. (2007) found five studies that evaluated the effectiveness of these programs on future postrelease criminality. The mean odds ratio across these five studies was nonsignificant and in the direction of *increased* criminality (mean odds ratio of 0.84). The benefits of these programs, however, may be in their ability to reduce drug use and risky injection behaviors in prison (Stallwitz & Stöver, 2007).

Pearson and Lipton (1999) also included substance abuse education programs in their review. These programs teach inmates about the harms of drug use. Pearson and Lipton (1999) found two evaluations of such educational programs. They did not meta-analyze the findings across these two studies, although they concluded that the evidence was promising. As Pearson and Lipton (1999) pointed out, we would not expect these programs to show much benefit. The methodological quality of these studies was also weak. Thus, no meaningful conclusions can be drawn regarding drug education programs in an incarceration context.

Overall, most of the evidence regarding prison-based substance abuse treatment programs is discouraging with the exception of therapeutic communities, although some group counseling programs may be beneficial. Therapeutic communities have demonstrated consistent evidence of effectiveness, including from methodologically rigorous studies. Unfortunately, therapeutic communities are the least likely program to be widely available to substance dependent inmates.

Cognitive-Behavioral Therapy Programs

Cognitive-behavioral therapy (CBT) represents a diverse collection of programs and practices based on the cognitive-behavioral model. There is no single therapeutic approach that defines CBT. The cognitive-behavioral model that underlies CBT posits that cognitions (thoughts), emotions, and behaviors are all interrelated and that altering any one of these can lead to changes in the others (Kendall, Krain, & Henin, 2000). In contrast to prior purely behavioral theories, the cognitive-behavioral model assumes that a person's reaction to the environment around them is mediated by cognitive processes. As stated by Kendall et al. (2000, p. 135), it is "not only the situation, but also what one *thinks* of the situation [that] drives his or her response." Change how a person interprets a situation and you change their behavioral response to that situation.

Psychological problems are presumed to arise from biased processing of information that leads to negative affective responses (e.g., depression and anxiety) or maladaptive behaviors (e.g., aggression, illicit drug use, and criminal behavior) (Kendall et al., 2000). Biased processing and the negative affective or behavioral responses are thought to reflect either *distortions* or *deficits*. Distorted thinking is a misinterpretation of the environment and social interactions and these distortions are the focus of many CPTs, such as Beck's cognitive-therapy for depression or Ellis' rational-emotive therapy (Kendall et al., 2000). Within the criminal justice context, distorted thinking represents the cognitive biases that provide rationalizations for criminal behavior (i.e., criminogenic thinking within the RNR framework). Thus, addressing distortions through cognitive-restructuring methods is a common focus of CBT programs for offenders (Landenberger & Lipsey, 2005). In contrast, deficits reflect limited cognitive skills or a restricted behavioral repertoire. Examples of cognitive and behavioral deficits include a lack of forethought, acting impulsively, or a lack of behavioral control (Kendall et al., 2000, p. 136), all common among the criminal justice population. A CBT program focusing on deficits may focus on the learning of new skills, such as interpersonal problem solving.

CBT based programs are generally structured, often manualized, and short-term. Within the criminal justice system, they are almost exclusively group-based.

Activities and methods vary substantially across the various CBT programs but most actively engage the participants in activities and discussion. Landenberger and Lipsey (2005) coded eleven distinct program elements across the various CBT studies identified in their review: cognitive skills, interpersonal problem-solving, social skills, cognitive restructuring, anger control, substance abuse, moral reasoning, relapse prevention, behavior modification, individual attention, and victim impact. This is by no means an exhaustive list of CBT methods but does represent the more common elements of CBT within the criminal justice system.

Five meta-analyses were identified that addressed the effectiveness of cognitive-behavioral programs for offenders (Dowden, Antonowicz, & Andrews, 2003; Landenberger & Lipsey, 2005; Pearson, Lipton, Cleland, & Yee, 2002; Tong & Farrington, 2008; Wilson, Bouffard, & Mackenzie, 2005). The details of these reviews are shown in Tables 7.1 and 7.2 and Fig. 7.1.

The most recent and methodologically sophisticated meta-analysis of cognitive-behavioral programs as a class of interventions is that by Landenberger and Lipsey (2005). This review included any variant of a cognitive-behavioral program for adult and juvenile offenders either in custody or in the community. The only restriction was that the program had to be for a general offender population and not for a specific offense type. The overall mean odds ratio was 1.53 and translates in a ten-percentage point reduction in recidivism from a 50% base rate. That is, overall, these programs reduced recidivism from roughly 50–40%. The findings were highly variable across studies; this is not surprising given the diverse collection of programs included. The primary focus of the Landenberger & Lipsey (2005) meta-analysis was exploring this variability through moderator analysis.

The methodological characteristics of the studies were only weakly related to the observed effect sizes (Landenberger & Lipsey, 2005). RCTs produced results that were, on average, very similar to less rigorous designs. The only exception to this was whether the studies performed an intent-to-treat analysis or an as-treated analysis. The latter produced larger effects, as would be expected. This finding establishes that the finding is robust to the methodological quality of the study and that the most rigorous studies support the effectiveness of CBT.

The moderator analyses found that no particular brand of CBT was superior to the others and most program elements produced roughly similar results with only a few exceptions. Cognitive-behavioral programs that included an anger control or an interpersonal problem-solving element produced larger effects. Smaller effects were observed for programs that included behavior modification or a victim impact component.

The Pearson et al. (2002) review also examined cognitive-behavioral programs of any type. The findings from this meta-analysis are in basic agreement with the Landenberger and Lipsey (2005) review. In particular, they also found smaller effects for programs that used traditional behavior modification methods and did not incorporate the cognitive aspects of cognitive-behavioral programs.

Two popular manualized group-based cognitive-behavioral programs for offenders are *Reasoning and Rehabilitation*, developed by Ross, Fabiano, and Ewles (1988), and *Moral Reconation Therapy*, developed by Little and Robinson (1988).

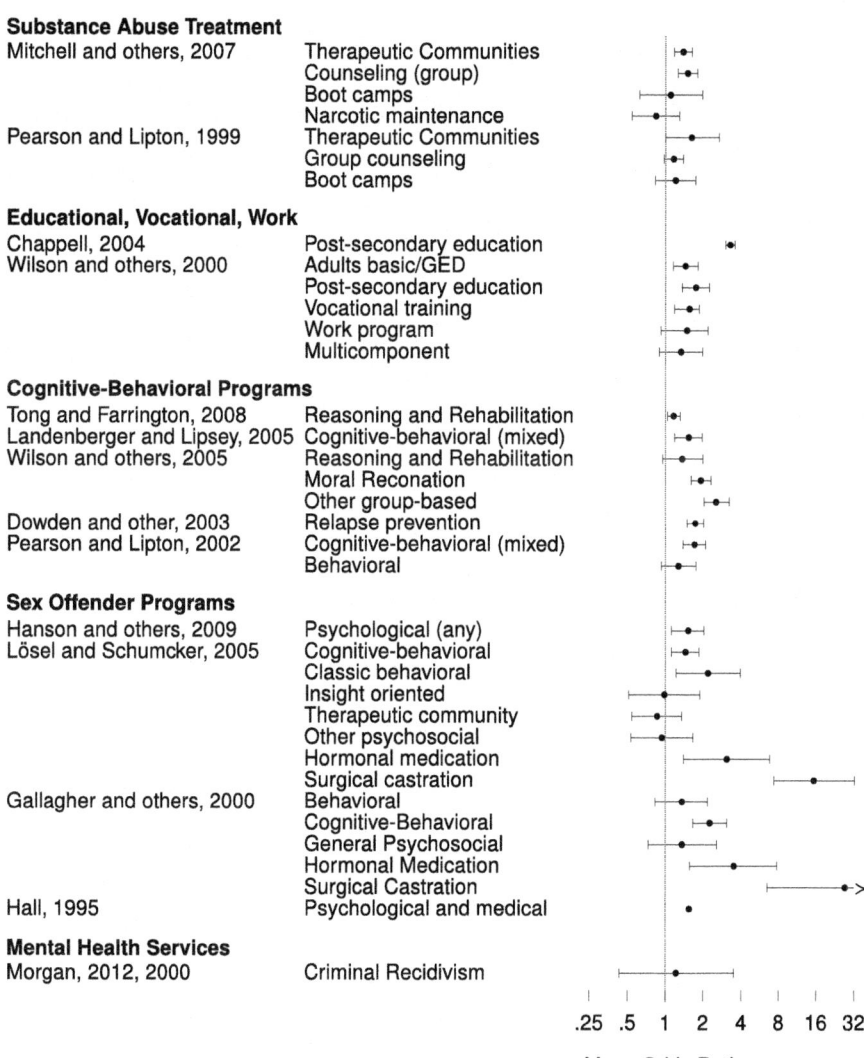

Fig. 7.1 Forest plot of mean odds ratio and 95% confidence interval by program type for the reviewed meta-analyses

Two meta-analyses examined the effectiveness of the former (Tong & Farrington, 2008; Wilson et al., 2005) and one of the latter (Wilson et al., 2005). The Tong and Farrington (2008) analysis is the most recent and comprehensive assessment of the evidence of the effectiveness of the Reasoning and Rehabilitation program. This meta-analysis identified 19 studies, several of which were unpublished. Eight of these 19 studies used random assignment to conditions (i.e., were RCTs). The findings suggest a small but positive effect. The mean odds ratio was 1.16 and statistically significant. This translates into a reduction in reoffending of four percentage points

(46% relative to a base-rate of 50%). The meta-analysis by Wilson et al. (2005) found similar, but slightly larger effects for this program (mean odds ratio of 1.36, based on seven studies). The moderator analyses by Tong and Farrington (2008) showed that randomized controlled designs produced slightly larger effects. Interestingly, the findings for low-risk and high-risk offenders were roughly similar, contrary to what would be expected from the RNR model. The RNR model posits, with some empirical support, that treatment resources should be focused on high-risk offenders.

Wilson et al. (2005) meta-analyzed evaluations of the effectiveness of Moral Reconation Therapy on offender recidivism. Six studies were identified, one of which was an RCT1 (with statistically significant results). The overall mean odds ratio was statistically significant and large by criminal justice standard (1.92). This translates into a reduction in reoffending from a base-rate of 50–34%. It is important to note, however, that four of the six studies were demonstration projects that involved the program developers. Unlike Reasoning and Rehabilitation, this program has not been tested "at scale" within the criminal justice system.

The final CBT specific meta-analysis was conducted by Dowden et al. (2003) and specifically examined the effectiveness of relapse prevention. Although initially developed for addictive behaviors, such as substance abuse (Dowden et al., 2003), the approach has been expanded to be suitable for a general offender population. Relapse prevention focuses on "teaching an individual how to identify high-risk situations, circumvent habitual coping styles, and enhance feelings of self-efficacy in dealing with these situations" (Dowden et al., 2003, p. 516). The studies reviewed were not solely relapse prevention programs but cognitive-behavioral programs that included a relapse prevention component. As such, effects cannot be interpreted as solely due to relapse prevention. This reflects that relapse prevention is typically used as an adjunct or add-on to other treatment approaches to help maintain therapeutic gains and to assist individuals in recovering from "lapses" into drug use or criminal behavior. Unfortunately, Dowden et al. (2003) did not indicate whether a subset of the study designs isolated the relapse prevention effect (i.e., compared CBT with relapse prevention to CBT without). However, the findings are encouraging. The overall mean odds ratio was 1.73 and was statistically significant. Moderator analyses showed that larger effects were associated with programs that incorporated helping offenders identify the offense chain (triggers or precursor cues for offending or substance use behaviors), that trained significant others in the program models, and that involved active relapse rehearsal. These findings must be interpreted cautiously because this meta-analysis analyzed multiple effect sizes per study without taking into account the statistical dependencies among those effects.

Overall, the empirical evidence for the effectiveness of CBT programs is relatively strong with numerous high-quality randomized trials demonstrating positive results across a diversity of approaches and therapeutic elements. This is consistent with the general recommendation of the RNR model to use cognitive-behaviorally based methods (Andrews & Bonta, 2010). It is also consistent with the strong empirical support that CBT has received in clinical psychology for a range of disorders, including depression, anxiety, eating disorders, sexual dysfunctions, and addictions (Kendall et al., 2000).

Sex Offender Programs

The public is understandably outraged by sexual crimes and is dubious regarding the rehabilitative potential of the offenders involved. In a survey of public attitudes in Melbourne, Florida, Levenson, Brannon, Fortney, and Baker (2007) showed that the public was skeptical regarding the effectiveness of sex offender treatment and believed, contrary to current data, that sex offenders recidivated at a high rate. The reviews summarized below, however, show that sex offender treatment programs can be effective, particularly those that use cognitive-behavioral methods and/ or hormonal medication. Four meta-analyses were identified (Gallagher, Wilson, Hirschfield, Coggeshall, & MacKenzie, 1999; Hall, 1995; Hanson, Bourgon, Helmus, & Hodgson, 2009; Lösel & Schmucker, 2005), the details of which are shown in Tables 7.1 and 7.2 and Fig. 7.1.

The meta-analysis by Lösel and Schmucker (2005) is the largest, including 69 studies representing 80 independent comparisons. A unique feature of this meta-analysis is its inclusion of German language studies. Seven of the studies included in the meta-analysis were RCTs. The studies were a mix of incarceration-based (e.g., prison, jail, forensic psychiatric facility, etc.) and community-based programs. Studies with adult and juvenile samples were included although most of the studies involved adults.

The findings showed that cognitive-behaviorally based programs, classic behavioral programs (e.g., aversion therapy), hormonal medication, and surgical castration all produced positive reductions in recidivism. As pointed out by the authors, the very large effect for surgical castration must be interpreted cautiously, as those studies were quasi-experimental and likely suffered from serious selection bias. Sex offenders receiving this treatment must volunteer for the procedure and are thus likely to differ in meaningful ways from nonvolunteers who typically make up the comparison condition. For hormonal medication studies it is important to note that this treatment generally also involved some form of psychological therapy, making it impossible to isolate the unique effect of hormonal therapy. However, the size of the effect relative to the effect of CPT without hormonal therapy strongly suggests an added benefit of the medical approach.

Most sex offender programs treat individuals convicted of any type of sexual offense, such as exhibitionist, rape, intrafamilial incest, etc. Surprisingly, most of the studies of these programs do not report results separately by offender type. Using a subset of studies that did, however, Lösel and Schmucker (2005) were able to test whether these programs were differentially effective for different sex offender types. All categories showed significant reductions in recidivism with the exception of intra-familial child molestation, suggesting that these programs may not be effective with this offender group.

Additional moderator analyses performed by Lösel and Schmucker (2005) found somewhat better results for community-based programs relative to institutional programs. Furthermore, programs for juvenile offenders produced slightly better results than programs for adults, although the difference was not statistically significant. Overall, Lösel and Schmucker (2005) stressed the importance of interpreting the findings with caution given that only seven of the studies used a randomized design and many of the remaining studies were of low quality.

The older meta-analyses by Gallagher et al. (1999) and Hall (1995) are in basic agreement with Lösel and Schmucker (2005) and the studies included in each of those earlier meta-analyses are subsumed by Lösel and Schmucker (2005). The newest meta-analysis by Hanson et al. (2009), however, examined directly whether the empirical evidence supported the application of the RNR principles to sex offenders.

Hanson et al. (2009) included 23 studies of sex offender programs that used a psychological treatment. The smaller number of studies relative to Lösel and Schmucker (2005) reflects the exclusion of studies that did not meet minimum quality standards. Overall, Hanson et al. (2009) found evidence of the effectiveness of sex offender treatment programs in terms of both sexual recidivism (mean odds ratio of 1.52) and general recidivism (1.64). The effect for violent nonsexual recidivism was smaller and not statistically significant (mean odds ratio of 1.23). The RNR principles tested were targeting high-risk offenders, focusing on criminogenic needs, and responsivity (emphasizing cognitive-behavioral methods and tailoring the intervention to the learning style and abilities of the offender). Although the moderator analyses were not statistically significant, the pattern of results was entirely consistent with predictions from the RNR model.

The findings from the meta-analyses of sex-offender programs are encouraging. There is consistency across the reviews in finding reduced risk of recidivism associated with both cognitive-behavioral programs and medical hormonal programs. Unfortunately, the research-base in this area is relatively weak with few RCTs. Those that do exist, however, established that sex offender programs can be effective. It is also important to recognize that these programs do not "cure" the offender. Some portion of treated offenders still recidivate, just fewer than would be the case without treatment. Thus, these programs should be part of the mix in how we address the problem of sexual offending but they are clearly not the sole solution to protecting the public.

Psychological Treatment for Mentally Ill Offenders

The offender population and the mentally ill population overlap to a surprising extent. As discussed by Morgan et al. (2012), it is estimated that one-quarter of the adult incarcerated population suffers from a mental illness. Within the USA, local jails have become the dominant institution for housing persons with mental illness. The criminal justice system has not been able to adequately address the mental health treatment needs of all of the offenders with mental illness (Morgan et al., 2012). However, jails and prisons do provide mental health services and it is worth examining the evidence on the effectiveness of these services at reducing future criminal behavior.

A meta-analysis by Morgan et al. (2012) found 26 studies examining the effectiveness of psychological and psychiatric services for offenders with mental illness. These studies examined a broad range of outcomes. Only four examined criminal recidivism, all of which found statistically significant effects, one finding increased recidivism and three findings reduced recidivism. The overall mean effect size was positive but not statistically significant (1.22). No information was provided on the methodological differences across these four studies, so it is impossible to assess the credibility of this finding. The meta-analysis did find positive effects of these services for mental health symptoms, coping, and institutional adjustment. Clearly more research is needed to better understand the role of mental health services in reducing criminal behavior for offenders with mental illness.

Discussion

This review has shown that correctional programs produce some benefit. The mean odds ratios across the included meta-analyses, as shown in Fig. 7.1, show a clear pattern of evidence in favor of correctional programs, with 36 of 40 mean odds ratios favoring the rehabilitative program being evaluated, although many are not statistically significant. Despite these mostly positive findings across reviews, the size of the effects tends to be small. The typical effect is roughly an odds ratio of 1.5. This represents a modest but arguably meaningful reduction in recidivism from 50 to 40 %. These programs help, but are by no means the solution to recidivism.

Clearly not all programs work and the evidence for some of the programs is weak. The existing evidence most strongly supports the effectiveness of the following programs: (1) group-based cognitive-behavioral programs for general offenders, (2) group-based cognitive-behavioral programs for sex offenders, (3) hormonal medication treatment for sex offenders, and (4) prison-based therapeutic communities for substance abusing offenders. Promising evidence supports the effectiveness of the following programs: (1) adult-basic and postsecondary educational programs for general offenders and (2) vocational programs for general offenders. Several other programs had encouraging findings, such as work programs and group counseling for drug abuse, but the weak methodological rigor of the research-base constrains the conclusions that can be drawn. No interventions were found to be clearly harmful, although the evidence suggests that a few are unlikely to be found effective even with more rigorous research, such as insight-oriented therapy for sexual offenders and specialized correctional boot camps for substance abusers.

It is important to interpret these effects in context. Most of the evaluation studies contributing to these reviews rely on comparison conditions that involved some level of rehabilitative effort. This is simplified to the phrase "treatment as usual" in the meta-analyses and primary studies and may reflect anything from a purely sanctions-based treatment (e.g., incarceration) to involvement in other programs designed to help the offender. This greatly complicates the interpretation of findings from these studies as the results generally do not reflect the pure effect of the program of interest but rather the added value of the program relative to the background noise of existing practices and services. For many programs, such as substance abuse or sex offender treatments, these alternatives will generally be nonspecific to substance abuse or sexual offending. For example, someone not participating in a substance abuse treatment may have more time available for participating in an educational or vocational program. It is reasonable to assume that an environment completely void of opportunities for an offender to improve him or herself would have worse outcomes then seen by most of the comparator conditions in the studies reviewed. The seriousness of this complication varies with the program type. For educational, vocational, and work programs, offenders in the program condition were often compared with offenders participating on other prison programming. For less routine treatments, such as a cognitive-behavioral program, offenders in both conditions may be participating in roughly similar collections of comparator programs, such as an educational program. The effect size from evaluations of the latter will more clearly isolate the added benefit of the program under investigation than the former. The bottom-line is that the nature of research in this area likely downwardly biases any estimate of effectiveness.

The methodological quality must also be considered in interpreting these findings. A clear minority of studies used a random assignment to conditions (RCT) design. The area with the largest number of such studies is the diverse collection of cognitive-behavioral programs. Most treatments examined had at least a few randomized studies. The evidence from these highest quality studies indicates that rehabilitation programs can produce reductions in postrelease criminal behavior. This does not establish, however, that routine practice within the field produces comparable results. An important lesson from researchers evaluating correctional programs is that quality implementation is difficult and weak implementation undermines program effectiveness. How best to ensure program quality implement has become an important area of research and scholarship (e.g., Taxman & Belenko, 2012). Additional research is clearly needed to better understand how to effectively implement rehabilitative programs in a correctional setting. This is particularly critical for treatments that will be delivered broadly in many locations and for numerous offenders.

A clear lesson from meta-analysis is the need for replications and multiple evaluations of a common program type. Additional RCTs are clearly needed for the treatments examined here to better establish the overall strength of the effect and the sub-populations, treatment variations, and program contexts associated with larger or smaller (including null) effects. In areas were the existing evidence establishes the general effectiveness of the program, such as with cognitive-behavioral programs, RCTs should be randomly assigning individuals to variations in the program or competing models.

A cornerstone of the RNR model is an emphasis on programs based on the cognitive-behavioral model. The meta-analyses of correctional programs reviewed here support this emphasis. Both general and specialized cognitive-behavioral programs produced reductions in reoffending. As demonstrated most clearly in the Landenberger and Lipsey (2005) review, this appears to be true across a diverse range of program models within the cognitive-behavioral framework.

As pointed out by Kazdin (2007), the field of clinical psychology has established the effectiveness of many therapeutic methods, particularly those based on the cognitive-behavioral model, but has yet to provide much insight into the mechanism that produce the positive behavioral changes. The various moderator analyses performed across these reviews that were focused on getting inside the "black-box" add little insight. Cognitive-behavioral programs that incorporate anger control and interpersonal problem solving elements appear to be more effective. At least within the substance abuse category, more mature programs and programs of longer duration appear to produce the larger effects. Clearly more research is needed to shed light on the effective change mechanisms.

Another lesson from these reviews is that providing offenders with opportunities to address skills deficits (e.g., educational, vocational, and interpersonal), increase self-control (e.g., anger management), and address ancillary problem behaviors (e.g., substance abuse) are meaningful pathways for facilitating crime-free behavior. It is worth noting that most rehabilitative programs are not targeting criminal behavior directly. That is, rehabilitation programs do not try to "teach" offenders how not to commit crime. The focus is on addressing deficits that prevent an individual from engaging in alternatives to crime, such as gainful employment, or addressing behaviors and cognitions that support criminal behavior, such as criminogenic thinking, association with deviant peers, substance abuse, and mental illness. Thus, correctional rehabilitation tries to foster change within an individual that will enable him or her to transition away from a life of crime. We need to better understand what the targets of rehabilitative interventions should be.

The introduction of the penitentiary system started us down a road of rehabilitative programming for criminal offenders, rather than simply inflicting corporal and capital punishments. Despite the mass incarceration binge in the USA during the 1980s and 1990s, the rehabilitative ideal that started roughly 200 years ago continues today. The tremendous quantity of scholarly work that contributed to the meta-analyses summarized in this chapter reflects continued progress in our understanding of how to facilitate change in persons convicted of crime.

References

Andrews, D. A., & Bonta, J. (2010). Rehabilitating criminal justice policy and practice. *Psychology, Public Policy, and Law, 16*(1), 39–55. http://doi.org/10.1037/a0018362.

Belenko, S., & Peugh, J. (2005). Estimating drug treatment needs among state prison inmates. *Drug and Alcohol Dependence, 77*(3), 269–281. http://doi.org/10.1016/j.drugalcdep.2004.08.023.

Bushway, S. D. (2011). Labor markets and crime. In J. Q. Wilson & J. Petersilia (Eds.), *Crime and public policy* (pp. 183–209). New York: Oxford University Press.

Chappell, C. A. (2004). Post-secondary correctional education and recidivism: A meta-analysis of research conducted 1990–1999. *Journal of Correctional Education, 55*(2), 148.

Clear, T. R., Hardyman, P. L., Stout, B., Lucken, K., & Dammer, H. R. (2000). The value of religion in prison an inmate perspective. *Journal of Contemporary Criminal Justice, 16*(1), 53–74. http://doi.org/10.1177/1043986200016001004.

Cullen, F. T., Fisher, B. S., & Applegate, B. K. (2000). Public opinion about punishment and corrections. *Crime and Justice, 27*, 1–79. http://www.jstor.org/stable/1147662.

Dodson, K. D., Cabage, L. N., & Klenowski, P. M. (2011). An Evidence-Based assessment of Faith-Based programs: Do Faith-Based programs "Work" to reduce recidivism? *Journal of Offender Rehabilitation, 50*(6), 367–383. http://doi.org/10.1080/10509674.2011.582932.

Dowden, C., Antonowicz, D., & Andrews, D. A. (2003). The effectiveness of relapse prevention with offenders: A meta-analysis. *International Journal of Offender Therapy and Comparative Criminology, 47*(5), 516–528. http://doi.org/10.1177/0306624X03253018.

Egli, N., Pina, M., Christensen, P. S., Aebi, M., & Killias, M. (2009). Effects of drug substitution programs on offending among drug-addicts. Campbell Systematic Reviews, Issue 3; The Campbell Collaboration (http://www.campbellcollaboration.org).

French, M. T., McGeary, K. A., Chitwood, D. D., McCoy, C. B., Inciardi, J. A., & McBride, D. (2000). Chronic drug use and crime. *Substance Abuse, 21*(2), 95–109. http://doi.org/10.1023/A:1007763129628.

Gallagher, C. A., Wilson, D. B., Hirschfield, P., Coggeshall, M. B., & MacKenzie, D. L. (1999). Quantitative review of the effects of sex offender treatment on sexual reoffendering. *Corrections Management Quarterly, 3*(4), 19–29.

Greenberg, E., Dunleavy, E., & Kutner, M. (2007). *Literacy behind bars: Results from the 2003 national assessment of adult literacy prison survey. NCES 2007–473*. Jessup, MD: National Center for Education Statistics. (ED Pubs. P.O. Box 1398, Jessup, MD 20794–1398. Tel: 877-433-7827; Web site: http://nces.ed.gov/help/orderinfo.asp)

Hall, G. C. N. (1995). Sexual offender recidivism revisited: A meta-analysis of recent treatment studies. *Journal of Consulting and Clinical Psychology, 63*(5), 802–809. http://doi.org/10.1037/0022-006X.63.5.802.

Hanson, R. K., Bourgon, G., Helmus, L., & Hodgson, S. (2009). The principles of effective correctional treatment also apply to sexual offenders: A meta-analysis. *Criminal Justice & Behavior, 36*(9), 865–891. http://doi.org/10.1177/0093854809338545.

Holzer, H. J., Raphael, S., & Stoll, M. A. (2003). *Employment barriers facing ex-offenders*. Washington, DC: The Urban Institute.

Karberg, J. C., & James, D. J. (2005). *Substance dependence, abuse, and treatment of jail inmates, 2002*. Washington, DC: Bureau of Justice Statistics. http://bjs.ojp.usdoj.gov/content/pub/pdf/sdatji02.pdf.

Kazdin, A. E. (2007). Mediators and mechanisms of change in psychotherapy research. *Annual Review of Clinical Psychology, 3*(1), 1–27. http://doi.org/10.1146/annurev.clinpsy.3.022806.091432.

Kendall, P. C., Krain, A. L., & Henin, A. (2000). Cognitive-behavioral therapy. In P. C. Kendall (Ed.), *Encyclopedia of psychology* (Vol. 2, pp. 135–139). New York: Oxford University Press.

Landenberger, N. A., & Lipsey, M. W. (2005). The positive effects of cognitive-behavioral programs for offenders: A meta-analysis of factors associated with effective treatment. *Journal of Experimental Criminology, 1*(4), 451–476. http://doi.org/10.1007/s11292-005-3541-7.

Levenson, J. S., Brannon, Y. N., Fortney, T., & Baker, J. (2007). Public perceptions about sex offenders and community protection policies. *Analyses of Social Issues and Public Policy, 7*(1), 137–161. http://doi.org/10.1111/j.1530-2415.2007.00119.x.

Lipsey, M. W., & Cullen, F. T. (2007). The effectiveness of correctional rehabilitation: A review of systematic reviews. *Annual Review of Law and Social Science, 3*, 297–320. http://doi.org/10.1146/annurev.lawsocsci.3.081806.112833.

Lipton, D., Martinson, R., & Wilks, J. (1975). *The effectiveness of correctional treatment: A survey of treatment evaluation studies*. New York: Praeger.

Little, G. L., & Robinson, K. D. (1988). Moral Reconation Therapy: A systematic step-by-step treatment system for treatment resistant clients. *Psychological Reports, 62*(1), 135–151. http://doi.org/10.2466/pr0.1988.62.1.135.

Lösel, F., & Schmucker, M. (2005). The effectiveness of treatment for sexual offenders: A comprehensive meta-analysis. *Journal of Experimental Criminology, 1*(1), 117–146. http://doi.org/10.1007/s11292-004-6466-7.

Mackenzie, D. L., Wilson, D. B., & Kider, S. B. (2001). Effects of correctional boot camps on offending. *The Annals of the American Academy of Political and Social Science, 578*(1), 126–143. http://doi.org/10.1177/000271620157800108.

Mattick, R. P., Breen, C., Kimber, J., & Davoli, M. (2009). Methadone maintenance therapy versus no opioid replacement therapy for opioid dependence. In The Cochrane Collaboration & R. P. Mattick (Eds.), *Cochrane database of systematic reviews*. Chichester: Wiley.

Mitchell, O., Wilson, D. B., & MacKenzie, D. L. (2006). The effectiveness of incarceration-based drug treatment on criminal behavior. Campbell Systematic Reviews, Issue 11; The Campbell Collaboration (http://www.campbellcollaboration.org). http://doi.org/10.4073/csr.2006.11.

Mitchell, O., Wilson, D. B., & MacKenzie, D. L. (2007). Does incarceration-based drug treatment reduce recidivism? A meta-analytic synthesis of the research. *Journal of Experimental Criminology, 3*(4), 353–375. http://doi.org/10.1007/s11292-007-9040-2.

Morgan, R., Flora, D., Kroner, D., Mills, J., Varghese, F., & Steffan, J. (2012). Treating offenders with mental illness: A research synthesis. *Law and Human Behavior, 36*, 37–50. http://doi.org/10.1007/s10979-011-9271-7.

Mumola, C. J., & Karberg, J. C. (2006). *Drug use and dependence, state and federal prisoners, 2004*. Washington, DC: Bureau of Justice Statistics. (Drug Use and Dependence, State and Federal Prisoners, 2004)

Pearson, F. S., & Lipton, D. S. (1999). A meta-analytic review of the effectiveness of corrections-based treatments for drug abuse. *The Prison Journal, 79*(4), 384–410. http://doi.org/10.1177/0032885599079004003.

Pearson, F. S., Lipton, D. S., Cleland, C. M., & Yee, D. S. (2002). The effects of behavioral/Cognitive-behavioral programs on recidivism. *Crime & Delinquency, 48*(3), 476–496. http://doi.org/10.1177/001112870204800306.

Petersilia, J. (2009). *When prisoners come home: Parole and prisoner reentry*. New York: Oxford University Press.

Prendergast, M., Farabee, D., & Cartier, J. (2000). The impact of in-prison therapeutic community programs on prison management. *Journal of Offender Rehabilitation, 32*(3), 63–78. http://doi.org/10.1300/J076v32n03_05.

Ross, R. R., Fabiano, E. A., & Ewles, C. D. (1988). Reasoning and rehabilitation. *International Journal of Offender Therapy and Comparative Criminology, 32*(1), 29–35. http://doi.org/10.1177/0306624X8803200104.

Rothman, D. J. (2002). *Conscience and convenience: The asylum and its alternatives in progressive America*. New York: Aldine de Gruyter.

Smith, P., Gendreau, P., & Swartz, K. (2009). Validating the principles of effective intervention: A systematic review of the contributions of meta-analysis in the field of corrections. *Victims & Offenders, 4*(2), 148–169. http://doi.org/10.1080/15564880802612581.

Stallwitz, A., & Stöver, H. (2007). The impact of substitution treatment in prisons—A literature review. *International Journal of Drug Policy, 18*(6), 464–474. http://doi.org/10.1016/j.drugpo.2006.11.015.

Sumter, M. (2006). Faith-based prison programs. *Criminology & Public Policy, 5*(3), 523–528. http://doi.org/10.1111/j.1745-9133.2006.00399.x.

Taxman, F. S., & Belenko, S. (2012). *Evidence-based implementation agenda* (pp. 275–314). New York: Springer.

Tong, L., & Farrington, D. (2008). Effectiveness of "Reasoning and Rehabilitation" in reducing reoffending. *Psicothema, 20*(1), 20–28.

Uggen, C. (2000). Work as a turning point in the life course of criminals: A duration model of age, employment, and recidivism. *American Sociological Review, 65*(4), 529–546. http://doi.org/10.2307/2657381.

Wells, E. (2009). Uses of meta-analysis in criminal justice research: A quantitative review. *Justice Quarterly, 26*(2), 268–294. http://doi.org/10.1080/07418820802119984.

Wilson, D. B., Bouffard, L. A., & Mackenzie, D. L. (2005). A quantitative review of structured, group-oriented, cognitive-behavioral programs for offenders. *Criminal Justice and Behavior, 32*(2), 172–204. http://doi.org/10.1177/0093854804272889.

Wilson, D. B., Gallagher, C. A., & MacKenzie, D. L. (2000). A meta-analysis of corrections-based education, vocation, and work programs for adult offenders. *Journal of Research in Crime and Delinquency, 37*(4), 347–368. http://doi.org/10.1177/0022427800037004001.

Chapter 8
Drug Interventions

Katy R. Holloway and Trevor H. Bennett

Drug Prevention

There has been no shortage of evaluations of the effectiveness of drug treatment. The main problem for criminology is that the majority of these studies do not include crime outcomes. Interest has focused instead on the reduction or elimination of drug misuse. Nevertheless, there is a growing body of treatment evaluations that have included crime outcomes and in recent years several systematic reviews have incorporated crime measures in their meta-analyses.

The early reviews tended to show that drug interventions had a favorable effect on crime and criminal behavior (Hough, 1996; Bennett & Holloway, 2005). However, they also showed some variability in outcomes across studies, even after controlling for the type of intervention. Until recently, there were insufficient numbers of systematic reviews to examine the reasons for these differences. This situation has changed and there is now a substantial body of systematic reviews on the effectiveness of drug interventions on crime. As a result, it is now possible to conduct systematic reviews of systematic reviews.

The phrase "systematic review of systematic reviews" is commonly used in the literature to refer to rigorous overviews of the results of several systematic reviews (Ernst, 2002; Derry, Derry, McQuay, & Moore, 2006). The principal elements of systematic reviews of systematic reviews are essentially the same as those of systematic reviews. These include rigorous and transparent methods, clear eligibility criteria, description of the search strategy, and documentation of the selection procedure and the attrition of studies (Ernst & Canter, 2006). Systematic reviews of systematic reviews are common in the areas of health care and medical science.

K. R. Holloway (✉)
University of South Wales, Pontypridd, UK
e-mail: katy.holloway@southwales.ac.uk

T. H. Bennett
University of South Wales, Pontypridd, UK
e-mail: trevor.bennett@southwales.ac.uk

They are less common in the areas covered by criminology. However, we found two recent systematic reviews of systematic reviews on the effectiveness of drug interventions on crime.

The first comprised a review of five Cochrane systematic reviews on substitution maintenance treatments for opioid dependence (Amato, Davoli, Perucci, Ferri, Faggiano, & Mattick, 2005). The authors investigated the effects of methadone maintenance treatment compared with waiting list patients or patients receiving heroin maintenance treatments on criminal behavior. The review concluded that there were no significant differences across the five comparisons in terms of percentage involved in criminal activity.

The second by Amato, Davoli, Vecchi, Ali, Farrell, & Faggiano, et al. (2011) evaluated the publications of the Cochrane Drugs and Alcohol Group held at the time of the research (January 2010). The authors examined 52 systematic reviews from the Cochrane database on the effectiveness of drug and alcohol interventions. They found that 39 of the 52 reviews used meta-analyses to pool the results. Forty-one of the 142 meta-analyses (29%) presented in the 39 reviews were classified as "beneficial" or "likely to be beneficial." The main finding relevant to criminology is that 1 of the 41 meta-analyses coded as having a beneficial effect examined the effectiveness of drug testing following court release on arrest at 90 days (OR 1.33 [1.04, 1.70]).

Clearly, the method of synthesizing the findings of systematic reviews in relation to drug interventions and crime outcomes is still in its infancy. The aim of the current paper is to summarize the contribution of systematic reviews to criminology in relation to drug interventions. The approach adopted is to examine the results of systematic reviews across a broad range of drug interventions and a broad range of crime-related outcome measures. It encompasses criminal justice interventions (e.g., drug testing, boot camps, and drug rehabilitation programs) as well as traditional prescribing and treatment methods (e.g., rapid detoxification, maintenance prescribing, prescription of opioid receptor antagonists, and psycho-social treatment programs). This chapter presents the results of a range of drug interventions in reducing crime and criminal behavior.

Methods

In practice, the same criteria are used for conducting the review as are used in systematic reviews of evaluations. In other words, the review uses rigorous and transparent methods for searching for studies and assessing them for eligibility. The main elements of this method are a search strategy for identification of relevant studies, criteria for inclusion and exclusion, a record of attrition of studies, and a description of the final sample selected for review.

Search Strategy

The search strategy was to some extent determined by the time available to conduct the review, and it was not possible in that time to conduct the most exhaustive versions of a search strategy. However, we used sources which we knew from experience held systematic reviews in the topic area of interest. The search strategy used several methods for identifying reviews: searching known sources of systematic reviews (e.g., Cochrane and Campbell Libraries), conducting database searches from other sources (e.g., Web of Science), selecting from documents already in our possession, and contacting researchers in the field (in practice only one was contacted).

The restriction on time meant that we had to limit our searches to just four data bases: Cochrane, Campbell, Web of Science, and Medline. The choice of database was guided by what we thought were likely to be the most productive in identifying relevant reviews. In addition, we already had in our possession five systematic reviews (three of which were conducted by the authors). We also contacted one researcher to obtain a more detailed version of a published summary of a systematic review.

The four databases were searched in slightly different ways due to their differing structures and search engines. The Cochrane Library was searched by focusing on the library of 60 reviews published by the Cochrane Drugs and Alcohol Group. The Campbell Library was searched by using all 69 of its published systematic reviews. Web of Science and Medline were searched using more traditional search techniques. The first round of searches focused on the title of the articles and searched for the terms "systematic review" AND ("drug* or substance*") AND (treatment or program* or intervention). The second round of searches was extended to include specified drugs, namely, "heroin" OR "cocaine" OR "opioid*".

Criteria for Inclusion

The criteria for initial inclusion of all studies were that it must be a systematic review, written in the English language, published between the period 1992 and 2012, accessible to us during the research period, and included a drug intervention and a crime outcome measure.

The only criterion of methodological adequacy used in the selection of systematic reviews to include in the review was whether the studies were analyzed using meta-analysis to synthesize the results. Hence, there was no variation across systematic reviews on this criterion. The main variation among the reviews was in the eligibility criteria used to assess the quality of the research design used in the evaluations. The large majority of reviews included accepted randomized control trials and quasi-experimental designs. However, some included pre–post designs without control and structured observation (see Table 8.2).

Attrition of Studies

The literature searches resulted in five separate lists of titles of potentially eligible papers ($n=370$). The lists were then carefully scrutinized independently by both authors. If the title clearly indicated that the paper was not a systematic review that evaluated a drug intervention designed for misusers, then it was considered ineligible and excluded from the review ($n=103$). If there was any uncertainty in what the study was about, then the paper was deemed potentially eligible and provisionally included in the review.

After excluding all duplicate publications, the next stage was to obtain copies of all reviews that had been deemed potentially relevant based on the initial analysis of titles ($n=80$). All 80 of the papers were obtained and then carefully reviewed independently by both authors. Papers were accepted for inclusion if they met the criteria for inclusion outlined above and if they included an outcome measure of criminal behavior. When papers were found to duplicate the results of another paper, the paper that presented the most up-to-date and thorough findings was selected for inclusion in the review. This resulted in 34 studies.

The 34 unique reviews that satisfied the above-mentioned criteria were then scrutinized to see whether the authors provided a summary measure of effectiveness across two or more studies. If no such summary measure was provided, the review was excluded. This left 14 studies. Six studies were excluded because they overlapped with other chapters in the book and three more were removed because they used unconvertible effect sizes. This left eight eligible reviews containing 23 relevant meta-analyses (see Table 8.1).

Results

A summary of all studies included in the review, along with some summary findings, is presented in Tables 8.2 and 8.3. The tables cover the same items covered in other chapters in the book and include information on the experimental and comparison conditions, the outcome variables and study design, method of searching for studies, the time period, types of participants and the number of studies included in the systematic review, followed by effect size, significance, and types of moderator analyses conducted.

The results section has been divided into two parts. The first examines the mean effect sizes for each study and determines the overall balance of the findings. The results are broken down by treatment type, and the most and least effective methods are discussed. The second summarizes the nature of the systematic reviews and the results obtained in a more descriptive manner with attention drawn to particular successful interventions.

8 Drug Interventions

Table 8.1 Attrition of eligible reviews

	Cochrane	Campbell	Web of Science	Medline	Other[a]	Total
Search results	37	69	140	119	5	370
Eligible publications (on title)[b]	37	5	34	22	5	103
Obtained publications	37	5	13	18	5	80
Duplicates (on title)			19	4		23
Not obtained	–	–	2	0	–	0
Total	37	5	34	22	5	103
Unique publications	37	5	13	17	3	77
Duplicates (on content)[c]	0	0	0	1	2	3
Total eligible	37	5	13	16	1	74
Eligible publications (on outcome)[d]	16	4	3	8	3	34
Ineligible publications (on outcome)	21	1	10	9	0	43
Eligible publications (on results)[e]	5	4	0	2	3	14
Ineligible publications (on results)	11	0	3	6	0	20
Total eligible meta-analyses[f]	13	8	0	2	9	32
Excluded due to overlap with other chapters[g]						6
Excluded due to effect size measure[h]						3
Total meta-analyses used						23

[a] Includes papers already held
[b] Review potentially relevant from reading the title and abstract
[c] The content of the review duplicates the content of a previous review
[d] Review includes a crime or criminal behavior outcome variable
[e] The results comprise a meta-analysis and include a weighted mean effect size for the outcome variable
[f] A meta-analysis is defined here as a statistical analysis of two or more evaluations of a non-duplicated drug intervention which includes a weighted mean effect size relating to a crime outcome measure
[g] The original search included systematic reviews on policing and drug courts which were excluded on the grounds that they were included in other chapters
[h] Three analyses used risk ratios as an effect size measure. The current analysis is based only on meta-analyses which used odds ratios or could be converted to odds ratios from the information provided

Quantitative Findings: Mean Effect Sizes

Each of the reviews included meta-analyses of the results of the individual evaluations and included a standardized mean effect size across all evaluations. The most common effect size measures were odd ratios (ORs) and only these studies, plus those whose effect sizes could be converted to an OR, are included in the following

Table 8.2 Study details of systematic reviews included in the review

Researcher, date	Intervention	Comparison group	Outcome	Design	Searches
Egli et al. (2009)	Heroin maintenance	Methadone or standard treatment	Criminal involvement	Systematic review RCT, QED, One group before and after studies	Abstracts, bibliographies, and databases
Egli et al. (2009)	Buprenorphine substitution treatment	MMT or placebo only	Criminal involvement	Systematic review RCT, QED, One group before and after studies	Abstracts, bibliographies, and databases
Egli et al. (2009)	Methadone maintenance treatment	No substitution treatment	Criminal involvement	RCT, QED, One group before and after studies	Abstracts, bibliographies, and databases
Egli et al. (2009)	Naltrexone treatment	Counseling or behavior therapy	Criminal involvement	Systematic review RCT, QED, One group before and after studies	Abstracts, bibliographies, and databases
Hesse et al. (2011)	Case Management	Other treatment	Re-incarceration and Criminal behavior	Systematic review RCT	Abstracts, bibliographies, and databases
Holloway et al. (2008)	Heroin prescribing	Other treatment	Recidivism	Systematic review RCT, QED	Databases, citations, and key researchers
Holloway et al. (2008)	Therapeutic community	Other treatment	Recidivism	Systematic review RCT, QED	Databases, citations, and key researchers
Holloway et al. (2008)	Supervision	Other treatment	Recidivism	Systematic review RCT, QED	Databases, citations, and key researchers
Holloway et al. (2008)	Methadone	Other treatment	Recidivism	Systematic review RCT, QED	Databases, citations, and key researchers
Holloway et al. (2008)	Drug testing	Other treatment	Recidivism	Systematic review RCT, QED	Databases, citations, and key researchers
Holloway et al. (2008)	Other drug-related crime interventions	Other treatment	Recidivism	Systematic review RCT, QED	Databases, citations, and key researchers
Holloway & Bennett. (2010)	Psycho-social interventions	Other treatment	Recidivism	Systematic review RCT, QED	Databases
Holloway & Bennett. (2010)	Reintegration drug treatment programs	Other treatment	Recidivism	Systematic review RCT, QED	Databases

8 Drug Interventions

Table 8.2 (continued)

Researcher, date	Intervention	Comparison group	Outcome	Design	Searches
Kirchmayer et al. (2002)	Naltrexone plus behavior therapy	Behavior therapy alone	Re-incarceration	Systematic review RCT, CCT	Databases, Cochrane trial register, periodicals, pharmaceutical producers, authors in the field, and reference lists.
Mattick et al. (2009)	Methadone maintenance therapy	No opioid replacement therapy	Criminal activity	Systematic review RCT, CCT	Databases, ongoing trials, conference proceedings, library catalogs, national organizations, and reference lists
Mitchell et al. (2006)	Therapeutic community	No treatment or minimal treatment	Recidivism	Systematic review RCT, QED	Databases, internet searches, reviews, and journals
Mitchell et al. (2006)	Narcotic maintenance	No treatment or minimal treatment	Recidivism	Systematic review RCT, QED	Databases, internet searches, reviews, and journals
Mitchell et al. (2006)	Boot camp	No treatment or minimal treatment	Recidivism	Systematic review RCT, QED	Databases, internet searches, reviews, and journals
Mitchell et al. (2006)	Counseling	No treatment or minimal treatment	Recidivism	Systematic review RCT, QED	Databases, internet searches, reviews, and journals
Perry et al. (2008)	Pre-trial release and drugs testing and sanctions	Routine pre-trial release	Arrest at 90 days	Systematic review RCT, QED, Controlled observation studies	Databases, reference lists, and consulting experts
Perry et al. (2008)	Therapeutic community and aftercare	Mental health program/waiting-list control	Incarceration at 1 year	Systematic review RCT, QED, Controlled observation studies	Databases, reference lists, and consulting experts
Perry et al. (2008)	Intensive supervision	Routine parole/probation	Recidivism at 1 year	Systematic review RCT, QED, Controlled observation studies	Databases, reference lists, and consulting experts
Perry et al. (2008)	Intensive supervision and increased surveillance	Other supervision	Recidivism at 1 year	Systematic review RCT, QED, Controlled observation studies	Databases, reference lists, and consulting experts

Table sorted in the alphabetical order of the first named author
RCT randomized controlled trial; *QED* quasi-experimental design; *CCT* Ccinical controlled trial

Table 8.3 Study results of systematic reviews included in the review

Researcher, date	Time period	Participants	number of studies	OR, statistical significance (p)	Moderators
Egli et al. (2009)	1968–2008	Drug addicts, adults and adolescents, males and females.	5	2.44, 0.007	Treatment type
Egli et al. (2009)	1968–2008	Drug addicts, adults and adolescents, males and females	3	2.78, 0.1	Treatment type
Egli et al. (2009)	1968–2008	Drug addicts, adults and adolescents, males and females	10	1.40, 0.12	Treatment type
Egli et al. (2009)	1968–2008	Drug addicts, adults and adolescents, males and females	2	3.21, 0.02	Treatment type
Hesse et al. (2011)	1993–2007	Drug misusers, people with mental disorders	15	1.09, ns	Model of care, treatment type, mental illness
Holloway et al. (2008)	1980–2008	Drug misusers, voluntary and criminal justice, males, females, juveniles, adults	2	1.12, ns	Treatment type, comparison type, referral type
Holloway et al. (2008)	1980–2008	Drug misusers, voluntary and criminal justice, males, females, juveniles, adults	10	2.06, sig.	Treatment type, comparison type, referral type
Holloway et al. (2008)	1980–2008	Drug misusers, voluntary and criminal justice, males, females, juveniles, adults	5	1.89, sig.	Treatment type, comparison type, referral type
Holloway et al. (2008)	1980–2008	Drug misusers, voluntary and criminal justice, males, females, juveniles, adults	9	1.14, ns	Treatment type, comparison type, referral type
Holloway et al. (2008)	1980–2008	Drug misusers, voluntary and criminal justice, males, females, juveniles, adults	6	0.85, ns	Treatment type, comparison type, referral type
Holloway et al. (2008)	1980–2008	Drug misusers, voluntary and criminal justice, males, females, juveniles, adults	3	0.84, ns	Treatment type, comparison type, referral type
Holloway & Bennett (2010)	1995–2010	Drug misusers, drug-misusing offenders, males, females, juveniles, adults	3	1.05, ns	Treatment type, intensity of intervention, length of intervention
Holloway & Bennett (2010)	1995–2010	Drug misusers, drug-misusing offenders, males, females, juveniles, adults	8	1.14, ns	Treatment type, intensity of intervention, length of intervention

Table 8.3 (continued)

Researcher, date	Time period	Participants	number of studies	OR, statistical significance (p)	Moderators
Kirchmayer et al. (2002)	1973–2002	In- and outpatients dependent on heroin	2	0.30, sig	Treatment type.
Mattick et al. (2009)	earliest-2008	Heroin dependent, males, females, juveniles, adults	3	0.39, 0.11	None
Mitchell et al. (2006)	1999–2004	Incarcerated substance misusers	30	1.38, 0.05	Treatment type, method of analysis
Mitchell et al. (2006)	1999–2004	Incarcerated substance misusers	5	0.84, ns	Treatment type, method of analysis
Mitchell et al. (2006)	1999–2004	Incarcerated substance misusers	2	1.10, ns	Treatment type, method of analysis
Mitchell et al. (2006)	1999–2004	Incarcerated substance misusers	25	1.50, <0.05	Treatment type, method of analysis
Perry et al. (2008)	1980–2008	Drug-using offenders	2	1.33, 0.02	Treatment type
Perry et al. (2008)	1980–2008	Drug-using offenders	2	0.37, 0.02	Treatment type
Perry et al. (2008)	1980–2008	Drug-using offenders	4	1.98, 0.05	Treatment type
Perry et al. (2008)	1980–2008	Drug-using offenders	3	2.09, 0.1	Treatment type

Table sorted in the alphabetical order of the first named author

OR odds ratio, *p*=*p* value. Where possible *p* values have been provided. When *p* values were not provided in the reviews the direction of the finding has been reported (i.e., *sig* significant, *ns* not significant)

analyses. The combined weighted mean effect sizes for all reviews (as calculated by the authors of the review) are shown in Table 8.4.

The table provides information on the 23 meta-analyses included in the current review. Six of the 23 analyses showed an overall significant and favorable effect of the experimental drug interventions on crime compared with the control (E>C). Fifteen of the analyses found no significant difference in the outcomes of the experimental drug intervention compared with the control with respect to crime. Two of the 23 analyses found an overall significant unfavorable effect of the experimental drug intervention on crime compared with the control (C>E).

The weighted mean ORs for the 23 analyses are shown in Fig. 8.1 as a forest plot, along with their confidence intervals. Overall, the results for all meta-analyses combined showed that the mean effect sizes of the majority of analyses ($n=17$) were on the favorable side of the "no effect" line and 6 were on the unfavorable side. However, only 6 of the 17 favorable results were statistically significant. Furthermore, those that were statistically significant were only just significant with small to medium effect sizes. The results are promising, but not overwhelming.

There are several possible explanations for these variations. Outcomes might be associated with features of the evaluation design and the quality of methods used. It is also possible that the results might vary by the characteristics of the clients entering the program or targeted by the intervention, or that the outcomes are correlated with the type of intervention included in the study. It is much more difficult to control the influence of extraneous factors when dealing with systematic reviews compared with evaluations because access to the original data is limited. However, it is possible to investigate differences in outcome by type of intervention as the type of intervention varied by systematic review.

The 23 meta-analyses were coded into intervention types, and the results of systematic reviews studying these types were analyzed. The coding identified five main types of intervention: supervision and surveillance, substitute prescribing, naltrexone treatment, therapeutic communities (TCs) and other psycho-social interventions, and reintegration and recovery programs. The results of the outcomes of reviews falling into these five categories are shown in Table 8.5.

There were notable differences in outcome effectiveness across the five types of interventions. The most consistently successful interventions were naltrexone treatment which was found to reduce criminal behavior significantly in both (100%) of the meta-analyses that investigated this method. Two-thirds (66%) of meta-analyses of TCs and other psycho-social interventions reported a favorable impact on crime. This increased to 100% among reviews of TCs.

The least successful interventions are defined as those that had less than 50% support from the meta-analyses. Reintegration and recovery programs resulted in none of the two (0%) meta-analyses showing a favorable crime outcome. Supervision and surveillance resulted in significant reductions in crime in just one of six (17%) analyses. Substitute prescribing was found to be effective in reducing criminal behavior in one of seven (14%) meta-analyses.

Overall, controlling for treatment type revealed substantial variations in treatment effectiveness. These differences in outcomes were also visible among ostensibly

Table 8.4 Weighted mean ORs for each review and crime outcome

	Authors (year)	Intervention	OR	CI low/ CI high	p	Effect in reducing crime
1	Egli et al. (2009)	Naltrexone treatment	3.21	1.23/8.31	0.02	E > C
2	Egli et al. (2009)	Buprenorphine substitution treatment	2.78	0.81/9.53	ns	No difference
3	Egli et al. (2009)	Heroin maintenance	2.44	1.27/4.69	0.007	E > C
4	Perry et al. (2008)	Intensive supervision and increased surveillance	2.09	0.86/5.07	ns	No difference
5	Holloway et al. (2008)	Therapeutic community	2.06	1.73/2.45	sig.	E > C
6	Perry et al. (2008)	Intensive supervision	1.98	1.01/3.87	0.05	C > E
7	Holloway et al. (2008)	Supervision	1.89	1.34/2.69	sig.	E > C
8	Mitchell et al. (2006)	Counseling	1.50	1.25/1.79	<0.05	E > C
9	Egli et al. (2009)	Methadone maintenance treatment	1.40	0.91/2.16	ns	No difference
10	Mitchell et al. (2006)	Therapeutic community	1.38	1.17/1.62	<0.05	E > C
11	Perry et al. (2008)	Pre-trial release and drugs testing and sanctions	1.33	1.04/1.7	0.02	C > E
12	Holloway et al. (2008)	Methadone	1.14	0.92/1.42	ns	No difference
13	Holloway & Bennett (2010)	Reintegration drug treatment programs	1.14	0.91/1.49	ns	No difference
14	Holloway et al. (2008)	Heroin prescribing	1.12	0.66/1.89	ns	No difference
15	Mitchell et al. (2006)	Boot camp	1.10	0.61/1.97	ns	No difference
16	Hesse et al. (2011)	Case management	1.09	not recorded	ns	No difference
17	Holloway & Bennett (2010)	Psycho-social interventions	1.05	0.73/1.51	ns	No difference
18	Holloway et al. (2008)	Drug testing	0.85	0.68/1.06	ns	No difference
19	Mitchell et al. (2006)	Narcotic maintenance	0.84	0.54/1.3	ns	No difference
20	Holloway et al. (2008)	Other drug-related crime interventions	0.84	0.58/1.2	ns	No difference
21	Mattick et al. (2009)	Methadone maintenance therapy	0.39	0.12/1.25	ns	No difference
22	Perry et al. (2008)	Therapeutic community and aftercare	0.37	0.16/0.87	ns	No difference
23	Kirchmayer et al. (2002)	Naltrexone plus behavior therapy	0.30	0.12/0.76	ns	No difference

Table sorted by OR (highest to lowest)

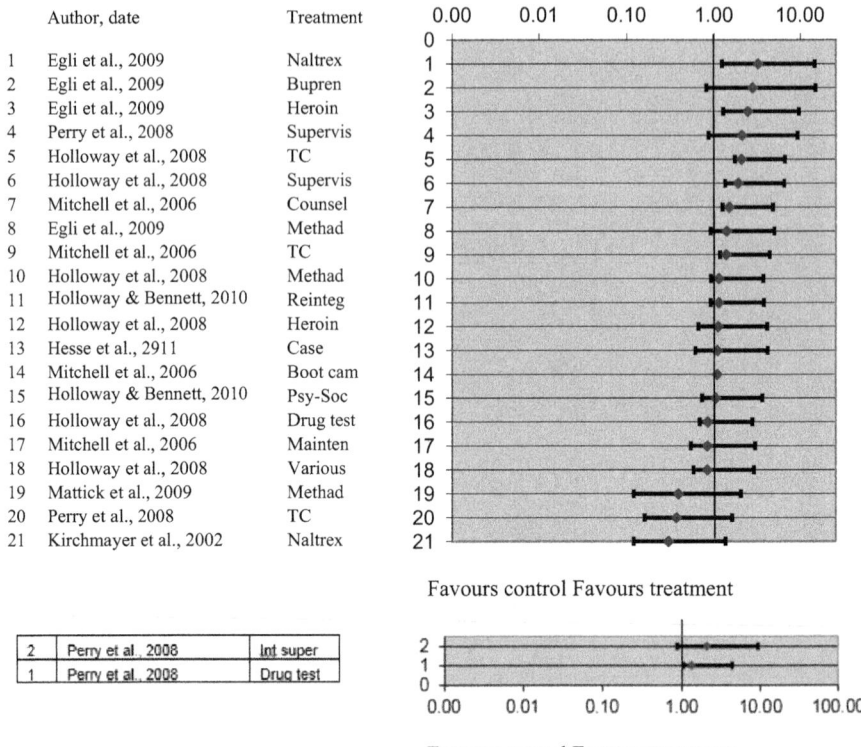

Fig. 8.1 Forest plot of weighted mean ORs by review. (Figure sorted by OR (highest to lowest))

similar interventions. Substitute prescribing and naltrexone treatment are both forms of drug treatment: the former an opioid agonist and the latter an opioid antagonist. In terms of effectiveness, substitute prescribing had the lowest percentage of favorable results compared with naltrexone which had the highest percentage. A similar comparison can be made in relation to the remaining three treatment types, which all fall under the heading of social/psychological approaches. These programs include TCs, which were found to be effective in two-thirds of meta-analyses, whereas supervision and surveillance, and recovery programs were found to be effective in 20% or fewer. It would appear that the factors impacting effectiveness in reducing crime are finer than simply the broad treatment type. It is likely that differences in the quality of staff, the readiness to change in the client population, the intensity of the program, and the duration of the program are all likely to be significant factors in determining outcome. Unfortunately, this kind of detail was not systematically collected or presented in the system reviews investigated. However, some insight into these variations can be identified from the qualitative descriptions of examples of programs investigated.

Table 8.5 Weighted mean effect sizes by type of intervention

Naltrexone treatment [4 evaluations]				
Egli et al. 2009	Naltrexone treatment (2)	OR=3.21	E>C	2 of 2 E>C
Kirchmayer et al. 2002	Naltrexone & behavoir therapy (2)	OR=0.30	E>C	
Reintegration and recovery programs [11 evaluations]				
Holloway and Bennett 2010	Reintegration programs (8)	OR=1.14	No difference	0 of 2 E>C
Holloway et al. 2008	Other drug interventions (3)	OR=0.84	No difference	
Supervision and surveillance [35 evaluations]				
Perry et al. 2008	Supervision and surveillance (3)	OR=2.09	No difference	1 of 6 E>C
Perry et al. 2008	Intensive supervision (4)	OR=1.98	C>E	
Holloway et al. 2008	Supervision (5)	OR=1.89	E>C	
Perry et al. 2008	Pre-trial release and drugs testing (2)	OR=1.33	C>E	
Holloway et al. 2008	Drug testing (6)	OR=0.85	No difference	
Hesse et al. 2011	Case management (15)	OR=1.09	No difference	
Substitute prescribing [37 evaluations]				
Egli et al. 2009	Buprenorphine substitution (3)	OR=2.78	No difference	1 of 7 E>C
Egli et al. 2009	Heroin maintenance (5)	OR=2.44	E>C	
Egli et al. 2009	Methadone maintenance (10)	OR=1.40	No difference	
Holloway et al. 2008	Methadone maintenance (9)	OR=1.14	No difference	
Holloway et al. 2008	Heroin treatment (2)	OR=1.12	No difference	
Mitchell et al. 2006	Narcotic maintenance (5)	OR=0.84	No difference	
Mattick et al. 2009	Methadone maintenance (3)	OR=0.39	No difference	
Therapeutic communities and other psycho-social interventions [72 evaluations]				
Holloway et al. 2008	Therapeutic community (10)	OR=2.06	E>C	4 of 6 E>C
Mitchell et al. 2006	Therapeutic community (30)	OR=1.38	E>C	
Perry et al. 2008	Therapeutic community (2)	OR=0.37	E>C	
Mitchell et al. 2006	Boot camp (2)	OR=1.10	No difference	
Holloway and Bennett 2010	Psycho-social interventions (3)	OR=1.05	No difference	
Mitchell et al. 2012	Counseling (25)	OR=1.50	E>C	

Table sorted by treatment type in the alphabetical order followed by OR (highest to lowest)
Figures in parentheses = total number of evaluations included per review. Figures in square brackets = total number of evaluations included in the group of reviews

Qualitative Findings: Description of Studies and Findings

In order to give greater insight into the nature of the interventions investigated and the outcome results obtained, some of the studies and findings are described in more detail below.

Supervision and surveillance. Six meta-analyses examined the effectiveness of supervision and surveillance programs in reducing criminal behavior. These were based on 3, 4, 5, 2, 6, and 15 evaluations, respectively (see Table 8.5). Supervision includes a range of interventions such as drug testing, monitoring, and surveillance. Drug testing can take place in all stages of the criminal justice system, including on arrest, in prison, on probation, and on parole. It is most commonly performed by urinalysis, although other methods are available, including the blood, hair, and saliva. The six analyses produced generally unfavorable results. Perry, Coulton, Glanville, Godfrey, Lunn, & McDougall, et al. (2008) noted that "Limited conclusions can be drawn about the effectiveness of drug treatment programs for drug-using offenders in the courts or the community. This is partly due to the range of studies and the heterogeneity of the different outcome measures used" (p. 2).

Substitute prescribing. Seven meta-analyses examined the effectiveness of substitute prescribing in reducing criminal behavior. These synthesized from 2 to 10 evaluation studies each. Substitute prescribing programs involve the prescription of synthetic opioid medication to heroin users. The main aim is to reduce the harms associated with heroin dependence (e.g., risks of overdose, spread of blood-borne viruses, and offending behavior) and to provide users with an opportunity to stabilize their drug intake while reducing the pain of heroin withdrawal. The drug most commonly prescribed as a substitute for heroin is methadone. Other substitutes include buprenorphine (also known as Subutex) and pharmaceutical heroin. The single positive findings in this section related to the prescription of pharmaceutical heroin. Egli, Pina, Christensen, Aebi, & Killias (2009) concluded that "Heroin maintenance has been found to significantly reduce criminal involvement among treated subjects, and it is more effective in crime reduction than methadone maintenance." (p. 6)

Naltrexone treatment. Two meta-analyses examined the effectiveness of naltrexone treatment, both based on the analysis of two evaluations. While the two evaluations were the same across the two reviews, each of the four meta-analyses used a different combination of intervention type (e.g., naltrexone alone or with a psycho-social intervention) or a different outcome measure (e.g., re-incarceration or any offence). Naltrexone is a synthetic opioid antagonist, which blocks the effects of opioids and takes away the euphoric effects experienced by heroin users (Adi, Juarez-Garcia, Wang, Jowett, Frew, Day, & Bayliss, et al., 2007). Both meta-analyses found that naltrexone, either alone or in combination with psycho-social treatment, was effective in reducing crime. Kirchmayer, Davoli, Verster, Amato, Ferri, & Perucci, (2002) concluded that the use of naltrexone in addition to behavioral treatment, "significantly reduced the probability of (re)-incarceration ..." (p. 1243). Similarly, Egli et al. (2009) concluded that naltrexone had "a significant and beneficial effect on criminal behavior ..." (p. 24).

Therapeutic communities and other psycho-social interventions. Six meta-analyses examined the effectiveness of TCs and other psycho-social interventions; the number of evaluations included in the analyses ranged from 2 to 30. Therapeutic communities are drug-free residential settings in which participants work together to overcome their drug dependence in a process of mutual self-help. Boot camps are similar to TCs in that they involve participants living and working in a residential setting with peers and staff members. However, boot camps are modeled on structured, military training and involve participants completing rigorous exercise programs, learning military drills, and wearing uniforms. Boot camps also involve considerable confrontation, which, unlike most TCs, is often between staff and participants (Mitchell, Wilson, & MacKenzie, 2006, p. 5).

Psycho-social interventions target the psychological and social factors that influence drug dependence. They include cognitive behavioral therapy, coping skills training, relapse prevention, contingency management, counseling, and motivational interviewing. The three meta-analyses that examined the effectiveness of TCs all produced positive results. They were also based on two of the three highest numbers of evaluations (30 and 10). Conversely, two of the three reviews of the remaining psycho-social interventions, which showed no intervention effect in comparison with the control, were based on the smallest number of evaluations (two and three, respectively).

Reintegration and recovery programs. Two meta-analyses examined the effectiveness of reintegration and recovery programs on offending behavior. These were based on eight and three studies respectively. Reintegration and recovery programs aim to help participants reenter society, often after a period of imprisonment or treatment. Such programs tend to run alongside more traditional drug treatment interventions and are usually delivered when the user has already made some progress in recovering from their drug problems. Reintegration and recovery programs include case management, which aims to link participants to appropriate services in the community, mentoring programs, and interventions designed to help participants enter education, training, or employment. None of the analyses found a difference between the experimental and comparison groups in terms of reduction in offending.

Conclusions

The findings of the review of systematic reviews were divided into two groups. The first was an analysis of all interventions combined, which aimed to determine whether drug interventions reduce criminal behavior. The results of this analysis were divided. Over half of the pooled results were associated with reductions in crime-related outcomes. However, less than half were associated with significant reductions. In other words, the results show an overall tendency toward favorable outcomes, but these were not always significant.

The second group broke down the meta-analyses by intervention type. These results were much clearer and demonstrated that intervention type was an important component of outcome variation. The analyses also showed that some interventions (such as naltrexone treatment and psycho-social interventions) were commonly associated with reductions in crime, while other interventions (such as reintegration programs, supervision, and substitute prescribing) were rarely associated with crime reduction effects.

As might be expected, there were no interventions that were always successful. This is likely to be because of variations due to differences in the nature of the program, the quality of implementation, and the characteristics and motivations of the clients. Nevertheless, there were some interventions which resulted in a higher proportion of successes and some a lower proportion. On these grounds, it is possible to draw some conclusions about the effectiveness on drug interventions in reducing criminal behavior.

The interventions most suitable to be included under the "What works?" category are "naltrexone treatment" and "therapeutic communities." In both the cases, there are clear mechanisms by which the intervention could be effective. Naltrexone makes it impossible for the users to experience the effects of their drug of misuse. The fact that this reduces criminal behavior provides support for the idea that drug misuse and crime are causally connected. Therapeutic communities provide social and psychological support during the period between abstinence and recovery.

The most suitable candidates for the "What's promising?" category would be those interventions that had small or medium ORs in a favorable direction, but failed to reach statistical significance. The only intervention that meets these criteria is buprenorphine substitution treatment. Reasons for buprenorphine being more effective than methadone have been discussed in the literature and include its longer-lasting effects and its convenience in allowing sublingual administration.

Under the heading of "No effect" are those interventions which produced a nonsignificant outcome. Apart from the case of buprenorphine treatment mentioned above, the category with the highest number of nonsignificant results was substitute prescribing (six of seven analyses were not significant). In addition, the category with the highest proportion of nonsignificant results was reintegration and recovery programs.

The category "What is harmful?" most appropriately applies to those interventions that resulted in a significant outcome in an unfavorable direction. In these cases, the comparison group was significantly more likely to have a favorable result than the experimental group. There were just two meta-analyses that produced this finding and both related to supervision and surveillance. It is difficult to estimate the mechanisms by which post-release supervision might be less productive than non-supervision. It is not wholly certain, therefore, whether this approach is actually harmful or whether other factors explain the relationship.

The final category that might be considered is "What's missing?" The total list of drug interventions is substantial and not all have been covered in the systematic reviews investigated. In terms of the major categories of interventions, no systematic reviews were found (that met our eligibility criteria) on prevention programs, such as school-based programs, further and higher education interventions, helplines, brief interventions, diversionary activities, and dissemination of substance misuse information. We excluded from the review enforcement interventions as these involved policing initiatives which are covered in other chapters in the book. Another major category of intervention not covered by the systematic reviews was harm reduction, such as needle-exchange and take-home naloxone. In short, systematic reviews to date have covered only a small part of drug interventions.

The results of the current systematic review of systematic reviews suggest that at least some drug interventions are effective in reducing criminal behavior. This finding is particularly striking in that drug interventions rarely have crime reduction as an aim. It is not wholly clear, therefore, how drug interventions reduce criminal behavior. It is unlikely that it is a direct effect of the intervention. It is more likely that the intervention first reduces drug misuse, which in turn reduces crime.

It could be argued that "What's missing?" is a better understanding of the role that drug interventions play, not only in reducing individual criminal behavior, but also in crime reduction more generally. Systematic reviews provide a good starting point for investigating this.

References

Adi, Y., Juarez-Garcia, A., Wang, D., Jowett, S., Frew, E., & Day, E., et al. (2007). Oral naltrexone as a treatment for relapse prevention in formerly opioid-dependent drug users: A systematic review and economic evaluation. *Health Technology Assessment, 11*(6), 1–55.

Amato L., Davoli M., Perucci, C.A., Ferri, M., Faggiano, F., & Mattick, R. P. (2005). An overview of systematic reviews of the effectiveness of opiate maintenance therapies: Available evidence to inform clinical practice and research. *Journal of Substance Abuse Treatments, 28,* 321–329.

Amato, L., Davoli, M., Vecchi, S., Ali, R., Farrell, M. & Faggiano, F.. et al. (2011). Cochrane systematic reviews in the field of addiction: What's there and what should be. *Drug and Alcohol Dependence, 113,* 96–103.

Bennett, T. H., & Holloway, K. (2005). *Understanding drugs, alcohol and crime.* Berkshire: Open University Press, McGraw-Hill Education.

Derry, C. J., Derry, S., McQuay, H. J., & Moore, R. A. (2006). Systematic review of systematic reviews of acupuncture published 1996–2005. *Clinical Medicine, 6*(4), 381–386.

Egli, N., Pina, M., Christensen, P. S., Aebi, M., & Killias, M. (2009). Effects of drug substitution programs on offending among drug addicts. *Campbell Systematic Reviews, 5*(3), 5–36.

Ernst, E. (2002). A systematic review of systematic reviews of homeopathy. *British Journal of Clinical Pharmacology, 54,* 577–582.

Ernst, E., & Canter, P. H. (2006). A systematic review of systematic reviews of spinal manipulation. *Journal of the Royal Society of Medicine, 99*(4), 192–196.

Hesse, M., Vanderplasschen, W., Rapp R., Broekaert, E., & Fridell, M. (2011) Case management for persons with substance use disorders. (Review). *The Cochrane Library, 10.*

Holloway, K., & Bennett, T. H. (2010). *A review of accredited substance misuse interventions.* Unpublished report commissioned by *the UK ministry of justice.* Pontypridd: University of Glamorgan.

Holloway, K., Bennett, T. H., & Farrington, D. P. (2008). *Effectiveness of treatment in reducing drug-related crime.* Sweden: Swedish National Council for Crime Prevention.

Hough, M. (1996). *Drugs misuse and the criminal justice system: A review of the literature.* London: Home Office.

Kirchmayer, U., Davoli, M., Verster, A. D., Amato, L., Ferri, M., & Perucci, C. A. (2002). A systematic review on the efficacy of naltrexone maintenance treatment in opioid dependence. *Addiction, 97,* 1241–1249.

Mattick, R. P., Breen, C., Kimber, J., & Davoli, M. (2009). Methadone maintenance therapy versus no opioid replacement therapy for opioid dependence (Review). *The Cochrane Library, 3,* 1.32.
Mitchell, O., Wilson, D. B., & MacKenzie, D. L. (2006). The effectiveness of incarceration-based drug treatment on criminal behavior. *Campbell Systematic Reviews, 2006*(11), 4–56.
Mitchell, O., Wilson, D. B., & MacKenzie, D. L. (2012). The effectiveness of incarceration-based drug treatment on criminal behavior. *Campbell Systematic Reviews, 2012*(18), 5–75.
Perry, A., Coulton, S., Glanville, J., Godfrey, C., Lunn, J., & McDougall, C.., et al. (2008). Interventions for Drug-Using Offenders in the Courts, Secure Establishments and the Community. (Review). *The Cochrane Library, 3.*

Chapter 9
Qualitative Data in Systematic Reviews

Mimi Ajzenstadt

An examination of systematic reviews conducted in disciplines such as public health, nursing, social work, and education indicates that recently, reviewers have started to use information generated in studies that were based on qualitative research, regarding it as able to provide valuable information, as well as enhancing decision-making processes (Sandelowski, Voils, & Barroso, 2007). An examination of the reviews published at the Campbell Crime & Justice Group website reveals, however, that almost all of these reviews excluded data gathered through qualitative studies (http://www.campbellcollaboration.org/reviews_crime_justice/index.php). A further analysis of the reviews on this website shows that of the 35 published reviews, 21 did not even refer to the possibility of using qualitative data, while six authors specifically declared that they did not use such data. Four authors acknowledged the important contributions that could be made to their reviews by the possible inclusion of qualitative data, but did not integrate this type of data into their current reviews (see, e.g., Murray, Farrington, Sekol, & Olsen, 2010). The authors of two other reviews included the results from qualitative studies within their literature reviews and discussions to support their theoretical frameworks and findings (Braga & Weisburd, 2012, p. 85; Mazerolle, Bennett, Davis, Sargeant, & Manning, 2013). Only two studies included qualitative works in their reviews. Van der Laan, Smit, Busschers, & Aarten (2011) assessed evidence on the effects of interventions aimed at preventing and suppressing trafficking in human beings. Their work also summarized results from qualitative studies that used questionnaires and interviews, and evaluated the attitudes of participants in various interventions. The authors concluded that these studies provided rich information about practices designed to contend with the phenomenon of international trafficking in human beings. However, since these works were noncontrolled studies, it is difficult to draw conclusions about actual outcomes and impacts (p. 19).

In their review of studies evaluating the outcomes of stress management, Patterson, Chung, and Swang (2012) integrated the interventions provided to

M. Ajzenstadt (✉)
Hebrew University of Jerusalem, Jerusalem, Israel
e-mail: mimi.ajzenstadt@mail.huji.ac.il

© Springer Science+Business Media New York 2016
D. Weisburd et al. (eds.), *What Works in Crime Prevention and Rehabilitation*,
Springer Series on Evidence-Based Crime Policy, DOI 10.1007/978-1-4939-3477-5_9

veteran police officers and recruits as well as data from focus groups and interviews. The qualitative data provided contextual information for the quantitative data that relates to the attitudes of participants in the intervention and their spouses (see discussion later). The authors concluded that the results of data obtained from qualitative studies "can add to the body of knowledge demonstrating the efficacy of stress management interventions for police officers and recruits, and help guide law enforcement organizations" (p. 26).

Such a research attitude, which judges as positive the inclusion of information generated in works utilizing qualitative research methods in systematic reviews, stems from two main sources: first, various scholars have recently challenged the polarization of quantitative and qualitative approaches to research, advocating their integration (see, e.g., Barbour & Barbour, 2003). In this vein, traditional systematic reviews have been criticized as being too narrow, and for ignoring the context within which evaluated interventions took place. Second, new theoretical insights in the study of policy design have been developed, focusing on the significance of such variables as opinions, perceptions, and cultural values, which cannot be measured by conventional statistical methods relative to the processes of policy formation and implementation (Béland, 2009; Stone, 1997). Studies have found that the examination of participants' characteristics and preferences influences the implementation of policies. In addition, the attitudes of participants in interventionist programs and the perceptions of practitioners administering treatments carry significant explanatory powers regarding the successes and failures of programs (Candy, King, Jones, & Oliver, 2011; Lipsky, 1980; Satterfield et al., 2009, p. 381). Thus, it is recognized that the decision-making process is complex, requiring reference to different types of evidence (Flemming, 2010). These developments have led scholars to incorporate information from diverse sources into the systematic review framework, to acquire a richer understanding of the evaluated phenomenon by embracing multiple ways of knowing (Dixon-Woods et al., 2006; Goldsmith, Bankhead, & Austoker, 2007).

Embracing this attitude, researchers in the areas of medicine, social work, education, and public health have set out to conduct systematic reviews, evaluating interventions from various angles (see, e.g., Hannes & Lockwood, 2012; The Joanna Briggs Institute (JBI) in Australia). Recognizing that the assembly of evidence from a variety of sources provides rich information that can inform policy and practice while assisting researchers to explore differences and similarities across settings, sample populations, and theoretical perspectives, scholars have modified traditional systematic review procedures to incorporate data generated by qualitative methods (Paterson, 2011; Weed, 2005).

Systematic reviews that examine evidence derived from a variety of sources carry with them important details that can significantly enlarge the knowledge base and contribute information to key questions within the perspective of "what works." The ability to reveal inner mechanisms of interventions by shedding light on the contextual variables in the examined policy can help researchers to understand how the examined program works. The integration of methods and data from various sources enables the researcher to address the complexity of the examined program by following the ways in which program attributes are experienced. In addition, qualitative research is essential in providing a fuller picture of areas that have not yet been examined.

In contrast to these methodological developments, the discipline of criminology remains almost static, hardly attempting to manage and analyze qualitative data in systematic reviews of effectiveness. The aim of this chapter is to try to bridge this gap by introducing some of the main issues in the arena of systematic review in order to encourage criminologists to participate in this new trend and give interpretive work a more central role within the criminological research sphere.

Bridging the Gap: Negotiating Evidence

The exclusion of data generated by studies using qualitative research methods originates in the different standpoints regarding the nature of data, its interpretation, and the position of the researcher in quantitative and qualitative research strategies. Each methodology is committed to different aims, has different ways of recording data, and has different expectations of what the study should reveal (Meekums & Daniel, 2011, p. 233).

The aim of systematic reviews, which use meta-analysis techniques, is to measure effect size of a range of studies, combining individual effect sizes of each separate study, giving greater power to the overall statistics. In general, quantitative studies are concerned with the measurement of change, addressing questions about the efficacy and cost-effectiveness of an examined policy or intervention (Satterfield et al., 2009, p. 378). These studies are regarded as providing the best objective and replicable quantitative evidence on the effectiveness of interventions. To furnish systematic reviews, detailed and explicit methods stemming from quantitative principles have been established to conduct a comprehensive search of the literature. In addition, quality appraisal procedures have been developed to identify and select relevant studies, and synthesis techniques have been created to extract and analyze data from original relevant works (Tricco et al. 2011, p. 11).

Qualitative research is a complex family of research methods—for example, case studies, interviews, observations, focus groups, ethnographies, documentary analyses, and life histories. While these research designs can generate quantitative data, the nature of the method, the questions the research aims to answer, and the way in which the data are collected differ from those used in quantitative methods. Moreover, the hallmark of qualitative research is that it emphasizes the significance of context and meaning. This type of research is concerned with understanding the ways in which people perceive their social worlds and with exploring the meanings of social phenomena as experienced by individuals in their natural contexts (Lincoln & Guba, 1985; Whyte, 1997). Its main aim is to find answers to questions such as how a specific intervention works or what the contextual dimensions of an examined intervention are.

At first sight, it seems that, due to the subjective nature of qualitative studies and their aims and work procedures, it is impossible to integrate qualitative methods within the rigid framework of systematic reviews. While there are many similarities between the quantitative and qualitative research strategies, most research procedures are very different, due to the special nature of and the assumptions underlying each method, the questions to be answered, the influence of the investigator on the study, the principles and consequences of sampling, as well as the process of interpretation during analysis. Moreover, the aggregation of data from multiple sites is unfamiliar to the anthropological discipline that stands at the core of qualitative research methods (Reis, Hermoni, Van-Raalte, Dahan, & Borkan, 2007, p. 215). In addition, scholars are concerned with the ability to integrate variations of methods and theoretical assumptions (Petticrew, 2001).

In terms of systematic review, the research question directing the synthesis can be created and tailored to address the data that have been generated during the data accumulation process. The question can be refined during the review process, while in a systematic review using a quantitative method the review question is set a priori. Similarly, since data interpretation in qualitative research depends on positions and perspectives, different researchers might develop different, although equally valid, representations of the examined situation. In qualitative research, these different ways of approaching the same subject contribute to an increased understanding of complex phenomena and not to a failure of reliability. This stands in sharp contrast to the research procedures of quantitative works that emphasize objective and replicable evidence. Indeed, Saini and Shlonsky (2012) explain: "qualitative approaches have traditionally been excluded from systematic reviews due in part to challenges confronting researches when they attempt to synthesize studies with diverse range of methodologies and epistemologies employed in the qualitative research field" (p. 9).

However, the new approach to systematic review challenges this perspective by criticizing the categorical exclusion of data generated by studies that use qualitative research methods. Both research perspectives share the belief that evidence is "derived from the systematic collection of data through observation and experimentation and the formulation of questions and testing of hypotheses" (Satterfield et al., 2009, p. 383). Both methods involve the systematic collection, organization, and interpretation of material derived from systematic research: thus they should be merged in a valid way, maintaining their own uniqueness and quality. Rather than considering quantitative and qualitative research strategies as incompatible, we should see them as complementary, contributing to the enhancement of knowledge regarding the examined phenomena (Malterud, 2001).

Data generated from studies utilizing qualitative methods can contribute to the improvement of knowledge in new areas (Weed, 2005). Indeed, researchers use systematic reviews based on qualitative methods to assess the nature and extent of knowledge—especially in areas that are understudied. This type of systematic review can also contribute to a broader understanding of the process and dynamics of the phenomenon under investigation, further contributing to theory-building (Schreiber, Crooks, & Stern, 1997). Findings from studies utilizing qualitative research design can generate a comprehensive understanding of a phenomenon, adding depth and breadth to systematic reviews of effectiveness by focusing on participants' views on the intervention (Atkins et al., 2008). Finally, qualitative research sheds light on the complexity of the examined phenomenon and facilitates the generation of new evidence relevant for practice and policy (see Discussion in Saini & Shlonsky, 2012).

I would now like to highlight a few specific issues discussed in works that use qualitative information in areas related to criminology, to illuminate the obstacles that might occur, and to suggest ways in which they might be overcome.

Inside the Box: An Examination of Systematic Reviews, Based on Qualitative Methods

To further examine systematic reviews using data generated by qualitative techniques and their relevance to criminology, a review of the literature was carried out, to identify studies using systematic reviews of topics related to crime, criminals, and the response to criminality, with information from qualitative research methods. Relevant studies were identified by conducting a general search in the following electronic databases: Criminal Justice Abstracts; Google Scholar; LexisNexis Academic; Medline; PsycNET; PsychInfo; Social Services Abstracts; Sociological Abstracts. The following keywords were used: (systematic review *OR metaanalys*) AND (qualitative*) AND (abuse* OR abuser* OR crime* OR criminal* OR offense* OR offender* OR *delinq*). Using this method, a total of 6541 studies were identified. At the next stage, 2396 reviews were eliminated because they presented literature reviews. Two researchers screened the remaining titles and the abstracts when titles were identified as relevant, excluding topics irrelevant to criminology or discussions about the use of qualitative methods in systematic reviews, leaving 146 works that appeared to be eligible for the review. They were retrieved as full-text articles for further inspection. At the final stage, there remained 12 works that conducted a systematic review or a synthesis of original studies evaluating a complete or partial intervention program relevant to criminologists. In addition, three articles that applied systematic review techniques to gain comprehensive knowledge of a new and understudied phenomenon were included (Douglas et al., 2008; Maher & Hudson, 2007; Rizo & Macy, 2011). These articles included a thorough description of the systematic procedures employed in an area central to the criminological enterprise and so for the purposes of this chapter were eligible for inclusion. I will now turn to a detailed examination of the reviewed articles, focusing on the systematic review process.

Characteristics of Reviewed Articles

Five articles reported on studies that conducted systematic research using data derived from both qualitative and quantitative research methods; nine articles reviewed original works that were based on qualitative research (see Table 9.1 for a description of the articles' characteristics). The inclusion of information from studies using qualitative techniques in the framework of a systematic review is a recent phenomenon: eight of the reviews were published in 2010–2011, five between 2006 and 2009, while the earliest one was published in 2001. The articles were published

Table 9.1 Details of included qualitative meta-analyses

Author/year	Topic	Aim	Participants	No. of studies	Methods of study	Main findings
Bair-Merritt et al. (2010)	Women's use of intimate partner violence	Identification of women's motivation for using intimate partner violence	Women in shelters, courts, and male and female participants in barterers' treatment programs, community members	23	Questionnaires with open-ended options, interviews, observations, documentary analysis of incident reports	Anger and not being able to get a partner's attention were the main motivations
Bilby et al. (2006)	Psychological interventions with sexual offenders	Measuring the effectiveness of interventions on sexual offenders	Programs' participants and programs' workers	21 quantitative works 4 qualitative works	Quantitative: quasi-experimental Qualitative: interviews	Contradictory findings about the effectiveness of treatment of sex offenders
Douglas et al. (2008)	Internet addiction	Studying the antecedent symptoms and negative effects of Internet addiction	Students, child pornography offenders, visitors of Internet cafes, therapists	10	Interviews, observations, case studies, surveys	Feelings of isolation, loneliness, low self-confidence and self-esteem are the main antecedents of Internet addiction
Feder et al. (2006)	The response of healthcare professionals to women exposed to intimate partner violence	Identification from health-care professionals of the experiences and expectations of women exposed to intimate partner violence from health-care professionals	Women with histories of intimate partner violence	25	Interviews, focus groups, participants' observations	Women's perceptions of appropriate responses depended on their readiness to address the issue and the relationships between the women and the heath-care professionals
Finfgeld-Connett and Johnson (2011a)	Substance abuse treatment for women who are under correctional supervision	Optimizing treatment effectiveness for substance abuse programs for women	Substance abuse program participants	5	Interviews, participant observation, focus groups	Gender-specific programs optimizing treatment

Table 9.1 (continued)

Author/year	Topic	Aim	Participants	No. of studies	Methods of study	Main findings
Finfgeld-Connett and Johnson (2011b)	Therapeutic substance abuse treatment for incarcerated women	Identification of attributes of optimal therapeutic strategies for treating incarcerated women who have a history of substance abuse	Current or former residents of prison and correctional facilities, treatment professionals	9	Focus groups, interviews, participant observation, telephone and mail exchanges	Trust-based relationships, individualized, just care and treatment in separate facilities enhance the effects of treatment programs
Flores and Pellicio (2011)	Women's experience of post-incarceration in the community	Identification of health and psychological needs women face upon release	Women formerly incarcerated in the USA	10	Interviews, focus groups	Women face major challenges when reentering the community. They also identified positive opportunities for personal growth
Kearney (2001)	Women's experience of domestic violence	Exploring women's responses to violent relationships	Women in shelters, justice centers, support groups, community services, and the community	13	Interviews, content analysis	Women normalized violent relationship while promoting idealized romance. This was linked to personal, sociopolitical, and cultural contexts
Maher and Hudson (2007)	Women in the drug economy	The nature of female participation in the drug economy	Women dealers, smugglers, women released from prison	15	Interviews, ethnographic observation	The drug economy is a gender-stratified labor market

Table 9.1 (continued)

Author/year	Topic	Aim	Participants	No. of studies	Methods of study	Main findings
Meekums and Daniel (2011)	Arts with offenders	The role of arts in therapeutic goals for offenders	Juvenile, male and female prisoners, and participants in treatment programs	4 quantitative studies 4 qualitative studies 1 mixed method	Quantitative: experimental design, surveys Qualitative: interviews, content analysis of participants' reports, ethnography	Arts and art therapies can have a positive, humanizing, and healing effect
Patterson et al. (2012)	Stress management interventions among police officers and recruits	Evaluating the effects of officer stress management interventions on stress outcomes	Police officers, spouses, and recruits	10 quantitative 2 mixed methods	Quantitative: experimental design, quasi-experimental design Qualitative: interviews, focus groups	Stress management interventions had no significant effect on psychological, behavioral, or physiological outcomes
Rizo and Macy (2011)	Help-seeking patterns of Hispanic partner violence survivors	Identify help-seeking behaviors and barriers	Hispanic intimate partner violence survivors; hospital patients; Hispanic community members, service providers, and nonabused community members	7 qualitative studies, 20 quantitative studies	Qualitative studies: interviews, focus groups, analysis of police reports Quantitative studies: analysis of national datasets, surveys, clinical record reviews, and analysis of calls to emergency centers	Limited language proficiency, Hispanic cultural tolerance of male violence, and fear of deportation prevent Hispanic women from seeking help for their partner violence abuse problem

9 Qualitative Data in Systematic Reviews

Table 9.1 (continued)

Author/year	Topic	Aim	Participants	No. of studies	Methods of study	Main findings
Robinson and Spilsbury (2008)	Responses of healthcare professionals to adult victims of domestic violence	Perceptions and experiences of accessing health services by adult victims of domestic violence	People from primary care services, domestic violence intervention services, health visiting services, mental health, and substance misuse services	10	Surveys, interviews, questionnaires, focus groups	Victims of domestic violence experience difficulties when accessing healthcare services
Sword et al. (2009)	Services addressing the needs of women with substance use issues and their children	Identification of the processes contributing to recovery of women using drugs	Women participating in addiction treatment programs	15	Interviews, focus groups	Programs need to focus on improving maternal health and social functioning in an environment characterized by empowerment, safety, and connections
Werb et al. (2011)	Drug law enforcement	The evaluation of the impact of drug law enforcement on drug market violence	Drug market participants	13 quantitative studies, 2 qualitative studies	Quantitative studies: linear regression, mathematical drug market models, Qualitative studies: interviews, observations, questionnaires	Increasing law enforcement is unlikely to reduce drug market violence. In some cases, it can increase it

mainly in public health and medical journals. It is not surprising that scholars of public health are in the forefront of research dealing with issues relating to the treatment of violence and abuse. During the past decade, the health promotion movement has begun to redefine crime and violence as health issues, thus bringing such areas as family violence, children-at-risk, and drug abuse within the sphere of public health (see, e.g., Kelly & Charlton, 1995; Parish, 1995). Qualitative methods frequently used interviews, participant observation, document analysis, and focus groups.

Research Aims and Questions

Many of the analyzed reviews based on quantitative analysis endorse research questions that assess available evidence of the effects of an intervention on a specific behavior or a specific group of people. Questions in systematic reviews using qualitative data and aiming to evaluate the various interventions span a wide panorama of aims and research questions, using a rich vocabulary of terms. These studies attempt to discover why a program or an intervention is successful in contrast to traditional systematic reviews that seek to assess whether the intervention works. Qualitative data are expected to provide information about participants' experiences and their perceptions, creating a focused observation on specific parts of the intervention that may contribute to its success or failure. These works try to develop a theory or build concepts, rather than test theories or concepts that have been predetermined.

Meekums and Daniel (2011) examined the role of art in therapeutic programs with offenders. Werb et al. (2011) sought to identify the impact of legal intervention—drug law enforcement on the drug market. Bilby, Brooks-Gordon, and Wells (2006) examined the success rates of psychological interventions in altering the behaviors or attitudes of adult sex offenders and abusers. Finfgeld-Connett and Johnson (2011b) set out to identify optimal therapeutic strategies for treating incarcerated women and to understand how prison-based substance abuse programs could be adapted to more effectively meet the needs of women prisoners. They also attempted to optimize substance abuse treatments for women in community settings (Finfgeld-Connett & Johnson, 2011a). The goal of the Finfgeld-Connett and Johnson study was to "more fully explicate therapeutic attributes of substance abuse treatment programs for non-incarcerated women who are referred for help through the criminal justice system" (2011a, p. 640). Feder, Hutson, Ramsay, and Taket (2006) systematically reviewed studies to identify participants' experiences of a program dealing with women exposed to intimate partner violence. Patterson et al. (2012), in their review of studies evaluating the outcomes of stress management, integrated the interventions provided to veteran police officers and recruits and data from focus groups and interviews. More specifically, they aimed to identify the attitudes of participants in the intervention as well as their spouses.

Finally, the systematic review approach aims to achieve a better understanding of current knowledge about a phenomenon that has previously not been studied sufficiently, by measuring it or learning about its symptoms and characteristics. Thus,

Douglas et al. (2008), aiming to identify the main symptoms of Internet addictions, explored the effects of this behavior on the abused and sought to identify coping strategies. Rizo and Macy (2011) explored help-seeking patterns of Hispanic survivors of partner violence, and Maher and Hudson (2007) described the nature of women's participation in the drug economy.

Criteria for Inclusion/Exclusion

Inclusion criteria utilized by authors of systematic reviews that applied qualitative methods can broadly be divided into two main groups: criteria relating to the study design and those relating to the intervention. In the first group, scrutinized articles had to meet the following requirements to be included in the review: reporting on systematic research, using qualitative design alone or with quantitative strategy, reporting on qualitative outcomes, or reporting on process evaluations of interventions, attempting to generate theories based on the study findings.

The second group referred to participants' characteristics and to the nature of the intervention. Among the criteria relating to participants' traits were age (young or adult), gender, and living in a specific geographical location. The programs' variables usually included requirements related to the program setting. For example, for treatment that had to be carried out in a criminal justice or mental health-care facility, participants had to be actively involved in the evaluated program, the program needed to have clear therapeutic goals, and there had to be verbal interaction between the researchers and the participants.

Exclusion criteria included articles that used randomized control trials, cohort studies, case-control studies, cross-sectional studies, and surveys. However, if the statistical settings included open-ended questions and had a qualitative component, they were potentially eligible for inclusion (see, e.g., Feder et al., 2006). Studies were excluded when the intervention was not the study's main focus. Many reviews excluded works that did not describe the analytical approach, or those utilizing non-theoretical descriptive techniques.

Quality Appraisal

The process of evaluating study quality in quantitative reviews is well established and aims to prevent the inclusion of poorly conducted work. In contrast, many different criteria for the assessment of qualitative studies have been proposed. The literature assessing the effectiveness of reviews based on qualitative studies that consider which criteria should be used for such assessments is quite varied (Blaxter, 1996; Goldsmith et al., 2007; Saini & Shlonsky, 2012).

For example, researchers are debating whether to apply criteria that are current in quantitative research, aiming for scientific rigor in qualitative studies. Lincoln and Guba (1985) advocate the assessment of qualitative works using the criteria of credibility, dependability, and transferability. Hamberg, Johansson, Lindgren, and Westman (1994) go on to claim that these criteria correspond to traditional ones, and thus they compare credibility with internal validity, conformability with objectivity, and transferability with generalizability. Mays and Pope (1995) encourage researchers to adopt a different set of criteria: the principles of triangulation and respondent validation; clear detailing of methods of data collection and analysis, reflexivity, and attention to negative cases. They further claim that relevance can be increased by the use of detailed reports and clear sampling techniques.

Others look for an open, transparent research procedure while examining the integrity and trustworthiness of the studies used for the systematic review. Researchers assess whether the studies present "thick" or "thin" descriptions of the program components, their mechanisms, and the study procedures (see discussion in Satterfield et al., 2009 about thick description in qualitative research). Thick description (the concept comes out of an anthropological tradition beginning with Geertz, 1973) provides a framework for reviewing whether enough information has been provided to judge how data accumulation and analysis was carried out. Such descriptions allow the reviewer to examine whether there were factors that might have affected program implementation and the reasons given for success or failure. It enables the reader to follow the process of analysis and the development of analytical categories, and to determine how rigorous or systematic the work has been (see discussion in Barbour & Barbour, 2003). Thin descriptions do not provide such details, nor do they describe the program's components and method of implementation, or engage in discussions about reasons for success or failure.

Scholars usually require that the reviewed studies include the following: an adequate description of the study aim and focus; a clear description of the sample, the size and characteristics of the sample, and explanations of how sampling and recruitment were conducted; an adequate description of the context/setting of the research; a clear description of the data analysis method and process, a description of how, and by whom, the analysis was conducted; a clear discussion of the research findings. Scholars require that original studies present sufficient original data to support the findings and demonstrate that these and the conclusions are grounded in the data (Attree, 2004). Rizo and Macy (2011) extended the criteria list to include at least one of the following strategies: the use of multiple coders; member checking (verification of findings with research participants); data triangulation (examination of the consistency of findings across different data collection sources); negative case analysis (intentionally searching the data for contradictory findings); and audit trail (leaving detailed records of coding and analysis decisions to allow for replication) (p. 254).

Some scholars use a list developed to assist in the assessment of the credibility and relevance of qualitative works: the Critical Appraisal Skills Program (CASP). The CASP contains ten questions, each with a number of subquestions to ensure consistency in reviewing and reporting results.

Clinical works set out additional requirements relating to the nature of the intervention, such as the quality of materials used to train the therapists, the quality of the materials that the therapists use, the quality of therapist training, and the quality of the intervention/therapy delivery (Bilby et al., 2006, p. 471). It is important to note that some scholars argue that using a checklist to evaluate quality contradicts the spirit of qualitative research as it adopts a technical reductionist perspective, thus ignoring the wealth of options available in this approach (Barbour, 2001). To increase the quality of the synthesis, some authors compare their findings with results from other individual studies. Thus Kearney (2001), for example, compared her findings regarding the responses of women abused by their partners to individual studies that examined the same phenomenon in other places.

Sampling

Discussions regarding quality-oriented analysis have usually entailed consideration of the sampling strategies employed by the original studies. Owing to the differences between qualitative and quantitative techniques, sampling strategies used by the researchers of both approaches result in differing evaluations of the sampling procedures. While researchers in quantitative studies are concerned with representation and empirical generalization, qualitative researchers look for information that reflects diversity within the groups or phenomena under investigation (Kuzel, 1992; Mays & Pope, 1995). Moreover, qualitative works aim to gain a comprehensive understanding of the phenomena from a variety of perspectives. Owing to these principles of research, validation by consensus or repeatability through the use of random sampling is seldom applicable in qualitative research (Malterud, 2001).

Many qualitative works use purposeful or theoretical sampling. This sampling procedure is based on the researcher's theory about what would constitute important characteristics in relation to the study question. While some data are collected prior to the analysis process, theorizing is "part of the qualitative research endeavor, even as data are generated and subjected to ongoing analysis, which may uncover unanticipated patterns related to the expression of particular perspectives or production of accounts/explanations by respondents" (Barbour & Barbour, 2003, pp. 180–181). In the qualitative research tradition, sampling partakes of the logic of the stepwise regression process associated with quantitative analysis: the researcher may include additional information from new sources as the research procedure develops, depending on what extra material is needed to answer the research question effectively. The aim of such a sampling method is to increase the breadth and depth of the findings, and to refine ideas (Charmaz, 2000).

Data Extraction

Data extraction processes usually involve multiple researchers independently extracting data for each article. In most studies, a protocol is created to facilitate the summarization of information on such issues as the aim of the research, participants' characteristics, methodologies, methods of data collection, methods of analysis, and key results.

Synthesis

An examination of reviews deriving their data from qualitative techniques points to a variety of synthesis techniques, such as meta-summary, meta-synthesis, meta-interpretation, meta-ethnography, and grounded theory. Meta-ethnography, developed by Noblit and Hare (1988), enables the development of a broader perspective while maintaining the specificity of individual studies. The meta-synthesis leads to a reconceptualization of key themes and concepts found in the raw material. The refining process occurs as the investigators re-read the original study, searching for key themes, keeping the study context in mind. The studies are compared and translated into one another by examining their similarities and contradictions. Key concepts are examined in relation to others in the original studies and across studies. The new concepts encompass more than any single one of the studies that are being synthesized. This is analogous to the method of constant comparison used in quantitative methods.

Generally, most of these techniques include two-three stages, providing multiple layers of accounts and interpretations. In the first stage, researchers map out each reviewed study to identify similar patterns in the various examined sources: documents, interview transcripts, field notes, and so on. This information is coded into themes/categories that are compared with similar categories extracted from other studies, using the original authors' terms. The categories are assembled and clustered as *first-order constructs*. First-order themes usually refer to such data as participants' views, beliefs, and desires. These are further refined and aggregated into a finite set of overarching constructs. Some reviewers rate these first-order constructs according to the quality level assigned to the original study from which the findings were extracted, prioritizing those from studies that scored higher in the quality appraisal procedure. In most cases, researchers construct the codes individually and resolve disagreements through discussion among themselves or with an additional researcher.

The next stage involves the identification of authors' inferences and conclusions about the first-order constructs, creating a set of *second-order constructs*, which group the findings into new, general themes. These new conceptual forms categorize the interpretation of the evidence on the basis of similarity in meaning. As with the first stage, these categories are synthesized and refined until they are reframed within a more abstract form. In the final stage, researchers produce *third-order constructs*, which synthesize both first- and second-order themes, creating a combination of primary evidence and researchers' interpretations. This meta-synthesis produces a comprehensive set of synthesized findings, usually presented in the form of narratives. Some authors test the scientific strength of each of the third-order constructs upon the studies that score high in the quality scoring tests and further compare them with similar findings of other studies in relevant areas (Feder et al., 2006).

Results

Researchers conducting systematic reviews with data extracted from qualitative studies report that the findings from the synthesized data, which integrate information from different angles, yield rich material and contribute to their knowledge of the phenomena they set out to examine. In addition, the synthesized studies significantly expand the range of subjects studied. Flores and Pellicio (2011), for example, synthesize studies examining the experience of women post-incarceration. Their synthesis derives from ten studies that examine the experience of 288 formerly incarcerated women from the USA. This number of subjects is unique to qualitative studies. The systematic compilation of data from the separate studies enables researchers to test hypotheses across a wide range of settings in different cultural contexts (Attree, 2004; Hodson, 2004).

Researchers conducting systematic reviews with qualitative information identify specific components of the reviewed interventions that contribute to the success or failure of a program. Depicting the mechanisms of success, they develop conceptual models and build theories. They claim that understanding the context in which a program occurs is a key to assessing why and how programs work. Systematic reviews have encouraged researchers to acknowledge the variations in contexts that mediate the outcome of a program. Bilby et al. (2006), for example, argue that qualitative studies were illuminating in terms of understanding why people drop out of programs treating sex offenders. Since the participants were themselves victims of sexual abuse, they could not empathize with their victims—a difficulty that became an obstacle during the treatment. Moreover, the review highlighted difficulties encountered by therapists treating sex offenders in the context of their own personal reservations regarding the offences committed (pp. 479–480). The reviewed studies illuminate the difficulty of offering effective treatment aimed at encouraging sex offenders to claim responsibility for their actions, while over a quarter of the professionals involved viewed sex offenders as suffering from a mental abnormality. These attitudes clarify the obstacles that exist in the treatment of sex offenders and may explain the failure of some treatments to have statistically significant effects on their behavior or attitudes (p. 477). Finfgeld-Connett and Johnson (2011a) report that the studies they reviewed led them to conclude that women agreed to participate in substance abuse programs only after they felt they were in a safe, caring environment. Health-care professionals are being asked to provide personalized care in various areas of acute care. The review expands the interpersonal aspects of personalized care. It suggests that women participating in substance abuse programs seek opportunities to hope, trust, attain, and preserve personal integrity (p. 647). The Patterson et al. (2012) review showed that the absence of significant improvement in reducing excessive alcohol consumption, smoking, and stress symptoms among police officers who participated in the studied intervention was due to their lack of trust toward the law enforcement organization's involvement in health issues. In addition, participants felt that alcohol consumption was a private matter and that the use of alcohol was an accepted coping mechanism in the context of police work and a central part of the police culture for bonding among officers (p. 25). Similarly, the qualitative data showed that officers did not feel that experiencing stress symptoms made officers less prepared for police work. At the same time, officers' "significant others" reported observing positive changes in their spouses following participation in the stress management interventions (p. 24).

Kearney (2001) systematically reviewed studies examining the responses of women to abusive relationships. She found that most women who stayed in such relationships developed a set of rationalizations that minimized or redefined violence as a sickness. Her review uncovered a four-phase process that women from various ethnic groups and different places undergo while responding to violent relationships: discounting early violence; seeing it as a romantic commitment; submerging one's own self-worth for the sake of the relationship; increasing realization of the intolerability of the situation; and seeking a life outside the relationship. In addition, the synthesis identifies the rationalization adopted by women to justify their situations in each one of these phases. Each one of these processes was linked to personal, sociopolitical, and cultural contexts.

Flores and Pellicio (2011) unearth the various obstacles women contend with after being released from jail. The aggregation of the findings from the various studies points to four main types of experience: tenuous relations with family members and the need to regain their mother role; the need to struggle with the stigma of being an ex-prisoner—which is experienced in various forms of life; the need to struggle with the realities of poverty, drugs, and blocked opportunities; and the need to abide by strict parole and probation requirements. The studies describe various reactions to these different sets of experiences, the decisions the women make, and the ways they choose to see themselves.

Sword et al. (2009) identify two processes that are central to women's addiction recovery: individual growth and transformative learning. Both lead to a higher quality of life and better interaction with their children. They point to the important role of an empowering environment, one that provides feelings of safety and experiences of empathy received respect, and compassion from the treatment staff. The presence of children in the treatment program is found to be highly motivating, facilitating the development of parenting skills, which contributes to the reestablishment of positive relationships with those children.

The integration of quantitative and qualitative methods pointed to a detailed review of victims' experiences. Thus, Rizo and Macy (2011) discovered that Hispanic survivors of intimate partner violence in the USA faced various barriers to accessing help, which were linked to the cultural experiences of Hispanic women. For example, the cultural expectations of Hispanic women that emphasize family loyalty and self-sacrifice prevented them from seeking help. In addition, they lacked relevant knowledge about potential support resources. Beyond that, the reviews indicated that when Hispanic survivors sought help they approached multiple sources and often multiple times; this usually involved family members, friends, and coworkers. They approached medical clinics, shelters, social workers, or counselors, but rarely sought help from lawyers, police, or clergy.

While researchers see the reviews as a stepping stone toward the development of theories or conceptual models, others believe that information gained from the systematic review can for a basis informing policy. Flores and Pellicio (2011), for example, claimed that the findings of their meta-synthesis could lead to the development of practices used by nurses to identify the health and psychological needs of women released from prison and develop interventions addressing challenges they face. Kearney (2001) claims that the phases she discovered and the set of arguments used by the women in abusive relationships give health professionals insights that better identify women's situations even if they choose to conceal them and to offer help during the various phases. Feder et al. (2006) claimed that their findings would provide data that supported recommendations in a series of national guidelines instructing health-care professionals how to deal with survivors of intimate partner violence.

Finally, researchers who used this technique to expand knowledge about a new area usually concluded that the systematic review helped in their assessment of current knowledge, helped to determine critical gaps in existing knowledge, and helped to create an holistic picture of a phenomenon that was still in its infancy (Douglas et al., 2008; Maher & Hudson, 2007; Rizo & Macy 2011).

Limitations

The systematic review of qualitative methods carries with it a number of limitations, most of them originating in the nature of this research technique. First, there are a small number of published original works using qualitative methods. Mitchell and MacKenzie (2004), examining narrative reviews of the relationships between race/ethnicity and sentencing outcome, explain that research in various areas of study has "consistently demonstrated that studies reporting statistically significant results are more likely to be published" (p. 3), thus excluding the publication of reports that do not include such strategies. This shortcoming can lead to a "publication bias," with negative influences on the ability to produce a comprehensive review (see discussion in Rothstein, Sutton, & Borenstein, 2005).

Second, the synthesis of findings from various studies can lead to a mixture of "experiences that are culturally or historically incomparable for reasons undetectable to the subsequent analyst" (Kearney, 2001, p. 279). Third, according to the principles of the qualitative research method, the synthesis process is characterized by a dynamic relationship between method and researcher. Qualitative research involves the interpretation of the data gathered and the outcomes, but is not detached from the process of data analysis. This requires a detailed, thick account of research procedures, to enable the reviewer to assess their trustworthiness by following the decision-making process through the entire study. However, many original articles lack this important information. In many studies, participants' experiences are not evident and only a few sentences are quoted, making it almost impossible to generate first-order constructs or to differentiate between their accounts and the researchers' interpretations.

Fourth, due to concerns about anonymity within small, context-rich samples, qualitative reports frequently do not include comprehensive demographic information, and thus important details are omitted. Fifth, some reviews reported that the original studies did not provide adequate information about data preparation or analytic procedures, thus limiting the ability to evaluate study rigor (Rizo & Macy, 2011, p. 254). The secondary analysis entails integration of data from various sources and their representation in an abstract form. The aggregation of data can lead to the isolation of the findings from the original context in which the study took place and the qualitative findings can lose their original meaning, individual differentiations, and their richness. This reinterpretation lacks the context in which the primary interpretation occurred (see discussion in Weed, 2005). Mays, Pope, and Popay (2005) warn that "attempts at aggression destroy the integrity of individual studies" (p. 7). To avoid this, researchers should develop a synthesis method that would allow for the inclusion of details regarding individual cases within the integrated framework (Doyle, 2003).

Finally, the majority of the studies were conducted in the USA. Such geographically focused research excludes knowledge about similar issues from other parts of the world.

Systematic Reviews of Qualitative Research in Criminology

The aim of this study was to show that the use of qualitative data is effective for the development of an overarching explanatory framework, linking together information from various sources. The inclusion of data derived from qualitative research methods is founded on an approach that sees the art of research as a systematic and reflective process for the development of knowledge that can be accumulated within, and then applied beyond a particular study setting. Drawing on these assumptions, researchers are able to deepen their analyses by synthesizing findings across primary studies, from different contexts and research platforms, while simultaneously discerning their points of commonality and uniqueness.

Systematic reviews, examining evidence derived from a variety of sources, generate important details that can significantly enlarge relevant knowledge bases and contribute information to key questions within the "what works" perspective. Their ability to reveal the inner mechanisms of interventions by shedding light on the contextual variables in the examined policy could enable researchers to understand how the examined program works. The triangulation of methods and data from various sources enables the researcher to address the complexity of the examined program, by following the ways in which program attributes are experienced. In addition, qualitative research is essential for providing a fuller picture in areas where there is a lack of previous examination.

An evidence-based approach that measures effectiveness would be enriched by a synthesis of multifaceted evidence. This would entail a redefinition of evidence that should now be understood within a broader framework, in which the contextual insights of the studied phenomenon would be considered. In addition, researchers should be more methodologically inclusive and seek ways to include information gathered from diverse sources in systematic reviews. This would facilitate the addition of new components to the systematic review arena.

The discipline of criminology should understand the added value of qualitative research, which, as a basis for policy design and implementation, is not new to the discipline of criminology. As early as the 1920s, members of the Chicago School considered the city a laboratory, and used such research methods as interviews, participant observation, and document analysis to understand the links between the experiences of new immigrants to the USA and their decisions to engage in criminal activity (Shaw, Zorbaugh, McKay, & Cottrell, 1929; Park, Burgess, & McKenzie, 1967). These findings formed the basis for extensive policy interventions, aiming to eliminate crime in various areas of the city.

During the 1970s, labeling theorists attempted to understand crime and crime control "from within," producing accounts by crime control agents about their work. More recently, through the use of qualitative paradigms, a growing number of studies in criminology have gathered important information regarding crime and interventionist programs in the criminal justice system (Davies, 1999; Chalmers & Altman, 1995; Mosteller & Boruch, 2002). Others integrate qualitative data with quantitative findings to obtain a comprehensive account of the examined phenomenon, thus adding another dimension to their analysis (Hagan & McCarthy, 1997; Nurse, 2002; Mastrofski, Parks, & McCluskey, 2010; Sampson & Laub, 2003; Weisburd et al., 2006).

It is important to note that many programs targeting offenders are being carried out by multidisciplinary teams, and thus experimental designs that are not sensitive to this rich context are irrelevant for their evaluation (see discussion in Bull, 2005, p. 224). In addition, many programs serve small-sized clients and involve complex interventions, which can be best assessed by qualitative research procedures.

Indeed, in 2005, the National Institute for Justice's solicitation for studies evaluating the outcome of violence prevention programs included a declaration that "as one aspect of a comprehensive evaluation, assessments of program processes should include objective measurements and qualitative observations of programs as they are actually implemented and services are delivered. These may include assessment of such aspects as adherence to program content and protocol, quantity and duration, etc." (p. 4). However, most criminologists conducting systematic reviews treat these data as still ineligible for inclusion.

The introduction of systematic reviews could lead to the improvement of the quality of the original studies, and should form the basis for the next generation of systematic reviews, paving the way to a shift in the analytical paradigm in criminology.

In conclusion, the inclusion of qualitative data in studies reviewing issues relating to criminology has rarely been adopted by criminologists, in spite of the accumulated evidence that qualitative research enhances systematic reviews, contributing to their ability to expand knowledge and extend the evidence-based terrain that supports policy formation and implementation.

Acknowledgments The author would like to thank Dr. Shomron Moyal for his comments on earlier drafts and the editors for their helpful suggestions in revising the original chapter.

References

Atkins, S., Lewin, S., Smith, H., Engel, M., Fretheim, A., & Volmink, J. (2008). Conducting a meta-ethnography of qualitative literature: Lessons learnt. *BMC Medical Research Methodology, 8,* 21–31.

Attree, P. (2004). Growing up in disadvantage: A systematic review of the qualitative evidence. *Child: Care, Health and Development, 30*(6), 679–689.

Bair-Merritt, M. H., Crowne, S. S., Thompson, D. A., Sibinga, E., Trent, M., & Campbell, J. (2010). Why do women use intimate partner violence? A systematic review of women's motivations. *Trauma, Violence & Abuse, 11,* 178–189.

Barbour, R. S. (2001). Checklists for improving rigor in qualitative research: A case of the tail wagging the dog? *British Medical Journal, 322,* 1115–1117.

Barbour, R. S., & Barbour, M. (2003). Evaluating and synthesizing qualitative research: The need to develop a distinctive approach. *Journal of Evaluation in Clinical Practice, 9*(2), 179–186.

Béland, D. (2009). Ideas, institutions, and policy change. *Journal of European Public Policy, 16*(5), 701–718.

Bilby, C., Brooks-Gordon, B., & Wells, H. (2006). A systematic review of psychological interventions for sexual offenders II: Quasi-experimental and qualitative data. *The Journal of Forensic Psychiatry and Psychology, 17*(3), 467–484.

Blaxter, M. (1996). Criteria for evaluation of qualitative research. *Medical Sociology News, 22,* 68–71.

Braga, A., & Weisburd, D. (2012). The effects of "Pulling Levers" focused deterrence strategies on crime. *Campbell Systematic Reviews, 8*(6).

Bull, M. (2005). A comparative review of best practice guidelines for the diversion of drug related offenders. *International Journal of Drug Policy, 16*(4), 223–234.

Candy, B., King, M., Jones, L., & Oliver, S. (2011). Using qualitative synthesis to explore heterogeneity of complex interventions. *BMC Medical Research Methodology, 11,* 124–133.

Chalmers, I., & Altman, D. G. (1995). *Systematic reviews.* London: BMJ Publishing.

Charmaz, K. (2000). Grounded theory: Objectivist and constructivist methods. In N. K. Denzin & Y. S. Lincoln (Eds.), *Handbook of qualitative research* (2nd ed., pp. 509–535). London: Sage.

Davies, P. (1999). What is evidence-based education? *British Journal of Educational Studies, 47*(2), 108–121.

Dixon-Woods, M., Bonas, S., Booth, A., Jones, D. R., Miller, T., Sutton, A. J., Shaw, R. L., Smith, J. A., & Young, B. (2006). How can systematic reviews incorporate qualitative research? A critical perspective. *Qualitative Research, 6*(1), 27–44.

Douglas, A. C., Mills, J. E., Niang, M., Stepchenkova, S., Byun, S., Ruffini, C., Ki Lee, S., Loutfi, J., Lee, J., Atallah, M., & Blanton, M. (2008). Internet addiction: Meta-synthesis of qualitative research for the decade 1996-2006. *Computers in Human Behavior, 24*(6), 3027–3044.

Doyle, L. H. (2003). Synthesis through meta-ethnography: Paradoxes, enhancements, and possibilities. *Qualitative Research, 3*(3), 321–344.

Feder, G. S., Hutson, M., Ramsay, J., & Taket, A. R. (2006). Women exposed to intimate partner violence: Expectations and experiences when they encounter health care professionals: A meta-analysis of qualitative studies. *Archives of Internal Medicine, 166*(1), 22–37.

Finfgeld-Connett, D., & Johnson, E. D. (2011a). Substance abuse treatment for women who are under correctional supervision in the community: A systematic review of qualitative findings. *Issues in Mental Health Nursing, 32*(10), 640–648.

Finfgeld-Connett, D., & Johnson, E. D. (2011b). Therapeutic substance abuse treatment for incarcerated women. *Clinical Nursing Research, 20*(4), 462–481.

Flemming, K. (2010). Synthesis of quantitative and qualitative research: An example using Critical Interpretive Synthesis. *Journal of Advanced Nursing, 66*(1), 201–217.

Flores, J. A., & Pellico, L. H. (2011). A meta-synthesis of women's postincarceration experiences. *Journal of Obstetric, Gynecologic, & Neonatal Nursing, 40*(4), 486–496.

Geertz, C. (1973). Thick description: Toward an interpretive theory of Culture. In C. Geertz (Ed.), *The interpretation of cultures: Selected essays* (pp. 3–30). New York: Basic Books.

Goldsmith, M. R., Bankhead, C. R., & Austoker, J. (2007). Synthesising quantitative and qualitative research in evidence-based patient information. *Journal of Epidemiology and Community Health, 61*(3), 262–270.

Hagan, J., & McCarthy, B. (1997). *Mean streets: Youth crime and homelessness.* Cambridge, Mass.: Cambridge University Press.

Hamberg, K., Johansson, E., Lindgren, G., & Westman, G. (1994). Scientific rigour in qualitative research: Examples from a study of women's health in family practice. *Family Practice, 11*(2), 176–181.

Hannes, K., & Lockwood, C. (Eds.) (2012). *Synthesising qualitative research: Choosing the right approach.* Chichester: Wiley.

Hodson, R. (2004). A meta-analysis of workplace ethnographies: Race, gender, and employee attitudes and behaviors. *Journal of Contemporary Ethnography, 33*(1), 4–38.

Kearney, M. H. (2001). Enduring love: A grounded formal theory of women's experience of domestic violence. *Research in Nursing & Health, 24*(4), 270–282.

Kelly, M. P., & Charlton, B. (1995). The modern and postmodern in health promotion. In R. Bunton, S. Nettleton, & R. Burrows (Eds.), *The sociology of health promotion: Critical analyses of consumption, lifestyle and risk* (pp. 78–90). London: Rutledge.

Kuzel, A. J. (1992). Sampling in qualitative inquiry. In B. F. Crabtree & W. L. Miller (Eds.), *Doing qualitative research* (pp. 31–44). Newbury Park: Sage.

Lincoln, Y. S., & Guba, E. G. (1985). *Naturalistic inquiry.* Beverly Hills: Sage.

Lipsky, M. (1980). *Street-level bureaucracy: Dilemmas of the individual in public services.* New York: Russell Sage Foundation.

Malterud, K. (2001). Qualitative research: Standards, challenges, and guidelines. *The Lancet, 358*(9280), 483–488.

Mastrofski, S. D., Parks, R. B., & McCluskey, J. D. (2010). Systematic social observation in criminology. In A. R. Piquero & D. Weisburd (Eds.), *Handbook of quantitative criminology* (pp. 225–247). New York: Springer.

Maher, L., & Hudson, S. L. (2007). Women in the drug economy: A metasynthesis of the qualitative literature. *Journal of Drug Issues, 37*(4), 805–826.

Mays, N., & Pope, C. (1995). Qualitative research: Rigour and qualitative research. *British Medical Journal, 311,* 109–112.

Mays, N., Pope, C., & Popay, J. (2005). Systematically reviewing qualitative and quantitative evidence to inform management and policy-making in the health field. *Journal of Health Services Research & Policy, 10*(1), 6–20.

Mazerolle, L., Bennett, S., Davis, J., Sargeant, E., & Manning, M. (2013). Legitimacy in policing: A systematic review. *Campbell Systematic Reviews, 9*(1).

Meekums, B., & Daniel, J. (2011). Arts with offenders: A literature synthesis. *The Arts in Psychotherapy, 38*(4), 229–238.

Mitchell, O., & MacKenzie, D. L. (2004). *The relationship between race, ethnicity, and sentencing outcomes: A meta-analysis of sentencing research*. Washington, DC: National Institute of Justice.

Mosteller, F., & Boruch, R. F. (2002). *Evidence matters: Randomized trials in education*. Washington, DC: Brookings Institution Press.

Murray, J., Farrington, D. P., Sekol, I., & Olsen, R. F. (2010). Effects of parental imprisonment on child antisocial behaviour and mental health: A systematic review. *Campbell Systematic Reviews, 5*(4).

Noblit, G. W., & Hare, R. D. (1988). *Meta-ethnography: Synthesizing qualitative studies*. Newbury Park: Sage Publications.

Nurse, A. (2002). *Fatherhood arrested: Parenting from within the juvenile justice system*. Nashville: Vanderbilt University Press.

Parish, R. (1995). Health promotion, rhetoric and reality. In R. Bunton, S. Nettleton & R. Burrows (Eds.), *The sociology of health promotion: Critical analyses of consumption, lifestyle and risk* (pp. 13–23). London: Routledge.

Park, R. E., Burgess, E. W., & McKenzie, R. D. (1967). *The city*. Chicago: University Of Chicago Press.

Paterson, B. L. (2011). 'It looks great but how do I know if it fits?': An introduction to meta-synthesis research. In K. Hannes & C. Lockwood (Eds.), *Synthesizing qualitative research: Choosing the right approach* (pp. 1–20). Chichester: Wiley.

Patterson, G. T., Chung, I. W., & Swang, P. G. (2012). The effects of stress management interventions among police officers and recruits. *Campbell Systematic Reviews, 8*(7).

Petticrew, M. (2001). Systematic reviews from astronomy to zoology: Myths and misconceptions. *British Medical Journal, 322*, 98–101.

Reis, S., Hermoni, D., Van-Raalte, R., Dahan, R., & Borkan, J. M. (2007). Aggregation of qualitative studies–From theory to practice: Patient priorities and family medicine/general practice evaluations. *Patient Education and Counseling, 65*(2), 214–222.

Rizo, C. F., & Macy, R. J. (2011). Help seeking and barriers of Hispanic partner violence survivors: A systematic review of the literature. *Aggression and Violent Behaviour, 16*(3), 250–264.

Robinson, L., & Spilsbury. K. (2008). Systematic review of the perceptions and experiences of accessing health services by adult victims of domestic violence. *Health & Social Care in the Community, 16*(3), 16–30.

Rothstein, H. R., Sutton, A. J., & Borenstein, M. (Eds.). (2005). *Publication bias in meta-analysis: Prevention, assessment and adjustments*. Chichester: Wiley.

Saini, M., & Shlonsky, A. (2012). *Systematic synthesis of qualitative research*. Oxford: Oxford University Press.

Sampson, R. J., & Laub, J. H. (2003). *Shared beginnings, divergent lives: Delinquent boys to age 70*. Cambridge: Harvard University Press.

Sandelowski, M., Voils, C. I., & Barroso, J. (2007). Comparability work and the management of difference in research synthesis studies. *Social Science & Medicine, 64*(1), 236–247.

Satterfield, J. M., Spring, B., Brownson, R. C., Mullen, E. J., Newhouse, R. P., Walker, B. B., & Whitlock, E. P. (2009). Toward a transdisciplinary model of evidence-based practice. *The Milbank Quarterly, 87*(2), 368–390.

Schreiber, R., Crooks, D., & Stern, P. N. (1997). Qualitative meta-analysis. In J. M. Morse (Ed.), *Completing a qualitative project: Details and dialogue* (pp. 311–326). Thousand Oaks: Sage.

Shaw, C., Zorbaugh, F. M., McKay, H. D., & Cottrell, L. S. (1929). *Delinquency areas: A study of the geographic distribution of school truants, juvenile delinquents, and adult offenders in Chicago*. Chicago: University of Chicago Press.

Stone, D. A. (1997). *Policy paradox: The art of political decision making*. New York: W.W. Norton.

Sword, W., Jack, S., Niccols, A., Milligan, K., Henderson, J., & Thabane, L. (2009). Integrated programs for women with substance use issues and their children: A qualitative meta-synthesis of processes and outcomes. *Harm Reduction Journal, 6*, 32–37.

Tricco, A. C., Tetzlaff, J., & Moher, D. (2011). The art and science of knowledge synthesis. *Journal of Clinical Epidemiology, 64*(1), 11–20.

Van der Laan, P. H., Smit, M., Busschers, I., & Aarten, P. (2011). Cross-border trafficking in human beings: Prevention and intervention strategies for reducing sexual exploitation. *Campbell Systematic Reviews, 7*(9).

Weed, M. (2005). 'Meta interpretation': A method for the interpretive synthesis of qualitative research. *Forum: Qualitative Social Research, 6*(1), Art. 37.

Weisburd, D., Wyckoff, L. A., Ready, J., Eck, J. E., Hinkle, J. C., & Gajewski, F. (2006). Does crime just move around the corner?: A controlled study of spatial displacement and diffusion of crime control benefits. *Criminology, 44*(3), 549–592.

Werb, D., Rowell, G., Guyatt, G., Kerr, T., Montaner, J., & Wood, E. (2011). Effect of drug law enforcement on drug market violence: A systematic review. *International Journal of Drug Policy, 22*(2), 87–94.

Whyte, W. F. (1997). *Creative problem solving in the field: Reflections on a career*. Walnut Creek: AltaMira Press.

Chapter 10
Evidence Mapping to Advance Justice Practice

Michael S. Caudy, Faye S. Taxman, Liansheng Tang and Carolyn Watson

The last two decades have seen an exponential growth in the popularity of systematic reviews (SRs) and meta-analyses across scientific disciplines, including the field of criminology (Pratt, 2010; Wells, 2009; Wilson, 2010). Research syntheses are relevant for informing theory, policy and practice, but more importantly they serve as a crucial building block for knowledge translation (Grimshaw, Eccles, Lavis, Hill, & Squires, 2012; Taxman & Belenko, 2012). This chapter provides an overview of the Evidence Mapping to Advance Justice Practice (EMTAP) project organized by the research team of Dr. Faye S. Taxman at the Center for Advancing Correctional Excellence (ACE!) at George Mason University. EMTAP enjoined support and contributions from scholars from around the United States and other countries. The EMTAP model provides a methodology for conducting "reviews of reviews" using high-quality, SR methods and provides a model for knowledge translation from existing SRs. This "collaboratory" of scientists was brought together to conduct a series of reviews of reviews to better understand the state of knowledge in behavioral health-related fields that affect justice populations, policies and practices. This research endeavor emanated from a need to summarize the existing SR evidence; to examine the impact of interventions on various health and justice-related outcomes, particularly substance abuse and recidivism; to identify

---

M. S. Caudy (✉)
The University of Texas at San Antonio, San Antonio, TX, USA
e-mail: michael.caudy@utsa.edu

F. S. Taxman
George Mason University, Fairfax, VA, USA
e-mail: ftaxman@gmu.edu

L. Tang
George Mason University, Fairfax, VA, USA
e-mail: ltang1@gmu.edu

C. Watson
George Mason University, Fairfax, VA, USA
e-mail: cwatson4@gmu.edu

gaps in the existing knowledge base where SRs are needed; and to establish guiding principles for conducting review of reviews in multidisciplinary areas.

This chapter has the following goals: (1) to explain the EMTAP project; (2) to provide an overview of the methodology used; (3) to highlight the development of tools designed to standardize the process of conducting reviews of reviews; and (4) to summarize the lessons learned from conducting "reviews of reviews." Given the importance of research synthesis methods, this chapter concludes with recommendations for strengthening the evidence base and improving the quality of primary SRs and "reviews of reviews" to advance practice in the areas of criminology and behavioral health.

The Importance of "Reviews of Reviews"

As observed during the design stage of the EMTAP process, the extant body of SR literature has sometimes produced conflicting findings. This raises challenges for interpreting and drawing conclusions about what the results of these studies mean and how they should be used to inform future research, theory development, and policy. SRs are further complicated when a diverse array of justice-and/or health-relevant outcomes (e.g., crime, recidivism, substance use, employment) are assessed. Methodological advancements and guidelines are needed to help consumers of research assess whether there is consistency in the evidence base. While research synthesis scholars have excelled at developing methodological guidelines for conducting SRs and meta-analyses (e.g., Higgins & Green, 2011; Moher, Liberati, Tetzlaff, & Altman, 2009), far less has been done to standardize procedures for conducting reviews of reviews (see Becker & Oxman, 2011 for an exception). Additionally, little research has been published concerning how to reconcile and summarize multiple SRs or meta-analyses of the same intervention or clinical question (Borenstein, Hedges, Higgins, & Rothstein, 2009; Jadad, Cook, & Browman, 1997).

The value of a "review of reviews" (synthesis of SRs or meta-analyses) is to highlight what is known on a particular topic or intervention, or what can contribute to a more complete understanding of the extant empirical evidence. The compilation of these reviews, given their scientific and policy value, calls attention to a need for standardizing the approach to conduct this type of research. Outside of the Cochrane Collaboration's overview of review procedures (Becker & Oxman, 2011), standardized review of review techniques have yet to be developed or adopted consistently. As illustrated in this book, various methods have been used across the chapters on justice-related topics. Ten teams of esteemed SR researchers were given the task of summarizing the SR literature on a given topic and, not surprisingly, all ten developed a slightly different approach to achieving this common goal. Also, several common barriers emerged. The importance of developing a methodology for addressing these methodological and conceptual issues became a central theme during the planning of this volume. In the developmental phases of the EMTAP process, similar issues were encountered and the current chapter discusses how these issues were handled to improve the transportability of research synthesis findings to practice.

The Evidence Mapping to Advance Justice Practice (EMTAP) Project

Motivation for EMTAP

Replication is a core building block of science. Assessing the consistency and robustness of findings across populations, settings, and contextual factors can help ensure that a practice is likely to produce similar results when it is implemented. A single study cannot determine, with certainty, that an intervention works or does not work. However, studies that are combined together, across different settings and conducted over time can establish a pattern of consistent findings that may be useful to justify new or refined practice. Several studies combined can establish both significance and repeatability of results (Arnqvist & Wooster, 1995; Cook & Leviton, 1980).

But the more studies that are conducted, the more difficult it can be to analyze and determine the cumulative findings from a body of literature. Traditional narrative literature reviews can be far too subjective to reflect the knowledge that has been gained through research. The use of quantitative research synthesis techniques such as meta-analysis overcomes many of the limitations of narrative reviews. Meta-analysis provides an objective and quantitative approach to research synthesis by taking into account factors such as sample size, effect size, magnitude and direction of relationships, and the methodological quality of the various studies analyzed (Borenstein et al., 2009; Egger & Smith, 1998; Egger, Smith, & Philips, 1997; Glass, 1977; Lipsey & Wilson, 2001; Wilson, 2001, 2010). Meta-analyses generally are not limited by a reliance on traditional indicators of statistical significance but instead rely upon effect sizes to give a picture of the size and scope of the impact of an intervention (Borenstein et al., 2009; Lipsey & Wilson, 2001; Wells, 2009; Wilson, 2001; 2010)

Despite the advantages of SRs and meta-analyses over traditional narrative review methods, these techniques are not without limitations. As is the case with primary studies, multiple SRs often produce conflicting findings even when they examine the same body of literature (Jadad et al., 1997; Pratt, 2010). SRs and meta-analyses have similar flaws as primary studies given the numerous methodological decisions that are made during the review process. These decisions affect the search strategy, coding of studies, moderators examined, inclusion/exclusion criteria, and the reporting of effect sizes—and each has the potential to impact the review findings. Despite the transparency of the method (a strength of SRs), there is always a certain degree of subjectivity in research synthesis (Borenstein et al., 2009; Wilson, 2010). As Wilson (2001, p. 72) posits, "the logical framework of meta-analysis is based on the assumption that the averaging of findings across studies will produce a more valid estimate of the effect of interest than that of any individual study." Similar arguments can be made about meta-analyses addressing the same topic; this logic guided the EMTAP process.

EMTAP Goals

The primary goal of EMTAP was to identify and summarize meta-analyses and SRs on behavioral health interventions applicable to people involved in the justice system. A secondary aim was to translate the knowledge from existing reviews to guide the field in the application of SR findings. Finally, the project was designed to identify areas where more research is needed to inform justice practice. The EMTAP project was devoted to building a knowledge base by systematically summarizing reviews related to: access to services or programs, effectiveness of interventions, organizational factors used to enhance effectiveness, and a myriad of proximal and distal justice and behavioral health outcomes.

The EMTAP project used a health services model as a framework for both the review process and identification of applicable areas of study. Given that people involved in the justice system have similar needs as others in society, the project was not limited to interventions delivered only to justice populations or delivered only in justice settings. Instead, the delivery process was embedded into the design of each review in order to expand knowledge about how to access interventions, engage people in interventions, deliver efficacious interventions, and implement interventions. The health services conceptual model considers interventions as a function of intake processes, organizational features, and systems of care. This conceptualization goes beyond efficacy and considers a wide range of individual client, organizational, and systems dimensions that are related to effective interventions.

The health services framework is built on the premise that there is more to understanding "what works" than examining the efficacy of interventions (Taxman & Belenko, 2012). Extant empirical research demonstrates the importance of understanding key intervention components and degrees of implementation fidelity (Dane & Schneider, 1998; Fixsen, Naoom, Blasé, Friedman, & Wallace, 2005; Glasziou et al., 2010; Green & Glasgow, 2006; Michie, Fixsen, Grimshaw, & Eccles, 2009; Schoenwald & Hoagwood, 2001; Taxman & Bouffard, 2000; 2002; Workgroup for Intervention Development and Evaluation Research [WIDER], 2012). Considering key intervention components, implementation fidelity, and organizational factors can assist in identifying the different processes that will lead to improved outcomes across settings. That is, a systematic review or meta-analysis can assess more than just the intervention and its outcomes—it often considers the inputs of the intervention such as system referral processes, techniques to engage people in the intervention, processes to match individuals to appropriate services (based on theory or on clinical expertise), and so on. This is recognition to the fact that the effectiveness of interventions is based on a wide array of inputs, not merely on the components of the intervention itself (Taxman & Belenko, 2012).

Integrating the health services conceptual model into the EMTAP review process afforded research teams the ability to assess the degree to which systematic or meta-analytic reviews considered factors affiliated with effective interventions or processes. That is, EMTAP reviews assessed the degree to which existing reviews can assist in understanding issues related to the implementation and sustainability of programs by answering critical questions that affect the uptake of innovations.

This approach provided a greater opportunity to identify gaps in the extant SR literature base.

Finally, an additional goal of the EMTAP project was to develop tools for conducting and disseminating synthesis findings from reviews of reviews. Tools were designed to standardize the process of synthesizing existing reviews and to increase the transportability of review findings to the field. With these knowledge translation goals in mind, the EMTAP project sought to address three broad research questions about the current state of knowledge in the areas of correctional programming, substance abuse treatment, and behavioral health interventions: (1) what are the criteria for determining whether practices are effective?; (2) how consistent are the findings across SRs in different thematic areas?; and (3) how can we best assess existing evidence and effectively apply it to justice practice? In essence, these questions allow us to answer questions about: what works for whom and in what setting?; in what areas are SRs/meta-analyses needed?; and, once efficacious practices have been identified, how can they be effectively implemented?

EMTAP Research Design, Methods, and Tools

The EMTAP methodology was guided by techniques developed and used by the Cochrane Collaboration as detailed in the *Cochrane Handbook for Systematic Reviews of Interventions* (Higgins & Green, 2011). These techniques were developed to minimize bias in the systematic search procedures and enhance the validity, objectivity, and inclusiveness of EMTAP searches and results. The primary steps in the EMTAP review process included: identifying a relevant review question, generating search terms and specifying inclusion criteria, comprehensively searching relevant databases, reviewing and documenting articles, coding articles, and reporting and synthesizing results across existing SRs. Each step of the EMTAP process was transparent and documented using CONSORT-like[1] documents (see Altman, 2001; Begg et al., 1996; Moher, Jones, & Lepage, 2001) developed specifically for the task of conducting reviews of reviews. All steps of the EMTAP process are documented and made available to users who access EMTAP reports through a specially designed web-based tool developed to disseminate project findings. Transparency of methods and decisions made during the review process is an essential element of research synthesis efforts. Incomplete reporting of SR methods, findings, and procedures is a major limitation of the extant SR literature base (Chan, Hrobjartsson, Haahr, Gotzsche, & Altman, 2004; Moher, Tetzlaff, Tricco, Sampson, & Alt-

---

[1] The Consolidated Standards of Reporting Trials (CONSORT) statement was developed by researchers to improve the reporting of Randomized Controlled Trials (Begg et al., 1996). The CONSORT statement is designed to ensure that adequate information is reported to assess the internal and external validity of a trial. The CONSORT model has been adapted for the reporting of systematic reviews and meta-analyses (see e.g., Delaney et al., 2005).

man, 2007; The PLoS Medicine Editors, 2007), and the EMTAP methodology was designed to limit the impact of these issues on project findings.

Search procedures: Similar to the specifications of SRs of primary studies, the EMTAP project employed a comprehensive and systematic search procedure to avoid reporting bias. This included searches to uncover published and unpublished grey material across multiple social science disciplines. The use of a systematic search procedure is essential for ensuring the comprehensiveness of a SR (Hammerstrom, Wade, & Jorgensen, 2010; Lefebvre, Manheimer, & Glanville, 2011). For example, Amato et al. (2011) recently observed that systematic search techniques identified 15% of published studies that would not have been identified through non-systematic search procedures, indicating the potential for bias associated with non-systematic searches (see also, Wilson, 2009).

The first step in the EMTAP search procedure was to identify relevant search terms. Search terms were identified through careful consideration of the extant literature on a given topic and through consultation with subject matter experts when appropriate. All search terms were generated through an iterative team process and approved by the EMTAP project manager. It was often necessary to adapt search terms after pilot testing search procedures. All generated search terms were combined with the terms "systematic review" and/or "meta-analysis" in Boolean searches to restrict the search results to reviews as opposed to primary studies. Non-reviews were often identified by EMTAP searches but were excluded during coding.

Consistent with Cochrane and Campbell guidelines, EMTAP searches were designed to ensure a high level of sensitivity (Hammerstrom et al., 2010; Lefebvre et al., 2011). All EMTAP searches queried nine primary databases to ensure the comprehensiveness of the search findings: PubMed, ScienceDirect, PsychArticles, PsychINFO, ProQuest Research Library, Criminal Justice Abstracts, Cambridge Journals Online, the Cochrane Database of Systematic Reviews, and the Campbell Systematic Review Library. Additionally, all EMTAP searches queried Google Scholar. When applicable, EMTAP searches included other more specialized databases that were topic appropriate. Searches for unpublished reviews were conducted within the ProQuest Research Library and Google Scholar.

To preserve the transparency and repeatability of EMTAP searches, a modified CONSORT-like flow chart was completed for every conducted review search (Fig. 10.1). These SEARCHSORTs were used to document: search terms used, databases searched, the number of hits from each search, the number of studies coded as relevant and irrelevant, rationale for exclusion of identified abstracts, and the total number of unique meta-analyses and SRs included. SEARCHSORT charts documented how articles progressed through the EMTAP coding process and provided users with a clear summary of the search procedure. The use of CONSORT-type documents has been identified as best practice (Altman, 2005) and research has found that such techniques are associated with improved quality of reporting of the findings of randomized controlled trials (RCTs) (Begg et al., 1996; Moher, Jones, & Lepage, 2001; Moher et al., 2007; Plint et al., 2006) and meta-analyses (Delaney et al., 2005). Empirical support has also been provided for the utility of modified

10 Evidence Mapping to Advance Justice Practice

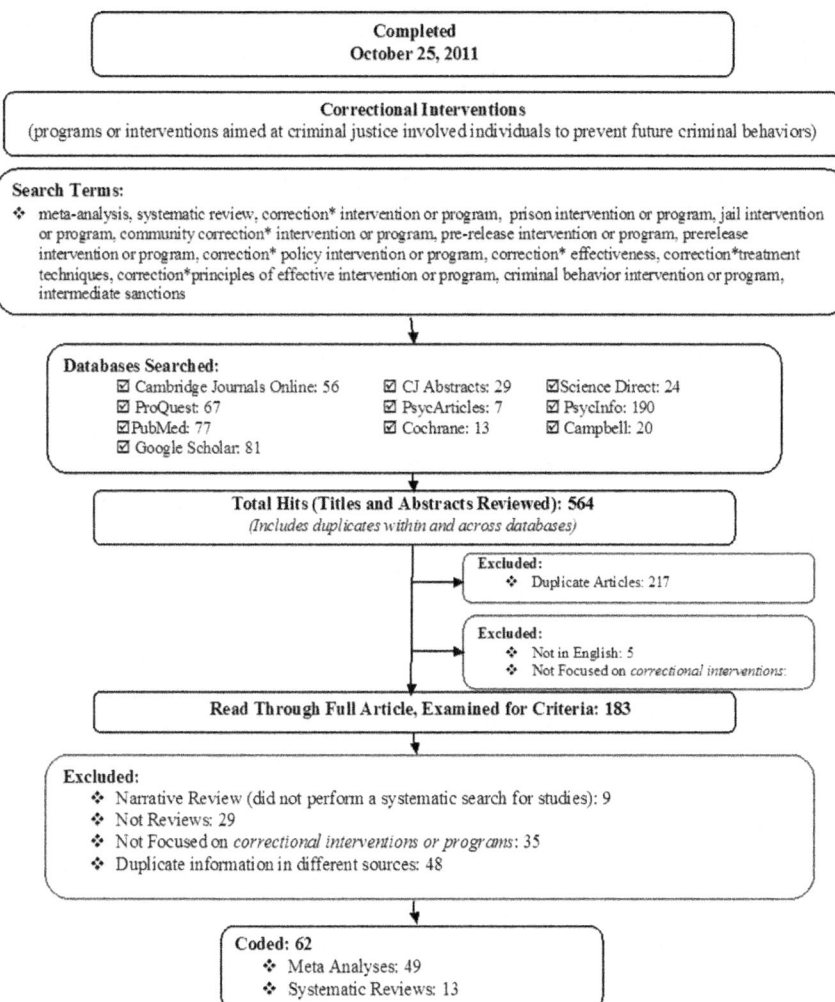

Fig. 10.1 Example EMTAP SEARCHSORT

CONSORT-like statements for reporting criminal justice research (Perry, Weisburd, & Hewitt, 2010).

Coding reviews: To standardize the data extraction process, the EMTAP research team developed a 68-item automated coding protocol.[2] The importance of using data extraction protocols is well documented as part of both the Cochrane and Campbell SR guidelines. For instance, Higgins and Deeks (2011) refer to the data collection form as the "bridge" between what is reported in the original studies and what is reported in the review (Higgins & Deeks, 2011, p. 7.5.1). This document

---

[2] A copy of the automated protocol is available upon request from the corresponding author.

guides the research team through the coding process and standardizes the information collected across reviews. Coding sheets provide documentation of the many decisions that are made during the process of determining if a review is eligible for inclusion and what information should be recorded from each review (Higgins & Deeks, 2011; Meade & Richardson, 1997). It is recommended as best practice that data collection/coding protocols be published or made available to research consumers to allow for replication and critical assessment (Silagy, Middleton, & Hopewell, 2002).

The development of a web-based EMTAP coding system was an iterative process that went through several revisions and refinements. As per the standard in the field (Higgins & Deeks, 2011), all coding and reporting documents were pilot tested before they were used in practice. The development of a web-based resource allowed other research teams interested in conducting EMTAP reviews to follow a common methodology. The final version of the EMTAP automated coding system covered all of the items identified by the Preferred Reporting Items for Systematic Reviews and Meta-Analyses (PRISMA) guidelines (Moher et al., 2009) plus additional items tailored specifically to reviews of reviews.

Information recorded in EMTAP automated coding system included: the types of outcomes examined, effect sizes reported (for each specific outcome), moderators/sub-groups examined, populations studied as well as the setting in which they were studied, methodological quality assessments, and key components of the interventions. Additionally, the authors of EMTAP searches coded information that allowed them to draw conclusions about implementation fidelity and transportability within each topic area. Transparency and transportability were the main concerns during the development of the EMTAP coding system.

Reporting findings: To standardize the reporting of findings from EMTAP reviews, all review teams completed a CONSORT-like (REVIEWSORT) flow chart (Fig. 10.2). REVIEWSORT documents summarized the information from the automated coding sheets and provided information about what outcomes were assessed, direction and number of effect sizes for each outcome, and key intervention components that contributed to positive or negative outcomes. In line with the project goal of developing standardized procedures that could be shared by the field, these REVIEWSORTs are appropriate for use in EMTAP reviews as well as reporting findings from SRs or meta-analyses of primary studies.

In addition to completing CONSORT-like documents, review teams provided narrative summaries of their findings and identified policy-relevant questions that were addressed by the existing research synthesis literature. All EMTAP reporting documents were entered into an online database as part of an interactive web tool that allows users to search and browse the study data and view user-friendly, informative summaries of the current knowledge in each topic area. Additionally, the EMTAP web tool provides a searchable database that allows users to identify existing SRs and meta-analyses and view summaries of their findings. This web-based reporting system was designed to aid knowledge translation efforts, to advance research to the field, and to provide a detailed picture of the areas that need further examination and review.

10 Evidence Mapping to Advance Justice Practice

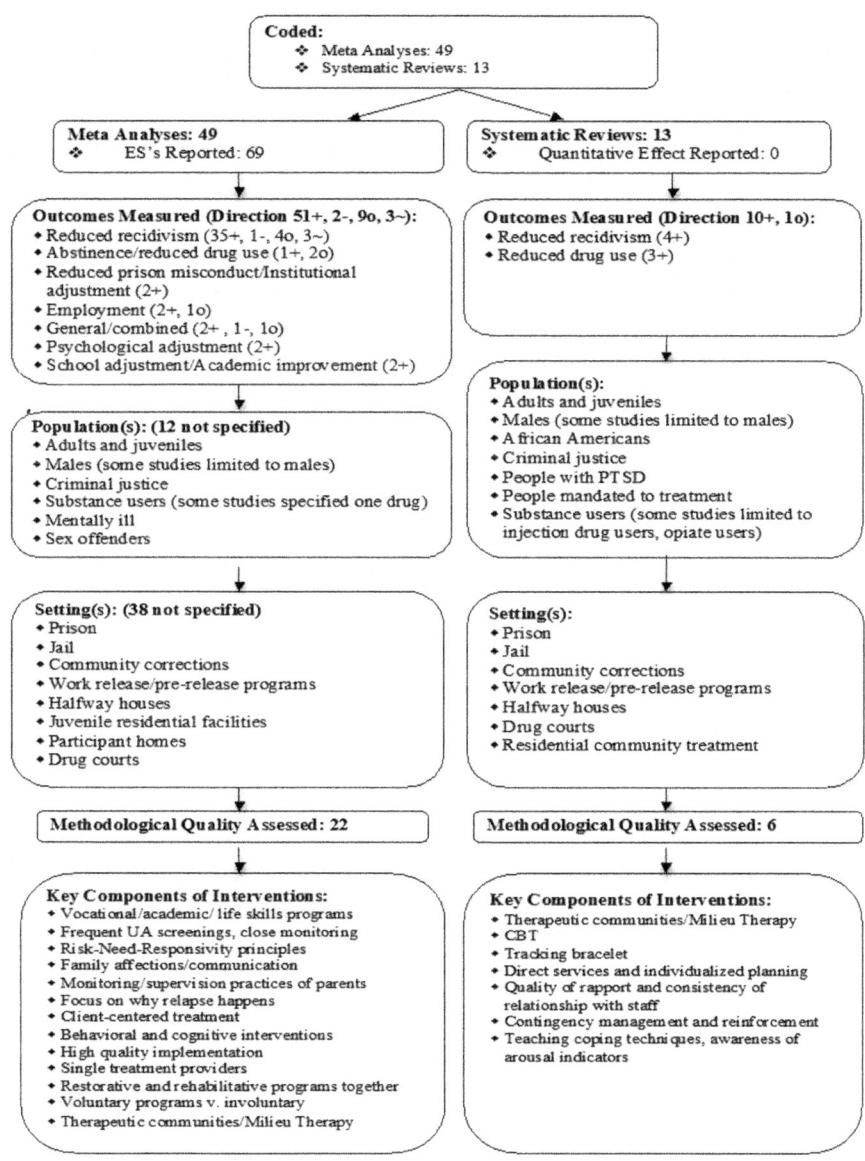

Fig. 10.2 Example EMTAP REVIEWSORT

Summary of EMTAP Reviews

Completed reviews: Since EMTAP began in 2010, over 18 reviews of reviews have been completed and another five reviews are currently in progress. A full review of the study findings is beyond the scope of this chapter, but the following section summarizes some preliminary findings. As of December 1, 2012, EMTAP research-

Table 10.1 Completed EMTAP reviews

Topic area	# of coded reviews	# of original studies*	# of primary outcomes assessed
Case management	69	3027	63
Community coalitions	2	81	No MA
Community intervention	8	131	4
Contingency management	3	111	1
Correctional intervention	62	3794	6
Family intervention	55	1566	16
HIV screening & testing	56	3046	13
Organizational culture	40	1922	37
PDSA (plan do study act)	0	–	–
Reentry	20	593	7
Referral	0	–	–
Risk assessment validations	4	135	No MA
School violence prevention	4	249	3
Sex offender treatment	18	329	3
Substance abuse treatment	14	542	3
Treatment length	42	2011	14
Treatment matching	5	110	1
Working alliance	3	173	No MA

[a] The number of primary studies was combined across coded studies and may contain duplicates
No MA No meta-analysis; primary outcomes were only coded from meta-analyses

ers have coded more than 340 SRs or meta-analyses; 300 of which are currently included in the online database. These coded reviews reported on findings from well more than 8000 primary studies assessing the effectiveness and implementation of interventions in corrections, public health, and substance abuse treatment. Since EMTAP had a focus on reviews related to health service issues within the justice system, the completed reviews extend beyond criminal justice interventions. Within each completed EMTAP review, numerous outcomes were assessed, and the results are presented for each outcome. Table 10.1 provides a summary of the completed EMTAP reviews and the full results of all completed EMTAP reviews can be accessed online at www.gmuace.org/tools/evidence-mapping.

Translational features: In addition to summarizing findings across existing reviews, EMTAP reviews explored the quality of the existing SR evidence base. Table 10.2 presents a summary description of some key features of the existing reviews that have been coded during the EMTAP project to date. Of the 300 reviews currently included in the EMTAP database, 164 (54.7%) include a quantitative meta-analysis. Consistent with existing findings indicating the growth in popularity of SRs in criminology and related fields (Pratt, 2010; Wells, 2009) a majority of the included reviews (57.7%) have been conducted since 2006. The findings reported in Table 10.2 also illustrate a great deal of variability in the size of existing SRs. The median number of primary studies included in the coded reviews was 25 with a range of 0–575. The median number of participants within the coded reviews

Table 10.2 Characteristics of coded systematic reviews and meta-analyses ($k=300$)

Review characteristic	Frequency/mean(SD)	%
Review design		
Systematic review	136	45.3
Meta-analysis	164	54.7
Publication year		
Pre-2000	35	11.7
2000–2005	92	30.7
2006– present	173	57.7
Specified study design for inclusion ($n=178$)[a]		
Experimental	141	47.0
Quasi-experimental	61	20.3
Controlled	26	8.7
Pre-post	19	6.3
Methodological quality assessed		
Not assessed	155	51.7
Inclusion criterion	60	20.0
Weighting	22	7.3
Discussion	63	21.0
Implementation fidelity assessed		
Not assessed	274	91.3
Inclusion criterion	6	2.0
Weighting	4	1.3
Discussion	16	5.3
Control/comparison condition specified ($n=78$)[a]		
No treatment	51	17.0
Treatment as usual	44	14.7
Other treatment	30	10.0
Moderators assessed[b]		
No	65	39.6
Yes	99	60.4
Publication bias assessed[b]		
No	103	62.8
Yes	61	37.2
Publication bias found	12	19.6[c]
# of primary studies (0–575)	46.4 (67.1)	median=27.0
# of participants (0–442,471)	14,073.7 (43,093.5)	median=2517.5

[a] Reported categories are not mutually exclusive
[b] Reported proportions are out of 164 coded meta-analyses only
[c] Reflects proportion within studies that assessed for publication bias

was 2518 with a range of 0–442,471. Among the 178 (59.3%) coded reviews that specified study design as an inclusion criterion, it was most common for reviews to prioritize experimental (79.2%) and quasi-experimental (34.3%) designs. Among studies that specified a control or comparison condition ($n=78$; 26.0%), it was most common for the efficacy of interventions to be tested against a comparison group not receiving treatment (65.4 %) or against treatment as usual (56.4 %). Comparative effectiveness was assessed in 38.5 % of the reviews that specified a comparison condition.

Summarizing Across Reviews

A key issue raised in the EMTAP process concerned the difficulty in synthesizing SR and meta-analysis findings. Attempting to make statements about the overall findings of a body of SR literature raised a number of emerging methodological questions. Part of the challenge was the lack of consistency in how authors report the findings of SRs and meta-analyses (Moher et al., 1999; 2007; 2009; The PLoS Medicine Editors, 2007). Since no standardized reporting procedures have been adopted, there is a great deal of variability in how SR and meta-analytic findings are reported both within and across academic disciplines. EMTAP review teams often found discrepancies in the reporting of inclusion/exclusion criteria, measures used to calculate effect sizes, whether and how summary effect sizes were calculated, and if moderators of intervention outcomes were assessed. It was also observed that many extant meta-analyses do not completely report effect sizes; confidence intervals, variance measures and precise p values were often omitted.

This lack of consistency and quality assurance is a major limitation of this body of research and potentially limits the transportability of SR and meta-analysis findings (The PLoS Medicine Editors, 2007). Like primary studies, SRs on similar constructs may differ from one another in many ways. To address this issue and make SRs and meta-analyses more compatible and therefore more appropriate for synthesis and better equipped to inform practice, it is apparent that the research community needs to continue to work toward adopting a set of standardized best practices for conducting and reporting SRs and meta-analyses in criminology and behavioral health (see e.g., Higgins & Green, 2011).

Reconciling Reviews: The summarizing of meta-analyses or SRs can be very challenging because existing reviews may be conflicting, may be reported differently or incompletely across studies, or may be more or less valid based on the quality of the research synthesis methods that were used in conducting the reviews. This is essentially the same issue researchers and practitioners face when attempting to summarize primary studies; the same issue that makes meta-analysis appealing. Accordingly, there is a considerable need to further develop techniques for reconciling findings across existing meta-analyses. This is not a new idea (Borenstein et al., 2009), but this is an area where more research is needed.

Several approaches for summarizing multiple SRs or meta-analyses of the same topic or intervention are currently available and they all have potential benefits and shortcomings. The Cochrane Collaboration has developed a set of recommended procedures for conducting overviews of reviews when multiple SRs exist regarding different treatments for the same clinical condition (Becker & Oxman, 2011).

Non-statistical approaches to summarizing multiple reviews, which may be used for either SRs or meta-analyses, include vote counting, and using decision algorithms to identify the review(s) that are most salient given the needs of the individual research consumer (Jadad et al., 1997). Statistical approaches for summarizing meta-analyses include conducting a new meta-analysis of all primary studies included in multiple meta-analyses; conducting a meta-analysis of summary effect sizes reported in existing meta-analyses; or using multiple-treatments meta-analysis techniques to assess the comparative effectiveness of interventions across existing reviews (see e.g., Cipriani et al., 2009).

What Works, What Is Promising, What Doesn't Work?

Given the aforementioned challenges to summarizing findings across such a large and diverse array of research syntheses, this discussion is limited to a general overview of what works, what is potentially promising, what needs more research, and what appears to not work based on existing reviews. As noted above, 300 SRs and meta-analyses had been coded and entered into the web-based reporting system designed to disseminate EMTAP project findings as of December 1, 2012. This section provides a general summary of the EMTAP findings that had been synthesized up to that date with a specific concentration on findings relevant to criminal justice populations. While the EMTAP project used a broad, interdisciplinary lens, this overview focuses primarily on correctional interventions and their impact on recidivism.

The EMTAP search for "correctional interventions" yielded 62 SRs or meta-analyses. Consistent with prior reviews (e.g., Lipsey & Cullen, 2007), the findings from these syntheses were generally positive suggesting that correctional treatment programs can effectively reduce recidivism and promote other positive outcomes (e.g., reduced substance use, improved vocational/educational skills). Cognitive-behavioral therapy, drug courts, therapeutic communities, and vocational/educational training programs were among the correctional interventions most consistently linked to reduced recidivism. These practices were generally associated with between a 10 and 30% reduction in recidivism with some meta-analyses reporting as much as a 50% reduction in recidivism (see Appendix A).

Incarceration/supervision only interventions were generally found to have limited or no effectiveness with one review finding that incarceration increased recidivism by 14% relative to community supervision (Smith, Goggin, & Gendreau, 2002). Faith-based programming, driving under the influence (DUI) counseling, post-traumatic stress disorder interventions, and relapse prevention models were identified among the interventions that needed more research to determine their effectiveness. Appendix A summarizes the quantitative findings from meta-analyses that were identified from the "correctional interventions", "sex offender treatment", and "substance abuse treatment" EMTAP searches.

Lessons Learned from EMTAP

The EMTAP process documented the importance of applying the standards associated with Cochrane and Campbell review methods to the field as a whole and in review of reviews. Findings from EMTAP are relevant for improving the quality of primary studies, SRs, and reviews of reviews. This section provides a discussion of the important lessons learned from this collaborative research effort.

Lesson 1: Multidisciplinary Searches

EMTAP search criteria allowed for the inclusion of reviews assessing non-criminal justice outcomes. This was an important design decision given the relevance of non-offending outcomes (e.g., substance abuse, treatment attendance, psychological functioning, etc.) to the overall functioning of justice populations. Restricting the focus of reviews to interventions that are targeted to offending outcomes overlooks a great deal of SR literature with important implications for people with various behavioral and mental health disorders, particularly if these outcomes are related to offending. Most EMTAP searches yielded SRs that assessed different primary outcomes within the same topic area (Table 10.1). For example, the EMTAP review of school violence prevention identified four SRs; two with bullying as a primary outcome, one on violence risk behaviors, and one on drug use. While a high-focused search design is sometimes appropriate, it is also important to consider the impact of interventions on an array of justice-relevant outcomes.

The health services conceptual framework allowed EMTAP reviews to identify interventions from fields outside of criminology (e.g., substance abuse treatment, mental health treatment, psychology) with relevance for justice-involved individuals. For instance, the EMTAP review on contingency management (CM) identified three meta-analyses from the substance abuse treatment field which found positive effects of CM on substance use outcomes, treatment attendance, and medication/methadone adherence (Griffith, Rowan-Szal, Roark, & Simpson, 2000; Lussier, Heil, Mongeon, Badger, & Higgins, 2006; Prendergast, Podus, Finney, Greenwell, & Roll, 2006). All of these outcomes are relevant to justice-involved individuals and the EMTAP findings suggest the potential efficacy of CM in the justice system. The CM reviews coded during EMTAP also identified key moderators of effective CM programs—such as access to CM, type of CM models, and type of population—that can be used to inform the design of interventions tailored to criminal justice populations. If EMTAP search criteria had been restricted to criminal justice populations, the three CM reviews would have been excluded. Given the similarity of CM to graduated sanctions and rewards, this would have limited the transportability of findings to justice settings (see Rudes, et al., 2012).

A key lesson learned from the EMTAP project is that multidisciplinary searches can yield relevant findings that are transportable to criminal justice populations. In evaluating the overall status of the SR literature on the efficacy of interventions, there is value in going beyond offender-specific studies and offending outcomes and using a wide, interdisciplinary lens. The EMTAP findings suggest that when conducting reviews of reviews, it is important to consider a wide range of proximal and distal outcomes and distinguish across outcomes when presenting summary findings.

Lesson 2: Comprehensive and Generalizable Searches

Like all research, SRs and meta-analyses vary in quality and generalizability. Given that not all reviews are the same, it is important to examine primary research methods and assess the impact of methodological quality on the overall SR findings. At the beginning of the EMTAP process, restricting the scope of systematic searches to only "high-quality" reviews was discussed. However, it was decided that doing so would limit search sensitivity and potentially overlook relevant reviews. And, in considering the degree to which the interventions or processes might be useful to the justice system, it was decided that the failure to include such reviews may have biased the findings or limited their utility for informing practice. While it is not uncommon for SRs and meta-analyses to limit includable studies to RCTs or high quality quasi-experimental designs, this may limit the transportability of review findings.

Similarly, during the planning of this book, the editors enjoined a discussion of whether the included reviews of reviews should be restricted to only SRs and meta-analyses that had been conducted under the auspices of either the Cochrane or Campbell Collaboration where standards are in place to limit bias and ensure the quality and validity of SR findings. While the decision to focus on higher quality reviews was appropriate for this book, the EMTAP project findings suggest that limiting the scope of review searches unnecessarily excludes many relevant SRs or meta-analyses. The overwhelming majority (97.3 %; 292/300) of the SRs coded as part of the EMTAP project to date were not published under the auspices of either the Cochrane or Campbell groups.

Within criminology and related fields where the SR literature is still relatively young and the use of RCTs is infrequent (but growing), it is important to allow for the inclusion of SRs of varying levels of methodological quality. There is empirical evidence suggesting that the findings from meta-analyses conducted on RCTs do not differ consistently from findings from meta-analyses of observational studies (Golder, Loke, & Bland, 2011). Additionally, an overreliance on highly controlled assessments of efficacy can lead to a lack of generalizability when interventions are translated into real world practice (Green & Glasgow, 2006)—in other words, the RCT might be useful for determining efficacy but not effectiveness. Researchers conducting reviews of reviews should undoubtedly be cognizant of the methodological quality issue and should report findings separately for higher and lower quality reviews but should not limit the potential transportability of their findings by focusing only on SRs of RCTs.

Lesson 3: Coding Issues in Reviews of Reviews

Clearly defining interventions and specifying their functional components is essential for understanding their effectiveness and potential transportability (Glasziou et al., 2010; Michie et al., 2009; Schoenwald & Hoagwood, 2001). Michie et al. (2009) identified numerous limitations of how interventions focused on behavioral change were reported in primary studies and SRs. These limitations included: a lack of well-defined intervention components; a lack of specification of study participants and study settings; inconsistent terminology in how interventions were described; a lack of consideration for the theory underlying interventions; and a lack of consideration of key moderating variables (Michie et al., 2009). The EMTAP findings support these observations. While the EMTAP automated coding system included prompts for coders to record the key components of interventions being assessed, in most cases, the primary reviews did not report sufficient information about the intervention (i.e., characteristics of individuals administering the intervention, characteristics of participants, key functional components of the intervention, setting, etc.) to draw meaningful conclusions from these fields. While it was common for SR authors to specify the name or type of the intervention, the reviews often did not describe the core components of the intervention in sufficient detail to better understand the mechanisms of action or allow for replication. This broad operationalization of interventions is problematic given the demands to identify guiding principles of effective interventions, to determine whether interventions are similar, to move research into practice, and to assess whether similar interventions generate similar findings across studies.

The importance of coding key elements of interventions and assessing the moderating impact of intervention features on effect sizes was another lesson learned from the EMTAP project. While scholars conducting reviews of reviews have no control over how well interventions are reported in SRs or primary studies, the EMTAP findings illustrate a need for improved reporting of interventions at all levels of research (Glasziou et al., 2010; Michie & Abraham, 2008; Michie et al., 2009). The lack of consideration of moderators of effect size is discussed below in the section on improving the SR evidence base.

The EMTAP project used a collaborative approach to coding SRs and assessing inter-rater reliability. Following the protocol of the Cochrane and Campbell Collaborations, the EMTAP reviews were always conducted by a team of researchers. Additionally, the EMTAP review teams often included at least one subject matter expert. This collaborative approach was essential for improving the reliability and validity of findings and maximizing the overall quality of the work that was done. To produce quality reviews, it is recommended that reviews of reviews be conducted by teams of researchers with at least a basic understanding of meta-analytic methods. A benefit of the team approach is that multiple parties can be involved in the data extraction process. Double-coding reviews (having multiple reviewers code the same review) to assess inter-rater reliability and the validity of coding procedures can help minimize errors and limit the threat of reviewer bias (Higgins & Deeks, 2011). As a best practice, it is recommended that review teams "double-code" reviews to improve reliability and limit bias. When complete double-coding is not feasible, periodic checks of inter-rater reliability should be conducted.

Finally, it is also important that the review teams spend a considerable amount of time before beginning their reviews developing protocols to guide the review process. All search and coding protocols should be pilot tested and published to ensure a systematic and transparent process and complete reporting of review findings (Higgins & Deeks, 2011). Empirical evidence suggests that publication of SR protocols reduces reporting bias by requiring authors to specify their hypotheses and procedures prior to having knowledge of review findings (Silagy, Middleton, & Hopewell, 2002).

Lesson 4: Implementation Fidelity

Effectiveness is often affected by the quality of the implementation. If implementation is faulty, programs will not deliver the expected outcomes. In many ways, this affects the external validity of SR findings (Dane & Schneider, 1998; Fixsen et al., 2005; Glasziou et al., 2010; Green & Glasgow, 2006; Taxman & Belenko, 2012). The EMTAP findings clearly document a lack of consideration of implementation fidelity within the reviewed SR literature on the efficacy of interventions. Across the 300 SRs entered into the EMTAP database to date, only 8.7% (26/300) included measures of implementation fidelity (Table 10.2). Of the 26 reviews that considered fidelity, six reviews excluded primary studies based on fidelity, four weighted effect sizes based on fidelity, and 16 discussed implementation fidelity as a possible explanation for their findings (Center for Advancing Correctional Excellence, 2012). When applicable, reviews assessing fidelity should be evaluated separately from reviews that fail to consider this construct. If the goal of SRs and meta-analyses is to determine "what works", it is essential to consider whether an intervention has been implemented as designed and what impact fidelity may have on SR findings (Michie & Prestwich, 2010). Implementation issues are essential for guiding the transportability of evidence-based practices (Glasziou et al., 2010; Schoenwald & Hoagwood, 2001; Taxman & Belenko, 2012).

Lesson 5: Transportability of Evidence-Based Practices

The preliminary findings from the EMTAP project illustrate the potential transportability of SR findings across disciplines. The EMTAP web tool provides a clearinghouse of SRs and meta-analyses from both criminal justice and health services fields and can serve as a valuable resource for guiding the translation of evidence-based practices to justice populations. All completed EMTAP reviews also include a narrative summary of key findings to aid knowledge translation (Box 10.1). EMTAP narrative summaries address three key questions: what are the essential elements of the intervention that make it effective?; what does it take to successfully implement?; and how can it be translated for adoption in justice settings? Considering these three questions throughout the process of conducting reviews of reviews can help guide the process and improve the quality of reporting.

> Box 10.1: Example Narrative Summary from EMTAP on Correctional Interventions

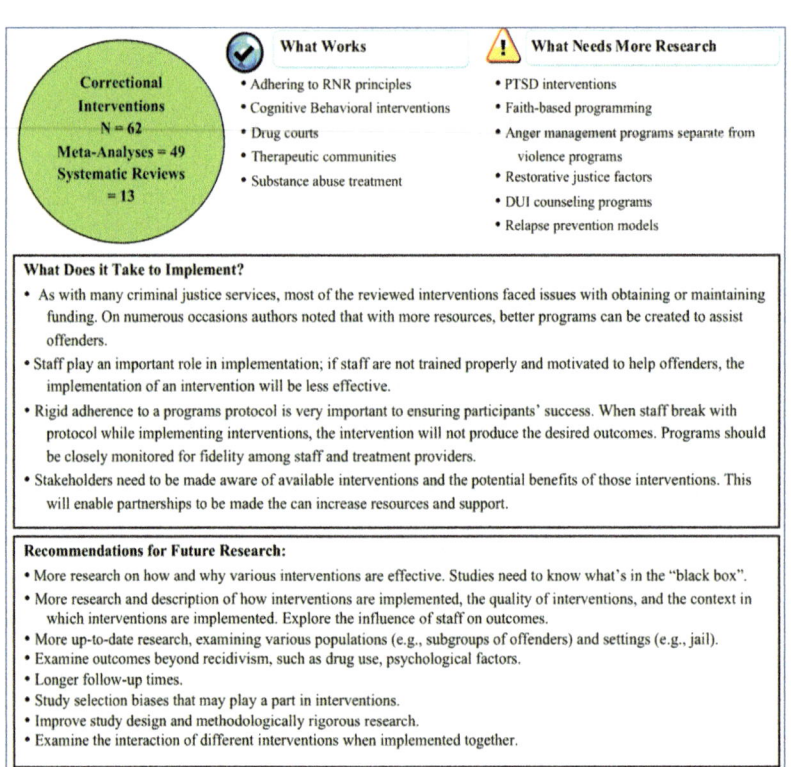

While the EMTAP findings suggest the potential transportability of SR findings to justice practice, they also indicate that there are numerous challenges to achieving transportability. The EMTAP findings clearly showed that implementation fidelity issues were not commonly considered and functional intervention components were not well described in primary reviews. Additionally, the EMTAP project found that the external validity of primary reviews was potentially limited because little attention was paid to the characteristics of the participants included in the studies being synthesized or the settings in which interventions were tested. Key participant characteristics (e.g., criminal risk level, mental health or substance use disorder diagnosis, drug of choice) were not discussed in the majority of the reviews coded during EMTAP. This limits transportability because research consumers do not know what interventions are most effective for which individuals and in which settings. Omitted information about implementation, intervention components, and study participants and settings is a major weakness of existing SRs and primary studies in criminology and related fields.

Despite the recent growth in the popularity of SRs in criminology and related fields, there are still many gaps in this evidence base. The EMTAP searches revealed a lack of SRs in many areas relevant to justice policy, evidence-based practices, and treatment provision within justice settings. Searchers found no SRs that met inclusion criteria for "Responsivity" or "Plan, Do, Study, Act (PDSA)" topic areas. Other potentially relevant topics (e.g., treatment matching and CM) were not found to have been tested within criminal justice populations. Within areas where systematic reviews were identified, there was a noticeable lack of reviews related to implementation (Table 10.2). For instance, while the EMTAP search on the effectiveness of correctional interventions yielded 62 reviews that met inclusion criteria and were coded, there was a lack of reviews found on topics related to access to care and organizational factors associated with improved intervention effectiveness. The EMTAP findings illustrate that more attention needs to be given to referral and access issues as well as the organizational and system factors that affect individual-level outcomes (based on the health services framework).

Improving the Quality of the Evidence from Systematic Reviews

As illustrated throughout the present volume, the ability to draw conclusions from reviews of reviews and use these techniques to aid knowledge translation is directly driven by the quality and completeness of the SRs and meta-analyses that are available to be summarized. Given this reality, we take the time in this section to call attention to several limitations of the extant SR literature included in the EMTAP project. The issues discussed here are by no means exhaustive, but they do call attention to some of the most common and problematic limitations of the existing SR literature that should be taken into account when conducting reviews of reviews. This section discusses several limitations of the SR literature reviewed during EMTAP and proposes strategies to improve the quality of future reviews and build a stronger, more transportable knowledge base.

During the EMTAP project, over 300 SRs and meta-analyses have been identified, reviewed, coded, and summarized. Throughout the project, EMTAP researchers spent time identifying limitations related to how SRs are conducted and how the findings of these reviews are reported (see Table 10.2). Consistent with prior research (Michie et al., 2009; Moher et al., 1999; 2007; 2009; The PLoS Medicine Editors, 2007), the primary concerns that arose during the EMTAP project generally centered on the amount of important information that was not reported in the reviewed research syntheses. Many of the SRs and meta-analyses that were coded during the EMTAP project suffered from methodological limitations that jeopardized the validity of their findings. The most common issues that arose during the EMTAP reviews were that SRs and meta-analyses frequently omitted: a consideration of potential moderating factors (66.0 %), assessments of implementation fidelity (93.4 %), assessments of the methodological quality of primary studies (54.0 %), and a consideration of publication bias (79.7 %).

Considering moderators of effect size enhances the value of meta-analysis. Moderator analyses allow researchers to explore how effect sizes vary based on differences in method, sample characteristics, settings, and intervention components (Borenstein et al., 2009; Lipsey, 2003; Lipsey & Wilson, 2001; Wilson, 2010). They go beyond assessing what works and can identify key components of interventions that are effective in certain settings or for certain sub-groups. They can help answer the question, "what works, for whom?" that has become a central focus of research on interventions across disciplines.

A majority of the meta-analyses coded during EMTAP (60.4 %, 99/164) did assess moderating factors; however, there was little consistency across reviews as to what moderators warranted inclusion or how they should be operationally defined. Considering moderators of intervention effectiveness is essential for guiding responsivity and improving the overall success of correctional and behavioral health interventions by matching clients to interventions in which empirical evidence indicates they are most likely to be successful. In the criminology literature, important moderators include gender, age, and risk level of the individual at a minimum. Further attention to moderating factors within SRs will help the field move beyond what works into what works for whom and in what setting. Empirical evidence suggests that responsivity can lead to more effective and cost-beneficial interventions in both corrections and substance abuse treatment (Bonta & Andrews, 2007; Pearson et al., 2012).

As noted above, another limitation of the existing SR literature is the lack of consideration of implementation fidelity in both primary and review studies. Implementation is an important issue for the field to consider when adopting findings from SRs or meta-analyses. The lack of consideration of fidelity is problematic given that the goal of most SRs of criminal justice and behavioral health interventions is to inform policy and practice; if fidelity is ignored, the utility of these findings is severely limited. Based on observations made during the EMTAP project, we recommend that fidelity items be added to standardized reporting documents for SRs and meta-analyses. As noted by Taxman & Belenko (2012) in their review of implementation factors, four levels of implementation should be considered: intervention issues, inner setting (the organization operating the intervention or process), outer setting (stakeholders and external partners), management factors, and sustainability.

Two additional limitations of the body of SR literature that were evident during the EMTAP project include a lack of consideration of methodological quality and a lack of consideration of publication bias. Aggregating results of primary studies with varying levels of methodological quality can potentially distort the findings of meta-analysis and therefore it is important to consider methodological quality and limitations of the primary studies that are included in any SR or meta-analysis (Lipsey & Wilson, 2001). Less than half (48.3 %) of the studies coded during EMTAP accounted for methodological quality either through inclusion criteria (20.0 %), weighting of effect size (7.3 %), or in the discussion of study findings (21.0 %).

The more problematic finding from the EMTAP process was that most of the coded SRs did not account for publication bias. Overall, only 20.3 % (61/300) of the coded reviews assessed publication bias and of the reviews that did assess it, 19.6 % found evidence of bias (Center for Advancing Correctional Excellence, 2012). Publication bias has been identified as a significant threat to the validity of SR and meta-analytic findings (Borenstein et al., 2009; Wilson, 2009; 2010), and methods have been developed to account for this bias and limit its influence on review findings (Borenstein et al., 2009; Sterne & Harbord, 2004). It is important that authors conducting SRs and meta-analyses assess and report on methodological quality and publication bias in order to enhance the validity of their findings.

Addressing these limitations and enhancing the quality and completeness of the SR evidence base is an important step in the process of using empirical evidence to inform justice and/or health practice. The quality of any meta-analysis or SR is directly driven by the quality of the primary studies that are included in the analysis (Lipsey & Wilson, 2001), and therefore it is important for reviewers to be cognizant of the limitations discussed in this section and take the necessary steps to account for and limit the influence of these validity threats during all stages of the research process—from primary studies to syntheses. Overall, attention to these details will strengthen studies and enhance their relevance to policy. The findings presented in this section further illustrate the need for more high-quality systematic reviews aimed at identifying and enhancing the quality of evidence-based interventions. Additionally, these findings suggest that there is a glaring need for both primary and review studies that adequately describe key intervention components and take into account implementation fidelity when considering the effectiveness of interventions.

Several important lessons were learned through the EMTAP initiative. EMTAP researchers learned about the process of conducting reviews of reviews and the EMTAP findings have illustrated the importance of taking an interdisciplinary, health services approach when designing and implementing evidence-based practices in justice settings. The lessons learned from EMTAP can help improve the quality of primary studies and SRs and meta-analyses across academic disciplines and can be used to guide the process of conducting reviews of reviews. Based on the preliminary findings presented in this chapter, there is a manifest need for the widespread adoption of standardized best practices (e.g., *Cochrane Handbook for Systematic*

Reviews of Interventions and *PRISMA*) for conducting and reporting SRs and meta-analyses. The EMTAP findings also identify a clear need for SRs that consider implementation fidelity and key moderators of intervention effectiveness. Finally, consistent with extant research (e.g., Glasziou et al., 2010; Michie et al., 2009), the EMTAP findings suggest that there are considerable limitations to how interventions are reported in SRs and meta-analyses. SRs are a "cornerstone of evidence-based practice" (The PLoS Medicine Editors, 2007, p. 399), but only when they are well designed, well executed, and transparently reported. Future research should continue to conduct SRs of reviews like the ones presented in this volume and should continue to take a critical look at the quality of the extant SR literature in criminology and related fields.

EMTAP as a Process

As the use of SR and meta-analytic techniques has rapidly expanded over the last two decades, the need to better understand this evidence base has also grown. The rapid growth of SR literature has raised questions about the state of our knowledge and how it can be translated for use in practice. In their recent article in *Implementation Science*, Grimshaw and colleagues (2012) identified "up-to-date systematic reviews" as the "basic unit of knowledge translation" (Grimshaw, Eccles, Lavis, Hill, & Squires, 2012, p. 1). This observation illustrates the importance of SRs and the need for continued growth and development of high-quality systematic reviews and meta-analyses in criminology and other behavioral sciences. The Evidence Mapping to Advance Justice Practice (EMTAP) project was implemented to facilitate the growth of the SR knowledge base by exploring what we know from extant SRs in the areas of behavioral health and correctional programming.

The EMTAP project has helped enhance the understanding of the current state of evidence in health services criminology. The EMTAP project is ongoing and the web-based resource can be accessed at http://www.gmuace.org/tools/evidence-mapping for more information about the reviews that have been conducted to date or to view the knowledge translation and evidence mapping resources that have been developed during the project. Through work on the EMTAP project, researchers at the Center for Advancing Correctional Excellence at George Mason University have developed several tools to standardize and improve SR and review of review search and reporting procedures; have compiled a large, updateable, web-based database that warehouses information on existing SRs and meta-analyses; have identified key limitations of extant reviews that limit their utility for informing justice practice; and have begun work on developing techniques to synthesize the knowledge base from existing SRs and meta-analyses. The EMTAP project is a collaboratory process where researchers can participate to build knowledge for the field. The EMTAP database will be updated and will serve as a valuable knowledge translation resource for both researchers and practitioners.

Appendix A: Summary of EMTAP Percent Reductions by Intervention Category (Source: Adapted from Caudy, Tang, Ainsworth, Lerch, & Taxman (2013))

Intervention	Control group	Recidivism reduction (%)	K[d]	N
Interventions for general offenders				
Cognitive behavioral therapy				
(Lipsey, Landenberger & Wilson, 2007)	NT or Non-CBT	25	58	–
Moral reconation therapy				
(Little, 2005)	Non-MRT	16[a]	9	10,139
(Wilson, Bouffard & MacKenzie, 2005)	NT, Non-CBT, or min tx	35	6	14,118
Reasoning and rehabilitation				
(Tong & Farrington, 2006)	–	14	25	18,234
(Wilson, Bouffard & MacKenzie, 2005)	NT, Non-CBT, or min tx	14	7	2753
Restorative justice				
(Latimer, Dowden & Muise, 2005)	No participation in restorative justice	14[b]	22	–
CBT for anger management				
(Beck & Fernandez, 1998)	–	51	50	1640
Intensive supervision probation w/ Tx				
(Drake, Aos & Miller, 2009)	Any, excluding non-completers	17.9	11	–
RNR supervision				
(Drake, 2011)	NT, TAU, Non-RNR	16	6	–
Electronic monitoring				
(Renzema & Mayo-Wilson, 2005)	Traditional or ISP Probation or Parole, Incarceration, or other	2[a]	3	879
Interventions for substance using offenders				
General drug treatment				
(Holloway, Bennett & Farrington, 2006)	NT	12[a]	22	–
(Prendergast, Podus, Chang & Urada, 2002)	NT, TAU, placebo tx, or tx not intended to produce change	22[a]	25	–
Therapeutic community				
(Lipton, Pearson, Cleland & Yee, 2008)	TAU or unrelated tx	16[a]	35	10,881
(Mitchell, Wilson & MacKenzie, 2007)	TAU, eligible but not referred, historical, other jurisdiction/ facility	27	30	–

Intervention	Control group	Recidivism reduction (%)	K[d]	N
Therapeutic community (Hard Drugs)				
(Holloway, Bennett & Farrington, 2006)	NT	45	7	–
Counseling (General)				
(Mitchell, Wilson & MacKenzie, 2007)	TAU, eligible but not referred, historical, other jurisdiction/ facility	20	25	–
Narcotic maintenance				
(Mitchell, Wilson & MacKenzie, 2007)	TAU, eligible but not referred, historical, other jurisdiction/ facility	9 INCREASE	5	–
Narcotic maintenance (Hard Drugs)				
(Holloway, Bennett & Farrington, 2006)	NT	27[a]	4	–
Boot camp				
(Mitchell, Wilson & MacKenzie, 2007)	TAU, eligible but not referred, historical, other jurisdiction/ facility	5	2	–
Intensive supervision program				
(Perry et al., 2009)	Randomly assigned: minimal, different, or NT	33[a]	24	8936
Post-release supervision				
(Dowden, Antonowicz & Andrews, 2003)	–	26[c]	24	–
Post-release supervision (hard drugs)				
(Holloway, Bennett & Farrington, 2006)	NT	33[a]	3	–
Interventions for offenders with mental illness				
Mental health treatment				
(Martin, Dorken, Wamboldt & Wootten, 2011)	Could not be from treatment refusals and dropouts	17[a]	36	15,512
Vocational/educational programs				
General vocation/education				
(Wilson, Gallagher & MacKenzie, 2000)	No educational, vocational, or work program	21	33	–
Ex-offender employment				
(Visher, Winterfield & Coggeshall, 2005)	TAU or NT	3[a]	8	–
Academic/educational				
(Wilson, Gallagher & MacKenzie, 2000)	No educational, vocational, or work program	18	14	–

Intervention	Control group	Recidivism reduction (%)	K[d]	N
Post-Secondary Correctional Education				
(Wilson, Gallagher & MacKenzie, 2000)	No educational, vocational, or work program	27	13	–
Vocational				
(Wilson, Gallagher & MacKenzie, 2000)	No educational, vocational, or work program	22	17	–
Correctional industries				
(Wilson, Gallagher & MacKenzie, 2000)	No educational, vocational, or work program	19	4	–
Supervision only interventions for general offenders				
Incarceration (vs. community)				
(Smith, Goggin & Gendreau, 2002)	Offenders sentenced to community	14 INCREASE	104	268,806
Intermediate sanctions				
(Smith, Goggin & Gendreau, 2002)	Lesser sanctions (e.g., regular probation)	2	167	66,500
Boot camp				
(Wilson, MacKenzie & Mitchell, 2008)	Probation or incarceration in an alternative facility	1	32	–
Interventions for domestic violence offenders				
General DV treatment (police report)				
*Experimental design only	NT, dropouts, other tx, or incarcerated	16	4	1480
(Babcock, Green, & Robie, 2004)				
(Feder & Wilson, 2005)	NT, TAU, Probation, or Jail	32	4	1962
General DV treatment (Partner Report)				
*Experimental design only	NT, dropouts, other tx, or incarcerated	0	4	1771
(Babcock, Green, & Robie, 2004)				
(Feder & Wilson, 2005)	NT, TAU, Probation, or Jail	10	3	1247
Interventions for Sexual Offenders				
Sex offender treatment (sexual recidivism)				
(Gallagher et al., 1999)	NT, TAU, non-participants, dropouts	37	22	–
(Hanson et al., 2002)	NT	16	38	8164
(Hall, 1995)	NT or other tx	28	12	1313
(Schmucker & Losel, 2008)	NT, TAU, or other tx	36	74[e]	22,181
Sex offender treatment (violent recidivism)				
(Schmucker & Losel, 2008)	NT, TAU, or other tx	44	20[e]	–

Intervention	Control group	Recidivism reduction (%)	K[d]	N
Sex offender treatment (gen. recidivism)				
(Hanson et al., 2002)	NT	31	38	8164
(Schmucker & Losel, 2008)	NT, TAU, or other tx	32	49[e]	–

[a] Calculation assumed 0.50 control recidivism base rate
[b] Standardized mean difference was converted to odds ratio. Phi coefficient was converted to an odds ratio with an assumed 0.50 control recidivism. Success/failure rates for treatment and control groups were used to calculate odds ratio
[c] Treatment and control group recidivism rates were converted to percent reduction
[d] K reflects number of studies included
[e] K reflects number of comparisons included

References

Altman, D. G. (2001). The revised CONSORT statement for reporting randomized trials: Explanation and elaboration. *Annals of Internal Medicine, 134,* 663–694.
Altman, D. G. (2005). Endorsement of the CONSORT statement by high impact medical journal: A survey of instructions for authors. *British Medical Journal, 330,* 1056–1057.
Amato, L., Davoli, M., Vecchi, S., Ali, R., Farrell, M., Faggiano, F., Foxcroft, D., Ling, W., Minozzi, S., Chengzheng, Z. (2011). Cochrane systematic reviews in the field of addiction: What's there and what should be. *Drug and Alcohol Dependence, 113,* 96–103.
Arnqvist, G., & Wooster, D. (1995). Meta-analysis: Synthesizing research findings in ecology and evolution. *Trends in Ecology and Evolution, 10*(6), 236–240.
Babcock, J. C., Green, C. E., & Robie, C. (2004). Does batterers' treatment work? A meta-analytic review of domestic violence treatment. *Clinical Psychology Review, 23*(8), 1023–1053.
Beck, R., & Fernandez, E. (1998). Cognitive-behavioral therapy in the treatment of anger: A meta-analysis. *Cognitive Therapy and Research, 22*(1), 63–74.
Becker, L. A. & Oxman, O. D. (2011). Overviews of reviews. In J. P. T. Higgins & S. Green (Eds.), *Cochrane Handbook for Systematic Reviews of Interventions* Version 5.1.0 (Chapter 22). www.cochrane-handbook.org.
Begg, C., Moher, D., & Schulz, K. F. (1996). Improving the quality of reporting of randomized controlled trials: The CONSORT statement. *Journal of the American Medical Association, 276*(8), 637–639.
Bonta, J. & Andrews, D. A. (2007). *Risk-Need-Responsivity model for offender assessment and treatment* (User Report 2007–06). Ottawa: Public Safety Canada.
Borenstein, M., Hedges, L. V., Higgins, J. P. T., & Rothstein, H. R. (2009). *Introduction to meta-analysis.* Hoboken: Wiley.
Caudy, M., Tang, L., Ainsworth, S. A., Lerch, J., & Taxman, F. S. (2013). Reducing recidivism through correctional programming: Using meta-analyses to inform the RNR Simulation Tool. In F. S. Taxman & A. Pattavina (Eds.), *Simulation Strategies to Reduce Recidivism: Risk Need Responsivity (RNR) Modeling in the Criminal Justice System* (pp. 167–193). New York: Springer.
Center for Advancing Correctional Excellence. (2012). *Evidence mapping to advance justice practice* [Data File]. http://www.gmuace.org/tools/evidencemapping.php
Chan, A., Hrobjartsson, A., Haahr, M. T., Gotzsche, P. C. & Altman, D. G. (2004). Empirical evidence for selective reporting of outcomes in randomized trials: Comparison of protocols to published articles. *Journal of the American Medical Association, 291*(20), 2457–2465.

Cipriani, A., Furukawa, T. A., Salanti, G., Geddes, J. R., Higgins, J. P. T., Churchill, R., Watanabe, N., Nakagawa, A., Omori, IM., McGuire, H., Tansella, M., Barbui, C. (2009). Comparative efficacy and acceptability of 12 new-generation antidepressants: A multiple-treatments meta-analysis. *The Lancet, 373,* 746–758.

Cook, T. D., & Leviton, L. C. (1980). Reviewing the literature: A comparison of traditional methods with meta-analysis. *Journal of Personality, 48,* 449–472.

Dane, A. V., & Schneider, B. H. (1998). Program integrity in primary and early secondary prevention: Are implementation effects out of control? *Clinical Psychology Review, 18,* 23–45.

Delaney, A., Bagshaw, S. M., Ferland, A., Manns, B., & Laupland, K. B. (2005). A systematic evaluation of the quality of meta-analysis in the critical care literature. *Critical Care, 9,* R575–R582.

Dowden, C., Antonowicz, D., & Andrews, D. A. (2003). The effectiveness of relapse prevention with offenders: A meta-analysis. *International Journal of Offender Therapy and Comparative Criminology, 47*(5), 516–528.

Drake E. K. (2011). *"What works" in community supervision: Interim report* (Document No. 11-12-1201). Olympia: Washington State Institute for Public Policy.

Drake, E., Aos, S., & Miller, M. (2009). Evidence-based public policy options to reduce crime and criminal justice costs: Implications in Washington State (No. 09–00-1201). Washington State Institute for Public Policy.

Egger, M., & Smith, G. D. (1998). Meta-analysis bias in location and selection of studies. *British Medical Journal, 361,* 61–66.

Egger, M., Smith, G. D., & Phillips, A. N. (1997). Meta-analysis: Principles and procedures. *British Medical Journal, 315,* 1533–1537

Feder, L., & Wilson, D. B. (2005). A meta-analytic review of court-mandated batterer intervention programs: Can courts affect abusers' behavior? *Journal of Experimental Criminology, 1*(2), 239–262.

Fixsen, D. L., Naoom, S. F., Blase, K. A., Friedman, R. M., & Wallace, F. (2005). *Implementation research: A synthesis of the literature.* Tampa: University of South Florida, Louis de la Parte Florida Mental Health Institute, The National Implementation Research Network (FMHI Publication #231).

Gallagher, C. A., Wilson, D. B., Paul Hirschfield, M. A., Coggeshall, M. B., & MacKenzie, D. L. (1999). Quantitative review of the effects of sex offender treatment on sexual reoffending. *Corrections Management Quarterly, 3*(4), 11.

Glass, G. V. (1977). Integrating findings: The meta-analysis of research. *Review of Research in Education, 5,* 351–379.

Glasziou, P., Chalmers, I., Altman, D. G., Bastian, H., Boutron, I., Brice, A., Jamtvedt, G., Farmer, A., Ghersi, D., Groves, T., Heneghan, C., Hill, S., Lewin, S., Michie, S., Perera, R., Pomeroy, V., Tilson, J., Shepperd, S., Williams, J. W. (2010). Taking healthcare interventions from trial to practice. *British Medical Journal, 341,* 384–387.

Golder, S., Loke, Y. K., & Bland, M. (2011). Meta-analysis of adverse effects data derived from randomised controlled trials as compared to observational studies: Methodological overview. *PLoS Medicine, 8*(5), 1–13.

Green, L. W. & Glasgow, R. E. (2006). Evaluating the relevance, generalization, and applicability of research: Issues in external validation and translation methodology. *Evaluation & Health Professions, 29,* 126–153.

Griffith, J. W., Rowan-Szal, G. A., Roark, R. R., & Simpson, D. D. (2000). Contingency management in outpatient methadone treatment: A meta-analysis. *Drug and Alcohol Dependence, 58*(1–2), 55–66.

Grimshaw, J. M., Eccles, M. P., Lavis, J. N., Hill, S. J., & Squires, J. E. (2012). Knowledge translation of research findings. *Implementation Science, 7*(50), 7–50.

Hall, G. C. N. (1995). Sexual offender recidivism revisited: A meta-analysis of recent treatment studies. *Journal of Consulting and Clinical Psychology, 63*(5), 802–809.

Hammerstrom, K., Wade, E. & Jorgensen, A. K. (2010). Searching for studies: A guide to information retrieval for Campbell systematic reviews. http://www.campbellcollaboration.org/resources/research/new_information_retrieval_guide.php

Hanson, R. K., Gordon, A., Harris, A. J. R., Marques, J. K., Murphy, W., Quinsey, V. L., & Seto, M. C. (2002). First report of the collaborative outcome data project on the effectiveness of psychological treatment for sex offenders. *Sexual Abuse: A Journal of Research and Treatment, 14*(2), 169–194.

Higgins, J. P. T., & Deeks, J. J. (2011). Selecting studies and collecting data. In J. P. T. Higgins & S. Green (Eds.), *Cochrane handbook for systematic reviews of interventions*, Version 5.1.0 (Chapter 7). www.cochrane-handbook.org.

Higgins, J. P. T., & Green, S. (Eds.). (2011). Cochrane handbook for systematic reviews of interventions, Version 5.1.0. www.cochrane-handbook.org.

Holloway, K. R., Bennett, T. H., & Farrington, D. P. (2006). The effectiveness of drug treatment programs in reducing criminal behavior: A meta-analysis. *Psicothema, 18*(3), 620–629.

Jadad, A. R., Cook, D. J., & Browman, G. P. (1997). A guide to interpreting discordant systematic reviews. *Canadian Medical Association Journal, 156*(10), 1411–1416.

Latimer, J., Dowden, C., & Muise, D. (2005). The effectiveness of restorative justice practices: A meta-analysis. *The Prison Journal, 85*(2), 127–144.

Lefebvre, C., Manheimer, E. & Glanville, J. (2011). Searching for studies. In J. P. T. Higgins & S. Green (Eds.), *Cochrane handbook for systematic reviews of interventions*, Version 5.1.0 (Chapter 6). www.cochrane-handbook.org.

Lipsey, M. W. (2003). Those confounded moderators in meta-analysis good, bad and ugly. *The Annals of the American Academy of Political and Social Science, 587*(1), 69–81.

Lipsey, M. W., & Cullen, F. T. (2007). The effectiveness of correctional rehabilitation: A review of systematic reviews. *Annual Review of Law and Social Science, 3*, 297–320.

Lipsey, M.W., Landenberger, N.A. & Wilson, S.J. (2007). Effects of cognitive-behavioral programs for criminal offenders. *Campbell Systematic Reviews, 3*(6). http://campbellcollaboration.org/lib/project/29/.

Lipsey, M. W., & Wilson, D. B. (2001). *Practical meta-analysis*. Thousand Oaks: Sage Publications.

Lipton, D. S., Pearson, F. S., Cleland, C. M., & Yee, D. (2008). The effects of therapeutic communities and milieu therapy on recidivism: Meta–analytic findings from the correctional drug abuse treatment effectiveness (CDATE) study. In J. McGuire (Ed.), *Offender Rehabilitation and Treatment* (pp. 39–77). John Wiley & Sons Ltd.

Little, G. L. (2005). Meta-analysis of moral reconation therapy recidivism results from probation and parole implementations. *Cognitive Behavioral Treatment Review, 14*(1/2), 14–16.

Lussier, J. P., Heil, S. H., Mongeon, J. A., Badger, G. J., & Higgins, S. T. (2006). A meta-analysis of voucher-based reinforcement therapy for substance use disorders. *Addiction, 101*(2), 192–203.

Martin, M. S., Dorken, S. K., Wamboldt, A. D., & Wootten, S. E. (2011). Stopping the revolving door: A meta-analysis on the effectiveness of interventions for criminally involved individuals with major mental disorders. *Law and Human Behavior, 36*(1), 1–15.

Meade, M. O., & Richardson, S. (1997). Selecting and appraising studies for a systematic review. *Annals of Internal Medicine, 127*(7), 531–537.

Michie, S., & Abraham, C. (2008). Advancing the science of behavior change: A plea for scientific reporting. *Addiction, 103*, 1409–1410.

Michie, S., Fixsen, D., Grimshaw, J. W., & Eccles, M. P. (2009). Specifying and reporting complex behaviour change interventions: The need for a scientific method. *Implementation Science, 4*(1), 40–45.

Michie, S., & Prestwich, A. (2010). Are interventions theory-based? Development of a theory coding scheme. *Health Psychology, 29*(1), 1–8.

Mitchell, O., Wilson, D. B., & MacKenzie, D. L. (2007). Does incarceration-based drug treatment reduce recidivism? A meta-analytic synthesis of the research. *Journal of Experimental Criminology, 3*(4), 353–375.

Moher, D., Cook, D. J., Eastwood, S., Olkin, I., Rennie, D., & Stroup, D. F. (1999). Improving the quality of reports of meta-analysis of randomised controlled trials: The QUOROM statement. *The Lancet, 354,* 1896–1901.

Moher, D., Jones, A., & Lepage, L. (2001). Use of the CONSORT statement and quality of reports of randomized trials: A comparative before-and-after evaluation. *Journal of American Medical Association, 285*(15), 1992–1995.

Moher, D., Liberati, A., Tetzlaff, J., & Altman, D. G. (2009). Preferred reporting items for systematic reviews and meta-analyses: The PRISMA statement. *PLoS Medicine, 6*(7), 1–6.

Moher, D., Tetzlaff, J., Tricco, A. C., Sampson, M., & Altman, D. G., (2007). Epidemiology and reporting characteristics of systematic reviews. *PLoS Medicine, 4*(3), 0477–0455.

Pearson, F. S., Prendergast, M. L., Podus, D., Vazan, P., Greenwell, L., & Hamilton, Z. (2012). Meta-analyses of seven of the National Institute on Drug Abuse's principles of drug addiction treatment. *Journal of Substance Abuse Treatment, 43,* 1–11.

Perry, A. E., Darwin, Z., Godfrey, C., McDougall, C., Lunn, J., Glanville, J., & Coulton, S. (2009). The effectiveness of interventions for drug-using offenders in courts, secure establishments and the community: A systematic review. *Substance Use & Misuse, 44*(3), 374–400.

Perry, A. E., Weisburd, D., & Hewitt, C. (2010). Are criminologists describing randomized controlled trials in ways that allow us to assess them? Findings from a sample of crime and justice trials. *Journal of Experimental Criminology, 6,* 245–262.

Plint, A. C., Moher, D., Morrison, A., Schulz, K., Altman, D. G., Hill, C., & Gaboury, I. (2006). Does the CONSORT checklist improve the quality of reporting randomized controlled trials? A systematic review. *The Medical Journal of Australia, 185*(5), 263–267.

Pratt, T. C. (2010). Meta-analysis in criminal justice and criminology: What it is, when it's useful, and what to watch out for. *Journal of Criminal Justice Education, 21*(2), 153–168.

Prendergast, M., Podus, D., Finney, J., Greenwell, L. & Roll, J. (2006). Contingency management for treatment of substance use disorders: A meta-analysis. *Addiction, 101*(11), 1546–1560.

Prendergast, M. L., Podus, D., Chang, E., & Urada, D. (2002). The effectiveness of drug abuse treatment: A meta-analysis of comparison group studies. *Drug and Alcohol Dependence, 67*(1), 53–72.

Renzema, M., & Mayo-Wilson, E. (2005). Can electronic monitoring reduce crime for moderate to high-risk offenders? *Journal of Experimental Criminology, 1,* 215–237.

Rudes, D. S., Portillo, S., Murphy, A., Rhodes, A., Stitzer, M., Luongo, P., & Taxman, F.S. (2012). Adding positive reinforcements in a criminal justice setting: Acceptability and feasibility. *The Journal of Substance Abuse Treatment, 42*(3), 269–270.

Schmucker, M., & Lösel, F. (2008). Does sexual offender treatment work? A systematic review of outcome evaluations. *Psicothema, 20*(1), 10–19.

Schoenwald, S. K., & Hoagwood, K. (2001). Effectiveness, transportability, and dissemination of interventions: What matters when? *Psychiatric Services, 52*(9), 1190–1197.

Silagy, C. A., Middleton, P., & Hopewell, S. (2002). Publishing protocols of systematic reviews: Comparing what was done to what was planned. *Journal of the American Medical Association, 287*(21), 2831–2834.

Smith, P., Goggin, C., & Gendreau, P. (2002). The effects of prison and intermediate sanctions on recidivism: General effects and individual differences. Ottawa, Canada: Department of Solicitor General Canada, Ottawa.

Sterne, J. A. C., & Harbord, R. M. (2004). Funnel plots in meta-analysis. *The Stata Journal, 4*(2), 127–141.

Taxman, F. S., & Belenko, S. (2012). *Implementing evidence-based practices in community corrections and addiction treatment.* New York: Springer.

Taxman, F. S., & Bouffard, J. A. (2000). The importance of systems in improving offender outcomes: New frontiers in treatment integrity. *Justice Research and Policy, 2*(2), 37–58.

Taxman, F. S., & Bouffard, J. A. (2002). Assessing therapeutic integrity in modified therapeutic communities for drug-involved offenders. *The Prison Journal, 82*(2), 189–212.

The PLoS Medicine Editors. (2007). Many reviews are systematic but some are more transparent and completely reported than others. *PLoS Medicine, 4*(3), 0399–0400.

Tong, J., & Farrington, D. P. (2006). How effective is the "Reasoning and Rehabilitation" programme in reducing reoffending? A meta-analysis of evaluations in four countries. *Psychology, Crime & Law, 12*(1), 3–24.

Visher, C., Winterfield, L., & Coggeshall, M. (2005). Ex-offender employment programs and recidivism: A meta-analysis. *Journal of Experimental Criminology, 1*(3), 295–316.

Wells, E. (2009). Uses of meta-analysis in criminal justice research: A quantitative review. *Justice Quarterly, 26*(2), 268–294.

Wilson, D. B. (2001). Meta-analytic methods for criminology. *The Annals of the American Academy, 587*, 71–89.

Wilson, D. B. (2009). Missing a critical piece of the pie: Simple document search strategies inadequate for systematic reviews. *Journal of Experimental Criminology, 5*(4), 429–440.

Wilson, D. B. (2010). Meta-analysis. In A. R. Piquero & D. Weisburd (Eds.). *Handbook of Quantitative Criminology* (pp. 181–208). New York: Springer.

Wilson, D. B., Bouffard, L. A., & MacKenzie, D. L. (2005). A quantitative review of structured, group-oriented, cognitive-behavioral programs for offenders. *Criminal Justice and Behavior, 32*(2), 172–204.

Wilson, D. B., Gallagher, C. A., & MacKenzie, D. L. (2000). A meta-analysis of corrections-based education, vocation, and work programs for adult offenders. *Journal of Research in Crime and Delinquency, 37*(4), 347–368.

Wilson, D. B., MacKenzie, D. L., & Mitchell, F. N. (2008). Effects of correctional boot camps on offending. *Campbell Systematic Reviews, 1*(6), 1–42.

Workgroup for Intervention Development and Evaluation Research. (2009). WIDER recommendations to improve reporting of the content of behavior change interventions. http://interventiondesign.co.uk/wp-content/uploads/2009/02/wider-recommendations.pdf

Chapter 11
Economic Analyses

Jacqueline Mallender and Rory Tierney

Analysis of programme spending of any Western government at federal or state level will show investments in interventions to keep communities safe, maintain law and order, prevent crime, reduce offending and reduce re-offending. This chapter explores what has been learned from systematic reviews about the costs and benefits of criminal justice interventions and how economic analysis can be used to inform investment and disinvestment decisions of policymakers.

The chapter is divided into five sections. The first section provides a brief overview of the background to economic evaluation in criminal justice. It then goes on to report the results of four systematic reviews of economic studies. This leads to a discussion of the current limitations of primary studies and indeed synthesis of economic evaluation. The penultimate section presents a complementary decision analytic approach which, while informed by reviews, enables jurisdiction-specific economic analysis of crime and justice programmes. A case study is presented from the Washington State Institute for Public Policy. The final section concludes with some recommendations for policymakers and researchers to build on the lessons learned so far.

Background to Economic Evaluation in Criminal Justice

Typically, when policymakers are thinking about costs and benefits they are asking the following questions:

- What are the resource costs of the intervention or programme compared with the value of the benefits it will deliver?

J. Mallender (✉)
Optimity Advisors, London, UK
e-mail: jacque.mallender@optimityadvisors.com

R. Tierney
Optimity Advisors, London, UK
e-mail: rory.tierney@optimityadvisors.com

- What is the return on investment for the public purse and the wider economy?
- How can spending on different interventions be prioritised?

The discipline of cost-benefit analysis has been developed to answer these questions (National Institute for Health and Care Excellence (NICE), 2011; Cohen, 2000). Models for economic analysis include:

- Cost-effectiveness analysis, designed to look at the technical efficiency of a decision and identify the least cost alternative to achieve any given outcome;
- Cost-utility analysis, designed to look at the costs of achieving a level of benefit measured on a utility scale (a good example of this in healthcare is the quality adjusted life year (QALY) or disability adjusted life year (DALY));
- Cost-benefit analysis, designed to compare costs and benefits in monetary terms
- Cost-consequence analysis, designed to look at costs and outcomes in discrete categories, without weighting or combining them. (See National Institute for Health and Care Excellence, 2011; National Information Center on Health Services Research and Health Care Technology, 2012; Welsh & Farrington, 2000.) The differences between these approaches are summarised in Table 11.1.

All of these models involve analysing economic data over time while adjusting for inflation and discounting future values. This enables consistent reporting of the real economic return in present value terms. Economic evaluation includes consideration of concepts such as opportunity cost, marginal and average costs, fixed and variable costs, current and future costs, tangible and intangible costs, and current and inflation adjusted costs (Cohen, 2000).

Cost-utility analysis is commonly used in healthcare, such as analyses for the National Institute of Health and Care Excellence (NICE) in the UK, which measure benefits in the form of QALYs, a composite measure of quality and quantity of life that allows comparison between health interventions (Marsh, 2010a). However, HM Treasury in the UK recommends cost-benefit analysis—which quantifies outputs in monetary terms—for public appraisal, as compared to cost-effectiveness analysis, which 'compares the costs of alternative ways of producing the same or similar outputs,' while noting that cost-utility analysis can be used if an appropriate human welfare benefit measure is available (HM Treasury, 2003). Comparability of studies

Table 11.1 Comparison of models for economic analysis

Type	Components
Cost-effectiveness analysis	Incremental cost (£)
	Given output/outcome/benefit
Cost-utility analysis	Incremental cost (£)
	Incremental benefit (units of benefit)
Cost-benefit analysis	Incremental cost (£)
	Incremental benefit (£)
Cost-consequence analysis	Incremental cost (£)
	Incremental benefit (£ or units of benefit—i.e. cases of x)

must be borne in mind—as cost–benefit studies produce outputs in monetary terms this allows evaluations to be measured against each other, while standardisation of outputs (e.g. QALYs) is needed to compare cost-utility analyses.

Economic analysis of crime and criminal justice aspires to use these techniques to answer questions about the value of investment in crime prevention programmes. The discipline has roots dating back to Becker's (1968) seminal work on the costs of crime. Since then there have been a variety of papers classifying and estimating costs of crime across a variety of perspectives, and in the last decade, the body of information has grown still further (see, for example, Welsh & Farrington, 2000; Cohen, 2005; Home Office, 2011—update of Dubourg, Hamed, & Thorns, 2005; Dhiri & Brand, 1999; Brand & Price, 2000; Godfrey, Stewart, & Gossop, 2004; Dolan, Loomes, Peasgood, & Tsuchiya, 2005; McCollister, French, & Fang 2010; Lee, Aos, & Pennucci, 2015).

Increasingly, governments are publishing comprehensive guides at federal and state levels to support those undertaking research into the costs and benefits of justice programmes. Examples include the Cost-Benefit Knowledge Bank for Criminal Justice, a project by the Vera Institute of Justice funded by the U.S. Department of Justice's Bureau of Justice Assistance (Cost-Benefit Knowledge Bank for Criminal Justice, 2015) and recent initiatives of the UK Home Office (Home Office, 2011, update of Dubourg, Hamed, & Thorns, 2005), and the Australian Institute for Criminology (Dossetor, 2011).

These resources are available to researchers and research funders to support the assessment of costs and benefits of criminal justice interventions and programmes. For instance, the UK Home Office (Home Office, 2011) makes public its 'unit costs of crime and multipliers' data, updated for 2010/2011 in the latest version. Unit costs, for a variety of different types of crime, reflect costs borne in anticipation, as a consequence, and in response to that crime. Multipliers reflect the disparity between the number of crimes recorded by police, and the estimated total numbers of crime.

As an example, unit costs at 2010 prices are given at £ 4970 for theft of a vehicle and £ 1034 for theft from a vehicle, with respective multipliers of 1.3 and 3.5 (suggesting most thefts of vehicles are recorded by police but most thefts from vehicles are not). The availability of these data provides a useful basis for research into the costs and benefits of criminal justice interventions (Home Office, 2011)

Findings from Systematic Reviews of Economic Studies

Given the four decades of established research in the costs of crime, policymakers who want to know whether investment in particular types of criminal justice interventions provides value for money might expect to find a bank of research from which they can draw conclusions, but sadly this is not the case. Good-quality economic studies available for review are still comparatively rare (Welsh & Farrington, 2000; Farrington, Petrosino, & Welsh, 2001; Swaray, Bowles & Pradiptyo, 2005;

McDougall, Cohen, Swaray, & Perry, 2008; Byford, Barrett, Dubourg, Francis, & Sisk, 2010; Marsh, 2010b).

The absence of primary research means that there are also only a limited number of published systematic reviews that report costs and benefits from real-world studies of interventions in crime prevention and criminal justice. In a review of the literature, Marsh (2010b) references four major reviews of crime prevention, sentencing and correctional interventions: Welsh and Farrington (2000), Farrington et al. (2001), Swaray et al. (2005) and McDougall et al. (2008). These are discussed sequentially in this section.

There is some overlap in primary studies (particularly between Welsh and Farrington (2000) and Farrington et al. (2001), where the latter is referred to by the authors as an update of an element of the former). However, the reviews are presented separately as they each take a slightly different approach to synthesis and reporting.

In their review of crime prevention studies, Welsh and Farrington's (2000) identified 26 candidates for economic analysis. The authors undertook a search of criminological, psychological, health, economic and medical literatures throughout the Western world to identify studies in crime prevention that had included economic analysis. They also consulted experts to identify relevant unpublished 'grey' literature.

From their research, the authors were able to look at four programme areas: situational crime prevention, developmental interventions, community prevention, and correctional intervention. A summary of findings is shown in Table 11.2.

Across each of these areas there were 'hopeful indications that benefits often exceed costs'. Of the 26 studies, 20 showed a positive benefit-cost ratio with some studies showing benefits in excess of five times the value of the investment.

The authors were unable to draw stronger conclusions because of the small number of studies and the lack of standardisation across the studies in terms of quality,

Table 11.2 Summary of findings from Monetary Costs and Benefits of Crime Prevention Programmes, Welsh and Farrington (2000)

	Situational crime prevention studies	Developmental prevention studies	Correctional intervention studies[a]	Community crime prevention programme
Number of studies included in the review	13	6	6 (*5 delivered in community settings*)	1
Number of studies where benefits exceeded costs (range of benefit: cost ratio)	8 (1.31–5.04)	5 (1.06–7.16)	6 (1.13–7.14)	1 (2.55)
Number of studies where costs exceeded benefits (range of benefit: cost ratio)	5 (0.32–0.78)	1 (0.38)	n/a	

[a] 5 of these studies were delivered in a community setting

scope or coverage. For example, they were not able to compare programmes or interventions within programmes.

In a more recent study by Farrington et al. (2001), economic studies of correctional services were selected for a more focused systematic review. The authors presented this as providing an update to the Welsh and Farrington (2000) study.

Criteria for inclusion in this review were that the studies:

- involved a clear definition of interventions—only interventions that went beyond punishment and modified behaviour were included;
- included reported outcomes in terms of re-offending in the community;
- were based on real experiments or quasi-experiments; and
- reported either a benefit-cost ratio or sufficient data to calculate one.

Searches included the Social Sciences Citation Index (1981–1998) of the Institute for Scientific Information database on the Internet-accessible Bibliographic Databases service, the most recent issues of major European and North American criminological journals, bibliographies of leading narrative and empirical (e.g. meta-analytic) studies, reviews of the literature on the effectiveness of correctional intervention programmes, and grey and yet unpublished literature were identified via leading researchers in the fields of correctional intervention and welfare economics.

A total of nine studies were identified. These included counselling, training, employment, drug treatment and other rehabilitative interventions delivered in both community and institutional settings and across an array of offender population types and age groups. All studies reported a positive benefit-cost ratio ranging from 1.13 to 7.14.

The authors did not draw conclusions about how specific interventions ranked comparatively from an economic perspective on account of the small number of studies and wide differences in methods used, scope of costs and benefits considered, and coverage and diversity of interventions. However, the consistent positive return on investment from correctional interventions which have a significant effect on reducing re-offending is to be noted.

The review by Swaray et al. (2005) covered published and grey literature on proactive and reactive criminal justice interventions. The authors describe their study as a hybrid between the more structured and rigorous methodology required in a systematic review study and the less rigorous but critical approach used in traditional literature. They identified only ten studies which distinguished themselves in: attempting to monetise intangible costs and benefits, using good-quality study designs, having appropriate internal validity measures and being backed by substantive content and rigorous study methodology. Interestingly, only one study (Knapp, Robertson, & McIvor, 1992) was experimental in design. The ten studies covered an array of interventions including situational crime prevention (residential electronic security, street lighting, etc.), and offender rehabilitative interventions and treatments (including for substance misuse and paedophiles). The authors commented on the potential for economic benefits from these type of interventions but did not report benefit to cost ratios. They did provide a comprehensive discussion about methodological differences between the studies. The authors concluded by calling for 'improvement in the methodological standards of study and data collection in projects that seek policy-relevant answers from economic analysis".

McDougall et al. (2008) report a systematic review of studies of the benefits and costs of sentencing. The study is published as a Campbell Collaboration systematic review and the full details of the search strategy and quality assessment protocols are reported in accordance with Campbell Collaboration requirements. The review covered studies published between 1980 and 2001 in a comprehensive array of databases and/or consulted experts for unpublished and grey literature in the field. Studies were assessed for inclusion in the review based on selection criteria which combined study design with economic quality requirements. The authors used the Benefit-Cost Validity Scale (Revised) developed by Cohen and McDougall (2008) to rate the quality of the economic information presented.

The authors found only nine benefit-cost studies meeting their selection criteria on study design and only six which met their economic quality requirements. Of these six, results varied both across and within studies. However, they were able to conclude that, from the studies they had examined, the following types of interventions were cost-beneficial: in-prison sex offender treatment, diversion from imprisonment to drug treatment, and imprisonment for high risk offenders (though not for less prolific offenders or for drug offenders).

As only a limited number of benefit-cost studies were identified, the authors also considered cost-effectiveness analyses (where benefits are not monetised), of which 11 were identified. However, they found the methodology in many of these studies to be poor. Frequently, the analyses did not take the key aims of the interventions under study, for example crime or re-offence reduction, as a major outcome measure. Seven studies were experimental or quasi-experimental, but only one of these was a randomised controlled trial (RCT, considered to be the strongest level of evaluation as per the Maryland Scientific Methods Scale of Sherman et al., 1997). Eight of the eleven studies found the target intervention to be cost-effective, but the authors advise caution when interpreting these results, especially from single studies. Four studies examined intensive supervision, but the results were contradictory: one showed it to be cost-effective versus imprisonment, one was inconclusive versus institutional placements or traditional probation, one showed mixed results against imprisonment and probation, and one—the RCT—found intensive supervision was not cost-effective versus traditional parole. Further, more rigorous analysis is needed to establish which variables are important for such an intervention to be considered cost-effective, and this is shown by the review.

Limitations of Primary Studies and Synthesis

The authors of all of the reviews discussed in the previous section were consistent in their reporting of limitations and shortcomings associated with economic studies.

Marsh (2010b) explored this further in his review of economic studies from a methods perspective. He undertook a review of all English language studies published between 2000 and 2006 across a range of criminal justice, economics and social science databases as well as consulting experts for unpublished and grey literature. He selected studies based on whether they reported an evaluation of an intervention in a real world setting, contained some form of economic analysis, and targeted a reduction in criminal behaviour as an outcome.

The author identified 61 studies: 39 from the USA, 19 from the UK, 2 from Australia, and 1 from Sweden. Of these 42 were cost-benefit analysis; 14 were cost-effectiveness studies and the remainder cost analysis.

Marsh (2010b) adopted a number of quality criteria for economic studies and he reviewed the UK and USA studies against each. Some of these were taken into consideration in the selection of studies and hence compliance scored highly. Studies were generally transparent in the recording of costs (95 % of UK studies and 93 % of US studies) and outcomes (100 %), and were clear about the economic perspective taken (100 %). However, there was significant variation in study design (only 32 % of the UK studies were experimental compared to 63 % of the US studies). The economic analysis varied too: in the UK, 67 % of studies measured costs from a 'bottom-up' analysis of resources; 47 % adjusted for inflation and 44 % used discounting techniques to compare costs over time. Similar figures for the USA were 47, 45 and 24 % respectively. Sensitivity analysis was only conducted in 11 % of the UK studies although the figure was much higher for US studies (42 %).

Strikingly, Marsh (2010b) compares the 61 studies he was able to identify and the 26 identified by Welsh and Farrington (2000), with the 3,736 economic evaluations identified by Kentaro, Duffy, and Tsutani (2004) in the UK National Health Service Economic Evaluation Database (NHS EED). According to the UK National Institute for Health Research, Centre for Reviews and Dissemination website, as of August 2015, there are currently over 17,000 health economic evaluations on NHS EED (Centre for Reviews and Dissemination, 2015).

Even where there is a wealth of good-quality primary economic analysis (such as healthcare), Anderson and Shemilt (2010) provide a strong set of arguments as to why systematic reviews of economic evaluations might still be of limited value to policymakers. The authors present a number of issues which challenge the premise that synthesis of economic evaluations is fit for purpose, namely to identify some generalisable estimate of the cost-effectiveness of an intervention. In summary they argue that not all variation in methods is due to lack of standards or compliance. Rather, international variation in methods is likely and justifiable (Sculpher & Drummond, 2006) and should be accepted as an inevitable consequence of this kind of analysis. Moreover, context matters: the resources required to deliver an intervention and their unit costs are likely to vary across geographies, time and the availability of existing infrastructure and services. This will impact on average and marginal costs, economies of scale, inter-country exchange rates, etc. (Sculpher et al., 2004). The same is true of benefits and their associated values (Shiell, Hawe, & Gold, 2008). Anderson and Shemilt (2010) do argue a role for systematic review of economic studies, if it is to: help provide data and information to populate new economic models, source relevant studies for a specific topic or intervention, help build theories about economic relationships, or simply map the existing evidence.

They reference different types of synthesis (see for example Hammersley's (2002) typology of evidence synthesis strategies) as providing a broader framework than has typically been adopted by those undertaking systematic reviews of economic studies.

Overall, the small number of studies, the rarity of experimental study designs, and the wide variations in methods of estimating costs and benefits limit the usefulness of synthesis (Byford et al., 2010). Until policymakers consistently fund cost-benefit analysis as an integral part of any impact evaluation of interventions or programmes then this huge shortage of primary studies will continue. To rely on systematic review of primary studies of the costs and benefits of criminal justice interventions to assess economic impact would be the equivalent of 'Waiting for Godot' (Beckett, 1954).

The Use of Decision Models to Estimate Costs and Benefits

Given the limited ability of researchers and policymakers to rely on reviews to provide evidence of the economic costs and benefits of crime and justice interventions, some policymakers have focused instead on the use of economic models or 'decision models'. For example, the NICE public health methods guidance (National Institute for Health and Care Excellence, 2012) recommends that, in addition to systematic reviews of economic evaluations, a "cost-effectiveness analysis could be modelled [either] on a single well-conducted randomised controlled trial (RCT), or using decision-analytic techniques to analyse probability, cost and health-outcome data from a variety of published sources". NICE began producing public health guidance after setting up the Centre for Public Health Excellence in 2005 (National Institute for Health and Care Excellence, 2009). As of analysis conducted in 2012, nearly 50 % of the NICE public health guidelines use either a static or dynamic decision model for economic analysis (Mallender et al., 2012).

In 2009, Health England commissioned research to assess whether it was possible or feasible to use this type of modelling to create a list of interventions which could be ranked or prioritised by policymakers (Matrix, 2009). Public health programmes were evaluated according to the number of people who benefit and the distribution of these benefits between population groups, as well as according to their cost effectiveness. Using multi-criteria decision analysis, the interventions were ranked on the basis of criteria defined by decision makers and their stated priorities. Cost-effectiveness was measured using decision models built using information derived from systematic review. Interestingly, using this approach, policymakers did not always prioritise those interventions which provided the greatest economic return; recognising that other criteria such as health inequalities, programme reach and affordability were also important (Matrix, 2009).

Economic decision models can be combined with systematic review to help policymakers understand the economic choices they are making when they invest in one intervention over another and/or one programme of interventions over another.

In criminal justice, perhaps the most widely known example is the analysis produced regularly by the Washington State Institute for Public Policy. First established in the mid-1990s to identify policies which are demonstrated as improving outcomes, it has developed since then and now provides estimates of the costs and benefits of programmes and policies across a wide range of topics including crime, education, child welfare, mental health and substance abuse. The Institute provides a regular report of the latest list of evidence-based interventions for reducing crime, which includes an independent assessment of the benefits and costs of each option from the perspective of Washington citizens and taxpayers (Lee, Aos, & Pennucci, 2015).

There is a risk of placing too much emphasis on these type of models. They are still reliant on primary studies (which we know to be scarce) and the complexity of the modelling and assumptions results in associated uncertainty. The Institute's model has not gone without criticism (Roman & Downey, 2010). However, the report includes a very comprehensive detailed technical appendix which outlines how the work is undertaken. Comparing these over time, it is possible to see continuous improvement in methods. For example, in the April 2012 update (Lee et al., 2012a) and technical appendix (Lee et al., 2012b), the authors draw attention to their solution to a biasing error (this change is described in the main report, and a full methodology is given in the technical appendix). Previously, when a number of outcomes were monetised through changes in a single measure (e.g. lifetime earnings), the highest value was allowed to 'trump' the others to avoid double counting. However, it was identified through Monte Carlo simulations that this favoured policies that measured multiple outcomes, as 'consistently selecting the highest of the [several] values biased the results in a positive direction'. As such, the methodology was adjusted to take a weighted average of all outcomes that are monetised from the same source, in order to correct this.

One of the main drivers of the work of the Institute is to prepare estimates which are internally consistent and can be used to compare one intervention with another and one programme over another; this overcomes the massive variability which is seen in any review of primary economic studies. The models are also built on a rigorous review of primary studies complemented with a clear and published meta-analytic strategy. The modelling enables an assessment of costs and benefits in the long run and associated risks and uncertainties. Detailed calculations are presented to show how the model estimates the marginal and capital costs of crime and the benefits to the state and to victims of crimes prevented by combining cost and prevalence data for adult and juvenile interventions, as well as prison and police policies. A summary of results is shown below.

Table 11.3 provides a summary of their findings for each type of intervention, ranked on the basis of the net financial benefit (benefits minus costs) discounted to present-day values.

As can be seen, the police interventions provide the highest return on investment by a large margin (in the order of $500,000). Of the 17 juvenile justice interventions, 16 provide positive benefits, and 15 provide a return on investment which outweighs costs (with benefit-cost ratios greater than 1). Interestingly, the interven-

Table 11.3 Washington State Institute for Public Policy Summary economic analysis of evidence-based public policies that affect crime: February 2015 (US$ Price). (From Lee, Aos, & Pennucci (2015), used with permission from the Washington State Institute for Public Policy)

Intervention	Benefits minus costs[a] ($)	Benefit to cost ratio[b] ($)	Chance benefits will exceed costs (%)
Juvenile justice			
Functional family therapy (youth in state institutions)	34,196	11.21	100
Aggression replacement training (youth in state institutions)	27,403	18.69	96
Functional family therapy (youth on probation)	26,587	8.94	100
Multisystemic therapy for substance abusing juvenile offenders	19,648	3.60	76
Multisystemic therapy	15,507	3.05	92
Aggression replacement training (youth on probation)	14,524	10.38	96
Family integrated transitions (youth in state institutions)	14,021	2.22	76
Functional family parole (with quality assurance)	10,000	3.24	79
Multidimensional treatment foster care	9175	2.13	67
Multidimensional family therapy (MDFT) for substance abusers	6380	1.82	67
Coordination of services	6040	15.90	76
Therapeutic communities for chemically dependent juvenile offenders	5788	2.27	76
Drug court	4159	2.32	65
Victim offender mediation	3790	7.37	88
Drug treatment for juvenile offenders	2388	1.64	70
Other chemical dependency treatment for juveniles (non-therapeutic communities)	(2973)	0.07	28
Scared straight	(13,557)	(204.33)	1
Adult criminal justice			
Electronic monitoring (probation)	28,465	n/a	94
Offender re-entry community safety program (dangerously mentally ill offenders)	25,245	1.76	95
Therapeutic communities for offenders with co-occurring disorders	23,994	7.56	100
Correctional education (basic or post-secondary) in prison	22,185	20.13	100
Vocational education in prison	19,757	13.22	100
Drug offender sentencing alternative (for drug offenders)	19,629	13.48	99
Mental health courts	17,245	6.75	100
Electronic monitoring (parole)	17,081	n/a	100

11 Economic Analyses

Table 11.3 (continued)

Intervention	Benefits minus costs[a] ($)	Benefit to cost ratio[b] ($)	Chance benefits will exceed costs (%)
Outpatient/non-intensive drug treatment (incarceration)	15,060	17.35	100
Inpatient/intensive outpatient drug treatment (incarceration)	14,861	10.45	100
Risk need & responsivity supervision (for high and moderate-risk offenders)	13,665	3.79	100
Therapeutic communities for chemically dependent offenders (community)	10,948	8.12	100
Cognitive behavioural treatment (for high- and moderate-risk offenders)	10,777	26.47	100
Case management: swift & certain/graduated sanctions for substance abusing offenders	10,755	3.20	96
Drug courts	9816	3.06	100
Drug offender sentencing alternatives (for property offenders)	9813	7.24	70
Sex offender treatment in the community	8728	6.36	85
Work release	6152	10.08	99
Employment training/job assistance in the community	6064	44.66	99
Therapeutic communities for chemically dependent offenders (incarceration)	5743	2.17	96
Correctional industries in prison	5491	4.77	100
Intensive supervision (surveillance & treatment)	4707	1.59	78
Sex offender treatment during incarceration	4436	1.87	78
Outpatient/non-intensive drug treatment (community)	4226	6.05	91
Inpatient/intensive outpatient drug treatment (community)	384	1.38	52
Case management: not swift and certain for substance abusing offenders	(1848)	0.62	34
Intensive supervision (surveillance only)	(7653)	(0.81)	7
Domestic violence perpetrator treatment (Duluth-based model)	(9864)	(6.29)	18
Strategies to reduce prison population			
For lower-risk offenders, decrease prison average daily population by 250, by lowering length of stay by 3 months	4445	n/a	98
For moderate-risk offenders, decrease prison average daily population by 250, by lowering length of stay by 3 months	240	n/a	53

Table 11.3 (continued)

Intervention	Benefits minus costs[a] ($)	Benefit to cost ratio[b] ($)	Chance benefits will exceed costs (%)
For high risk-offenders, decrease prison average daily population by 250, by lowering length of stay by 3 months	(4554)	n/a	18
Strategies to increase police presence (costs and benefits are presented per-officer)			
Deploy one additional police officer with hot spots strategies	552,066	6.94	100
Deploy one additional police officer with statewide average practices	488,375	6.52	100

N.B. Calculations are for Washington State. For instance, prison findings are estimated at current levels of crime and incarceration in Washington, and results would vary in jurisdictions with different crime-prison levels

Several programmes did not have benefits and costs calculated at this time, but past findings can be found in previous WSIPP publications

[a] Net present value

[b] Benefit-to-cost ratios cannot be computed in every case; 'n/a' is listed for those that cannot be reliably estimated

tion showing a negative return on investment is the scared straight programme for juvenile justice. This shows a significant negative cost-benefit ratio which is a direct result of the effectiveness evidence that shows it to increase crime and hence generate negative financial benefits. Of the 28 adult justice interventions, 26 provide a positive return on investment with benefit-cost ratios ranging from 0.62 to 44.66 for those calculated. Of these, 'Case management: not swift and certain for substance abusing offenders' is the only one with a (positive) ratio less than 1, indicating the return is not as great as the initial investment (by $1848). Intensive supervision with both surveillance only and domestic violence perpetrator programmes generated negative cost benefit ratios. Regarding strategies to reduce prison population, lowering length of stay by 3 months was cost-beneficial for lower and moderate risk offenders, but not high risk offenders (through the reduction in costs offsetting negative benefits).

Also included in Lee, Aos, and Pennucci (2015) are estimates of benefits from the taxpayers' perspective for each of these interventions. Using these estimates it is possible to calculate the percentage of the benefits which are attributed to the taxpayer and the associated net present value for taxpayers. Table 11.4 shows that across the majority of these interventions, between 20 and 30% of the overall benefit is attributable to taxpayers. Interestingly, the net present value is still positive for 27 of the 50 interventions even when ignoring other benefits. Interventions where the economic case would have changed from positive to negative if just the taxpayers' perspective was taken into account are mostly relatively expensive—the wider economic benefits (including victim benefits) must be included to demonstrate a case for investment from an economic perspective.

Table 11.4 Washington State Institute for Public Policy summary economic analysis of evidence-based public policies that affect crime: taxpayers perspective. (Authors' calculations using source data from Lee, Aos and Pennucci (2015))

Interventions	Taxpayer perspective	
	% Total benefit[a]	Benefit minus cost ($)
Juvenile justice		
Functional family therapy (youth in state institutions)	21	4654
Aggression replacement training (youth in state institutions)	21	4574
Functional family therapy (youth on probation)	26	4371
Multisystemic therapy for substance abusing juvenile offenders	19	(2343)
Multisystemic therapy	24	(2081)
Aggression replacement training (youth on probation)	26	2569
Family integrated transitions (youth in state institutions)	25	(5146)
Functional family parole (with quality assurance)	24	(1003)
Multidimensional treatment foster care	25	(3855)
Multidimensional family therapy (MDFT) for substance abusers	30	(3524)
Coordination of services	26	1287
Therapeutic communities for chemically dependent juvenile offenders	25	(1948)
Drug court	29	(1067)
Victim offender mediation	27	601
Drug treatment for juvenile offenders	32	(1797)
Other chemical dependency treatment for juveniles (non-therapeutic communities)	200	(2752)
Scared straight	25*	(3495)
Adult criminal justice		
Electronic monitoring (probation)	24	7793
Offender re-entry community safety program (dangerously mentally ill offenders)	33	(13,917)
Therapeutic communities for offenders with co-occurring disorders	27	3846
Correctional education (basic or post-secondary) in prison	26	4927
Vocational education in prison	26	4030
Drug offender sentencing alternative (for drug offenders)	26	3918
Mental health courts	27	2534
Electronic monitoring (parole)	25	5052
Outpatient/non-intensive drug treatment (incarceration)	26	3272
Inpatient/intensive outpatient drug treatment (incarceration)	27	2815

Table 11.4 (continued)

Interventions	Taxpayer perspective	
	% Total benefit[a]	Benefit minus cost ($)
Risk need & responsivity supervision (for high- and moderate-risk offenders)	29	405
Therapeutic communities for chemically dependent offenders (community)	27	1769
Cognitive behavioural treatment (for high- and moderate-risk offenders)	26	2460
Case management: swift & certain/graduated sanctions for substance abusing offenders	29	(387)
Drug courts	27	(951)
Drug offender sentencing alternatives (for property offenders)	27	1466
Sex offender treatment in the community	21	583
Work release	27	114
Employment training/job assistance in the community	25	1429
Therapeutic communities for chemically dependent offenders (incarceration)	32	(1565)
Correctional industries in prison	28	499
Intensive supervision (surveillance & treatment)	33	(3864)
Sex offender treatment during incarceration	25	(2709)
Outpatient/non-intensive drug treatment (community)	27	530
Inpatient/intensive outpatient drug treatment (community)	34	(551)
Case management: not swift and certain for substance abusing offenders	45	(3531)
Intensive supervision (surveillance only)	9*	(4563)
Domestic violence perpetrator treatment (Duluth-based model)	23*	(3353)
Strategies to reduce prison population		
For lower-risk offenders, decrease prison average daily population by 250, by lowering length of stay by 3 months	41*	5186
For moderate-risk offenders, decrease prison average daily population by 250, by lowering length of stay by 3 months	19*	4648
For high-risk offenders, decrease prison average daily population by 250, by lowering length of stay by 3 months	16*	4010
Strategies to increase police presence (costs and benefits are presented per-officer)		
Deploy one additional police officer with hot spots strategies	11	(23,819)
Deploy one additional police officer with statewide average practices	11	(26,966)

[a] Benefit may be negative, in which case a lower percentage is preferable. These percentages are indicated with an asterisk

Table 11.5 What public policies work to reduce crime: five evidence-based principles for crime. (Source: Aos (2011))

1	Risk: Focus on higher risk, not lower risk, populations
2	Treatment (delivered with fidelity): focus on research-proven prevention and intervention
3	Punishment: Strong evidence (for crime deterrence) for certainty, but not for severity of punishment
4	Economics: Benefits and costs need to be computed: not all things that "work" also have sound economics
5	"Good Cop Bad Cop": The combination often seems to be more effective

The Institute is going even further in the scope of its analysis and has begun seminal work on analysing the combined benefits and costs of a package or 'portfolio' of policies instead of judging each programme separately (Aos & Drake, 2013). Moreover, general lessons are being drawn from the work (e.g. the 'cheat sheet')—see Table 11.5.

In a 2012 assessment of the impact of this work, Urahn (2012) argues that, as a direct result of the work of the Institute, the initiatives now being adopted by Washington State policymakers have 'contributed to a greater improvement in crime rates and juvenile-arrest rates compared with the national average, an incarceration rate lower than the national average, and savings of $1.3 billion per 2-year budget cycle—eliminating the need to build new prisons and making it possible to close an adult prison and a juvenile-detention facility.' One important aspect of this work has been the move away from the use of crime intervention programmes as a 'political football', with the institute providing a bi-partisan perspective for all policymakers.

The Institute's model has attracted a great deal of research interest in the USA. The comprehensive technical appendices which are produced and the continual improvement and development of methodologies are rendering it an essential resource for anyone interested in cost-benefit analysis in criminal justice. (See for example the 'Resources on cost-benefit methods on our radar screen' blog (Henrichson, 2012)).

Perhaps more interesting is the attention the Institute is getting from US policymakers outside Washington State. Supported by the Pew Charitable Trusts and the John D. and Catherine T. MacArthur Foundation, eighteen states and four California counties are involved in a programme, called the Pew-MacArthur Results First Initiative. All are working to adapt the Washington State model to suit their own state perspectives (Pew-MacArthur Results First Initiative, 2015). It will be interesting to see how this work develops and the extent to which analysis and results vary across states.

Despite the paucity of high-quality primary studies of effectiveness and economic impact, the use of decision models to plug the gap is creating a demand for economic analysis, at least in the USA, which should trigger an improvement in research and associated funding.

Discussion and Conclusion

The purpose of economic analysis for investment in crime control, as in any other area of public policy, is to establish what a policymaker 'gets for their money'. Given that public funds are finite (and may be especially constrained in times of recession), evidence for the outcomes a programme will deliver, and whether a monetary valuation of the benefits outweighs the costs, is undoubtedly important, and if programmes can be ranked or compared against each other this information is even more useful. (Similarly, a policymaker may well be interested in the least damaging *disinvestment* they can make.)

Unfortunately, the field of crime control is still a long way from being able to achieve this. In large part, this is due to the lack of good-quality primary data on the costs of crime (and thus the benefits of preventing crime). Where studies have been conducted, their methodologies are often inconsistent, and rarely are they experimental in design.

The reviews covered in this chapter each compared a variety of cost-benefit studies, but no review was able to rank or weight the outcomes of these studies to compare interventions. Many of the studies found their intervention to be cost-beneficial, but the methodologies used were inconsistent, and experimental studies were rare. As such, systematic reviews like these may have limited use for policymakers.

Aside from the quality and quantity of primary studies, there are other reasons to suggest systematic reviews in crime economics may not perform well at informing policymakers' decisions: there is necessarily a great deal of variation between studies of crime, and context and sampling will naturally vary enormously (for justifiable reasons) (Sculpher et al., 2004; Sculpher & Drummond, 2006; Shiell et al., 2008). They can be useful as a summary of the current state of the art, including data gaps; to help build theoretical relationships; and for decision models, as detailed next (Anderson & Shemilt, 2010).

Until more research is carried out into the economics of crime, narrowing down some of the inherent variation and improving methodologies, this will continue to be the case. The field of health economics sets a good example, with public agencies like NICE consistently producing economic evaluation before making a decision on whether to recommend an intervention. As the body of economic research into crime begins to grow, systematic reviews will become more useful. Government agencies such as the UK Home Office are encouraging this process with their own contributions, but could do more in terms of funding analysis.

Decision models may offer a more immediate and useful approach to establishing the costs and benefits of crime interventions. We looked at the example of the Washington State Institute for Public Policy (Lee, Aos, & Pennucci, 2015), which creates comparable cost-benefit tables for major crime types. Although still reliant on primary studies, this method takes a more rigorous economic and statistical approach to comparing interventions, using decision analysis to establish probabilities, costs and outcomes. The methodology is continuously improving and this work has attracted attention, not just in Washington State but across the USA. Urahn

(2012) suggests it has already had a demonstrable effect on crime and public expenditure in Washington, in part due to its non-partisan, evidence-based policy recommendations.

Of all the studies reviewed in this chapter, the Washington State model has been the one that produces the clearest guidelines as to what works best in crime reduction, the five evidence-based principles detailed earlier. Combining a review of literature with decision-analytic models provides a more complete and consistent output across a range of crimes, and becomes a useful tool.

Overall, there is great potential for the use of economic analysis of crime to inform evidence-based policy. Studies so far show that there are benefits that greatly outweigh the costs of certain programmes, and that many interventions are cost-beneficial. The more these calculations can be refined, the more informed policymakers can be as to what they will 'get' for a given investment, and/or what to (dis)invest in. The work of the Washington State Institute of Public Policy shows perhaps the most thorough example of this so far. Systematic reviews, although not always directly useful for policymakers, can provide valuable information to be used as the basis for a decision model.

Ultimately, the key development needed is more and better primary data, ideally from experimental or quasi-experimental studies.

References

Anderson, R., & Shemilt, I. (2010). The role of economic perspectives and evidence in systematic review. In I. Shemilt, M. Mugford, L. Vale, K. Marsh, C. Donaldson (Eds.), *Evidence-based decisions and economics: health care, social welfare, education and criminal justice*. Oxford: Wiley-Blackwell.

Aos, S. (2011). *Crime trends, good news, what works, and analyzing options. Presentation to Washington Senate Human Services & Corrections Committee*. http://www.wsipp.wa.gov/ReportFile/1072/Wsipp_WSIPP-s-Benefit-Cost-Tool-for-States-Examining-Policy-Options-in-Sentencing-and-Corrections_Presentation-to-the-Senate-Human-Services-Corrections-Committee-January-21-2011.pptx.

Aos, S., & Drake, E. (2013). *Prison, police, and programs: Evidence-based options that reduce crime and save money*. Document NO. 13-11-1901. Olympia: Washington State Institute for Public Policy.

Becker, G. S. (1968). Crime and punishment: An economic approach. *Journal of Political Economy, 76*(2), 169–217.

Beckett, S. (1954). *Waiting for Godot: Tragicomedy in 2 acts*. New York: Grove Press.

Brand, S., & Price, R. (2000). *The economic and social costs of crime*. Research study 217. London: Home Office.

Byford, S., Barrett, B., Dubourg, R., Francis, J., & Sisk, J. (2010). The role of economic evidence in formulation of public policy and practice. In I. Shemilt, M. Mugford, L. Vale, K. Marsh, & C. Donaldson (Eds.), *Evidence-based decisions and economics: Health care, social welfare, education and criminal justice*. Oxford: Wiley-Blackwell.

Centre for Reviews and Dissemination. (2015). *About the CRD databases*. http://www.crd.york.ac.uk/crdweb/AboutPage.asp.

Cohen, M. A. (2000). Measuring the costs and benefits of crime and justice. In *Measurement and Analysis of Crime and Justice*, vol. 4 of *Criminal Justice 2000*, 263–315. NCJ-182411.

Washington, DC: National Institute of Justice, Office of Justice Programs, U.S. Department of Justice.

Cohen, M. A. (2005). *The costs of crime and justice*. New York: Routledge.

Cohen, M., & McDougall, C. (2008). Appendix 1: Benefit-cost validity scale—revised. In C. McDougall, M. Cohen, R. Swaray, A. Perry. Benefit-cost analyses of sentencing. *Campbell Systematic Reviews, 4*(10), 51–58.

Cost-Benefit Knowledge Bank for Criminal Justice. (2015). *About CBKB*. http://cbkb.org/about/.

Dhiri, S., & Brand, S. (1999). *Analysis of costs and benefits: Guidance for evaluators, crime reduction programme*. Guidance Note 1. London: Research Development and Statistics Directorate, Home Office.

Dolan, P., Loomes, G., Peasgood, T., & Tsuchiya, A. (2005). Estimating the intangible victim costs of violent crime. *British Journal of Criminology, 45*(6), 958–976.

Dossetor, K. (2011). *Cost-benefit analysis and its application to crime prevention and criminal justice research*. AIC (Australian Institute of Criminology) Reports: Technical and Background Paper 42. http://www.aic.gov.au/documents/A/4/F/%7bA4FA76DE-535E-48C1-9E60-4CF3F878FD8D%7dtbp042.pdf.

Dubourg, R., Hamed, J., & Thorns, J. (2005). The economic and social costs of crime against individuals and households 2003/04. *Online Report 30/05*, London: Research Development and Statistics Directorate, Home Office. http://webarchive.nationalarchives.gov.uk/20100413151441/http:/www.homeoffice.gov.uk/rds/pdfs05/rdsolr3005.pdf.

Farrington, D. P., Petrosino, A., & Welsh, B. C. (2001). Systematic reviews and cost-benefit analyses of correctional interventions. *The Prison Journal, 81*, 339–359.

Godfrey, C., Stewart, D., & Gossop, M. (2004) Economic analysis of costs and consequences of the treatment of drug misuse: 2-year outcome data from the National Treatment Outcome Research Study. *Addiction, 99*, 697–707.

Hammersley, M. (2002) *Systematic or unsystematic, is that the question? Some reflections on the science, art and politics of reviewing research evidence*. London: Health Development Agency Public Health Steering Group. http://guidance.nice.org.uk/nicemedia/pdf/sys_unsys_phesg_hammersley.pdf.

Henrichson, C. (2012). April focus: Resources on cost-benefit methods on our radar screen. *Cost-benefit knowledge bank for criminal justice*. http://cbkb.org/2012/04/april-focus-resources-for-cost-benefit-methods-on-our-radar-screen/.

HM Treasury. (2003). *The green book: Appraisal and evaluation in central government*. http://www.hm-treasury.gov.uk/d/green_book_complete.pdf.

Home Office. (2011). *Revisions made to the multipliers and unit costs of crime used in the integrated offender management value for money toolkit*. http://www.homeoffice.gov.uk/publications/crime/reducing-reoffending/IOM-phase2-costs-multipliers.

Kentaro, K., Duffy, S., & Tsutani, K. (2004). *Classification of FEE studies in NHS EED according to ICD-10 categories*. Paper presented at the Cochrane Collaboration Colloquium, Ottawa, October 2–6.

Knapp, M., Robertson, E., & McIvor, G. (1992) The comparative costs of community service and custody in Scotland. *Howard Journal, 31*(1), 8–30.

Lee, S., Aos, S., Drake, E., Pennucci, A., Miller, M., & Anderson, L. (2012a). *Return on investment: Evidence-based options to improve statewide outcomes, April 2012*. Document No. 12-04-1201. Olympia: Washington State Institute for Public Policy.

Lee, S., Aos, S., Drake, E., Pennucci, A., Miller, M., Anderson, L., & Burley, M. (2012b). *Return on investment: Evidence-based options to improve statewide outcomes, April 2012: Technical Appendix: Methods and User-Manual*. Olympia: Washington State Institute for Public Policy.

Lee, S., Aos, S., & Pennucci, A. (2015). *What works and what does not? Benefit-cost findings from WSIPP*. Document No. 15-02-4101. Olympia: Washington State Institute for Public Policy.

Mallender, J. (2012). *Economic modelling in public health*. Presentation to European Conference on Health Economics, July 20th, 2012.

Marsh, K. (2010a). The role of review and synthesis methods in decision models. In I. Shemilt, M. Mugford, L. Vale, K. Marsh, & C. Donaldson (Eds.), *Evidence-based decisions and economics: Health care, social welfare, education and criminal justice*. Oxford: Wiley-Blackwell.

Marsh, K. (2010b). Economic evaluation of criminal justice interventions: A methodological review of the recent literature. In J.K. Roman, T. Dunworth, & K. Marsh (Eds.), *Cost-benefit analysis and crime control*. Washington: The Urban Institute Press.

Matrix. (2009). Prioritising investments in preventative health. http://help.matrixknowledge.com/.

McCollister, K. E., French, M. T., & Fang, H. (2010). The cost of crime to society: New crime-specific estimates for policy and program evaluation. *Drug and Alcohol Dependence, 108*, 98–109.

McDougall, C., Cohen, M., Swaray, R., & Perry, A. (2008). Benefit-cost analyses of sentencing. *Campbell Systematic Reviews, 4*(10), 51–58.

National Information Center on Health Services Research and Health Care Technology. (2012). *HTA 101: IV. Cost analysis methods*. http://www.nlm.nih.gov/nichsr/hta101/ta10106.html.

National Institute for Health and Care Excellence. (2011). *National Institute for Health and Care Excellence: Supporting investment in public health: Review of methods for assessing cost effectiveness, cost impact and return on investment: Proof of concept report*. http://www.nice.org.uk/media/664/ac/cost_impact_proof_of_concept.pdf.

National Institute for Health and Care Excellence. (2012). *Methods for development of NICE public health guidance* (third edition, 2012). http://www.nice.org.uk/phmethods.

NICE. (2009). *National Institute for Health and Clinical Excellence: 10 years of excellence*. http://www.nice.org.uk/mediacentre/factsheets/NICEMilestones.jsp.

Pew-MacArthur Results First Initiative. (2015). *Overview*. http://www.pewtrusts.org/en/projects/pew-macarthur-results-first-initiative.

Roman, J., & Downey, P. M. (2010). *A Bayesian, meta cost-benefit model*. Presentation to the Brookings Institution. http://www.dccrimepolicy.org/costbenefitanalysis/images/Roman_DCPI_CBA-Final_1.pdf.

Sculpher, M., & Drummond, M. (2006) Analysis sans frontières: Can we ever make economic evaluations generalisable across jurisdictions? *Pharmacoeconomics, 24*(11), 1087–1099.

Sculpher, M. J., Pang, F. S., & Manca, A. et al. (2004). Generalisability in economic evaluation studies in healthcare: A review and case studies. *Health Technology Assessment, 8*(49), 1–192.

Sherman, L. W., Gottfredson, D. C., MacKenzie, D. L. et al. (1997). *Preventing crime: What works, what doesn't, what's promising*. Washington, DC: National Institute of Justice, US Department of Justice. https://www.ncjrs.gov/pdffiles1/Digitization/165366NCJRS.pdf.

Shiell, A., Hawe, P., & Gold, L. (2008) Complex interventions or complex systems? Implications for health economic evaluation. *British Medical Journal, 336*(7656), 1281–1283.

Swaray, R. B., Bowles, R., & Pradiptyo, R. (2005). The application of economic analysis to criminal justice interventions: A review of the literature. *Criminal Justice Policy Review, 16*, 141–163.

Urahn, S. K. (2012). The cost-benefit imperative. *Governing.com*. http://www.governing.com/columns/mgmt-insights/col-cost-benefit-outcomes-states-results-first.html.

Welsh, B. C., & Farrington, D. P. (2000). Monetary costs and benefits of crime prevention programs. *Crime and Justice, 27*, 305–361.

Chapter 12
Conclusion: What Works in Crime Prevention Revisited

David Weisburd, David P. Farrington and Charlotte Gill

In the Introduction to our book, we noted the role of Martinson's (1974) critique of crime prevention in corrections published four decades ago. We also pointed out that similar conclusions were being developed in other fields, though sometimes the basis of the evidence was cumulative across studies rather than from a single review (e.g., see Weisburd & Braga, 2006). The "nothing works" narrative came to dominate criminological thinking, and it was to have a very significant impact on crime policy across the world. Whether in New York or Tel Aviv, Berlin or London, Tokyo or Sydney, policymakers became aware that scientists had concluded that there was little they could do to prevent crime.

In this concluding chapter, we want to begin with this question: have systematic reviews, which have just begun to be developed with frequency over the past decade in criminology, changed our overall understanding of what works? In the 1970s and 1980s, the narrative of nothing works came to dominate criminological thinking and public policies about crime control. In the 1990s and into the new century, with crime rates declining across Western democracies (Baumer & Wolff, 2014), a new narrative has begun to develop that seems to imply that most things work. In the next section, we show that a review of systematic reviews brings us to a more sophisticated understanding of the potential of crime prevention programs. Our reviews of systematic reviews show that there is strong evidence of the crime prevention effectiveness of programs, policies, and practices across a wide variety

---

D. Weisburd (✉)
George Mason University, Fairfax, VA, USA
e-mail: dweisbur@gmu.edu

Hebrew University of Jerusalem, Jerusalem, Israel
e-mail: david.weisburd@mail.huji.ac.il

D. P. Farrington
University of Cambridge, Cambridge, UK
e-mail: dpf1@cam.ac.uk

C. Gill
George Mason University, Fairfax, VA, USA
e-mail: cgill9@gmu.edu

© Springer Science+Business Media New York 2016
D. Weisburd et al. (eds.), *What Works in Crime Prevention and Rehabilitation*,
Springer Series on Evidence-Based Crime Policy, DOI 10.1007/978-1-4939-3477-5_12

of intervention areas. That array of findings is broad and persuasive. It is time to abandon the "nothing works" idea not only in corrections, but also in policing, community interventions, and many other areas in crime and justice. The reviews also suggest that not everything works, and that criminologists, practitioners, and policymakers must look to the evidence to identify effective programs.

Having synthesized the evidence gained from our book, we turn to key gaps in the existing knowledge base. As we illustrate below, systematic reviews in crime and justice seldom get into the weeds. They give a general sense of whether crime prevention programs work, but they do not provide the kind of everyday guidance to practitioners and policymakers that an evidence base requires to be truly useful. A part of the reason for this, as we note below, is simply the paucity of primary research on key questions. But it is also time for systematic reviews to be considered carefully by criminologists so that gaps in the knowledge base can be focused upon. And it is time for criminologists to add new methods to their toolbox for developing systematic reviews. In particular, we will argue by drawing from chapters in this volume that they must pay more attention to cost-benefit analysis, qualitative studies, and descriptive validity.

What Have We Learned from a Review of Systematic Reviews?

It is natural in a volume on systematic reviews to begin with a review of the studies.[1] Our authors have summarized seven broad areas of criminological interventions:

Developmental and Social Prevention (Chap. 2: David Farrington, Maria Ttofi, and Friedrich Lösel)
Community Interventions (Chap. 3: Charlotte Gill)
Situational Prevention (Chap. 4: Kate Bowers and Shane Johnson)
Policing (Chap. 5: Cody Telep and David Weisburd)
Sentencing and Deterrence (Chap. 6: Amanda Perry)
Correctional Interventions (Chap. 7: David B. Wilson)
Drug Treatment Interventions (Chap. 8: Katy Holloway and Trevor Bennett)

Farrington, Ttofi, and Lösel examine developmental and social prevention. Their focus is on community-based programs (not clinical or institutional) targeted at children and adolescents up to age 18. They identify a number of systematic reviews covering general prevention ($N=3$) and individual ($N=5$), family ($N=8$), and school-based ($N=17$). The findings are positive overall across both broad dimensions examined. As Farrington et al. concluded, "[i]n general, developmental prevention is effective, whether targeted on individuals, families, or schools" (p. 67). They also develop important findings from a moderator analysis of the studies. For example, they report that more intensive and longer lasting programs are more effective, and programs that focus on higher risk children are more effective. This points to the importance of not just identifying whether programs

---

[1] We rely heavily on the authors' own comments in summarizing the studies below.

in a broad context work, but what types of programs work in reducing offending behavior.

Gill reviews community-based crime prevention, which includes a wide variety of potential interventions. As we will note in the next section, there are here, as in other areas, many realms of intervention for which we have little evidence. This deficit is particularly surprising given the broad scope of community interventions and their popularity in public policies. Gill assesses 15 reviews, of which 12 included quantitative meta-analyses. Her findings report very positive outcomes for primary prevention (e.g., mentoring or diversion programs), but the findings are much more ambiguous regarding secondary prevention programs. It is important to recognize the broad interventions included in this review, and that the studies reviewed do not say everything works, but often point to specific types of programs within domains that are successful.

Overall, Gill argues that there is good evidence that community-based programs designed to strengthen and restore positive social ties with at-risk youth are effective. In community corrections, she finds that research quality is strong, but results are mixed at best. The most effective programs target specific risk factors or directly re-engage the offender with the community. At the same time, general deterrence and punishment programs are at best ineffective and at worst harmful. Her review suggests that proactive engagement with the police and other civic partners to enhance legitimacy and build social cohesion are the most effective strategies to mobilize communities against crime. Finally, she concludes that the key mechanisms of effectiveness underlying effective community programs across all dimensions are efforts to enhance informal and supportive social controls and reintegration, and maintain or repair social bonds.

Bowers and Johnson conclude in their review of situational prevention programs: "[t]he general message from this chapter is a positive one; the existing systematic reviews of situational crime prevention tend to indicate significant, albeit modest reductions in levels of crime or victimization as a consequence of this type of activity" (p. 133). Situational crime prevention (SCP) measures are defined here as those that aim to prevent crime by reducing opportunities for offending and by increasing the effort and risk to offenders (Clarke, 1995). SCP interventions are based on one or more of five general strategies: increasing the effort, increasing the risk, decreasing the rewards, reducing the excuses, and reducing provocations to commit crime (Cornish & Clarke, 2003). They mainly consider seven systematic reviews that have examined the impact on crime of improvements to street lighting on crime (Welsh & Farrington, 2008a); closed-circuit television cameras (Welsh & Farrington, 2008b); repeat victimization strategies (Grove, Farrell, Farrington, & Johnson, 2012); public area surveillance (Welsh, Peel, Farrington, Elffers, & Braga, 2011); neighborhood watch schemes (Bennett, Holloway, & Farrington, 2008); counter-terrorism measures (Lum, Kennedy, & Sherley, 2006); and designated driver initiatives (Ditter, Elder, Shults, Sleet, Compton, & Nichols, 2005). All of these reviews report important crime prevention effects.

Telep and Weisburd report on systematic reviews in policing. They note that there has been a very large increase in policing reviews, particularly those conducted under the auspices of the Campbell Collaboration. A key reason for this is generous funding from the National Policing Improvement Agency (NPIA). Telep and Weisburd identify 17 completed and in progress reviews for which they could gain information. Their findings suggest the effectiveness of a number of policing strategies for addressing crime, including hot spots policing, problem-oriented policing, directed patrol to reduce gun violence, focused deterrence approaches, and using DNA in investigations. In addition, they find little evidence that focused policing approaches displace crime to areas nearby. Moreover, their review reports that information-gathering interrogation methods seem promising for reducing false confessions, and programs to increase procedural justice show promise for increasing citizen satisfaction, compliance, and perceptions of police legitimacy. Community policing programs have a small impact on crime and a more substantial impact on improving citizen satisfaction and perceptions of legitimacy.

The review also points to programs that do not work. Second responder programs, though considered an important innovation in policing, provide little evidence of effectiveness. Similarly, existing studies do not support Drug Abuse Resistance Education, despite its popularity as an intervention in the USA, nor do they provide evidence of benefits from police stress management programs.

Amanda Perry reviewed systematic reviews on sentencing and deterrence-based interventions. For the purpose of her review, sentencing interventions referred to any sanction imposed by a judge via legal proceedings. She identified 16 reviews, of which only six reported on outcomes of effectiveness using meta-analytic techniques (Coben & Larkin, 1999; Feder & Wilson, 2005; Mitchell, Wilson, Eggers, & MacKenzie, 2012; Petrosino, Turpin-Petrosino, & Buehler, 2003; Sarteschi, Vaughn, & Kim, 2011; Wilson, MacKenzie, & Mitchell, 2005). Twelve of the reviews focused on different sentencing options and four reviews focused on strategies using or applying deterrence theory as part of the intervention. Non-custodial sentences, jail-based court interventions (including assertive forensic mental health and ignition interlocking devices for the reduction of drink driving) were found to work in the reduction of criminal behavior. Promising initiatives included mental health courts and mental health schemes. Interventions showing no evidence of any effect included those relating to the severity of the sentence and deterrence. Mandated substance abuse programs for women, juvenile drug courts, and use of the death penalty were found to have uncertain conclusions.

One deterrence intervention (Scared Straight) for juvenile offenders did more harm than good. This is a particularly important because it points to the reality that sometimes cures can harm (McCord, 2003). The Scared Straight programs have much popularity around the world, and have been commonly applied in the USA. Indeed, they are the subject today of a popular American reality TV series, *Beyond Scared Straight*. But Petrosino et al.'s (2013) updated Campbell review showed overall that such programs lead to higher rates of criminality. Too often criminal justice agents view what they do as leading only to good outcomes and at its worst having no impact. They look to see whether programs work without consideration of whether they might harm offenders. In criminal justice, as in medical treatments, interventions can do harm.

Martinson's (1974) paper summarizing the review conducted by Lipton, Martinson, and Wilks (1975) concluded that focused offender-based rehabilitation programs provided little hope of effectiveness, and led him to look to larger societal changes to reduce crime (see also Martinson, 1976). David B. Wilson's review of 15 systematic reviews examining 36 different correctional treatments debunks Martinson's (1974) key narrative by providing a clear and unambiguous portrait of the potential for positive outcomes in rehabilitation in prisons. Most importantly, Wilson's study again points to the importance of systematic reviews in identifying which programs work best, which are promising, and which have no evidence of effectiveness. As Wilson notes in summarizing his findings: "[c]learly not all programs work and the evidence for some of the programs is weak" (p. 213).

Typically, programs reviewed by Wilson focus on educational or vocational deficits or address problems that contribute to crime, such as criminogenic thinking or substance abuse. The existing evidence most strongly supports the effectiveness of (1) group-based cognitive-behavioral programs for general offenders, (2) group-based cognitive-behavioral programs for sex offenders, (3) hormonal medication treatment for sex offenders, and (4) prison-based therapeutic communities for substance abusing offenders. Promising evidence supports the effectiveness of (1) adult basic and post-secondary educational programs for general offenders and (2) vocational programs for general offenders. Several other programs had encouraging findings, such as work programs and group counseling for drug abuse, but the weak methodological rigor of the research-base constrains the conclusions that can be drawn. The evidence suggests that insight-oriented therapy for sexual offenders and specialized correctional boot camps for substance abusers are not effective.

The final review in our book examines what has been learned from systematic reviews on the effectiveness of drug treatment interventions in reducing crime. Katy Holloway and Trevor Bennett identify 8 systematic reviews containing 23 different meta-analyses in this area. Six of the twenty-three analyses showed an overall significant and favorable effect of the experimental drug interventions on crime. Fifteen of the analyses found no significant difference in the outcomes of the experimental drug intervention compared with the control with respect to crime. Two of the twenty-three analyses found an overall unfavorable significant effect of specific experimental drug interventions on crime. Again, these findings points to the importance of considering backfire effects in crime and justice interventions.

The largest and most consistent treatment effects were found in terms of both naltrexone drug treatment and therapeutic communities. The authors note that this is important because it means that both medication-based and social interventions can successfully reduce drug use and recidivism. The single treatment type described as promising was buprenorphine substitution. Programs defined as having no effect or a negative effect included other forms of substitute prescribing (excluding buprenorphine), reintegration and recovery programs, and supervision and surveillance.

A very interesting finding in this review is that at least some drug interventions are effective in reducing criminal behavior. Holloway and Bennett note that this is striking in part because drug interventions rarely have crime reduction as an aim. They argue that the impact may be indirect, as reducing drug involvement may in turn lead to less involvement in criminal behavior. But we think that this fits more generally into a growing recognition of the unintended benefits of social intervention programs. For example, increased police presence to deter terrorism has been found to have crime prevention benefits (DiTella & Schargrodsky, 2004), as have security barriers (Gunaratna, 2008). And programs such as those to increase healthy childbearing, for example, have been found to have strong benefits as well (Olds et al., 1998). This suggests the importance of considering crime outcomes in many other types of social programs that might be expected to have indirect influences on crime.

What Can We Learn from a Quantitative Summary of the Reviews?

Our narrative review of the chapters provides a view of the effectiveness of crime prevention and rehabilitation programs that is directly at odds with narratives of "nothing works" that dominated thinking in this area for most of the last quarter of the previous century. There is simply a good deal of evidence that crime prevention practices and programs are effective. Nevertheless, as we noted earlier, not all such programs are effective, and indeed there are some programs that harm. This reinforces the importance of the evidence-based policy movement that has been growing in crime and justice since the turn of the century. We can reduce crime and prevent reoffending. But it is key to develop solid evidence on programs or practices so that we can identify whether they work, which are most effective and which cause harm.

A quantitative summary of the chapters reinforces this conclusion (see Fig. 12.1). We want to emphasize that a meta-analysis of these results is not appropriate. Many times studies are used across systematic reviews in one chapter, and appear more than once across the chapters, violating assumptions of statistical independence. At the same time, we think that we can learn from looking across the reviews more generally for patterns, or at least for a broad understanding of the types of effects we are observing in crime and justice reviews. We have summarized across each area of intervention identified by our authors the average weighted mean effects of programs. We recognize the statistical problems in taking this approach, given the overlap of studies, but we think it provides a broad portrait of the findings across the various crime prevention domains represented in our book.

Most striking in Fig. 12.1 is the weighting of the studies on the right side of the plot, representing odds ratios (OR) greater than 1. In all the chapters, OR>1 indicated that the program or intervention reduced crime relative to comparison or control groups. This shows that there is a clear weighting of effects toward interventions reducing crime and anti-social behavior. This figure simply depicts what our narrative review above implies. There is very significant evidence today of the ability of programs and practices to have desirable impacts on offenders and places. If we ask, "what works in crime prevention?" our answer overall is that there is much that works. And many interventions have large effect sizes. There are many here,

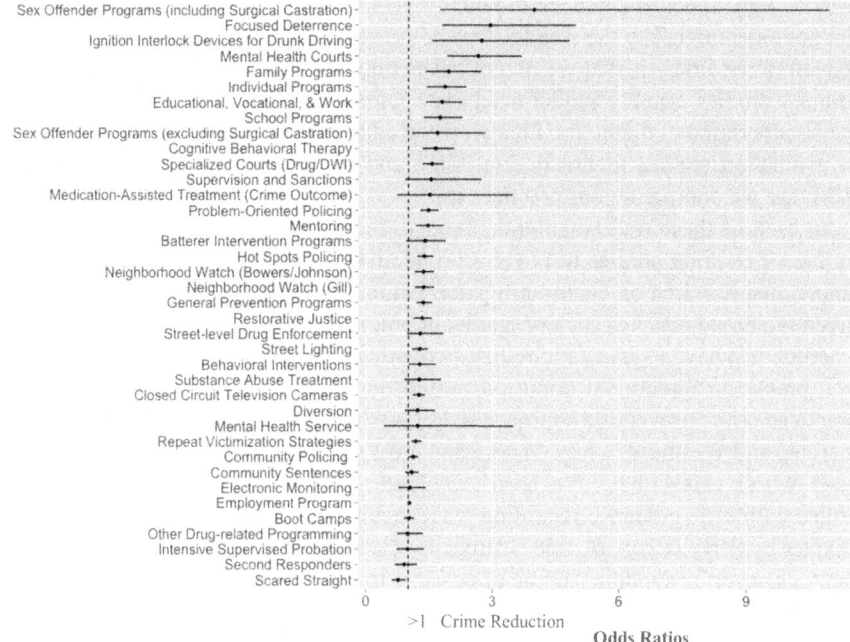

Fig. 12.1 Odds Ratios of Crime Prevention and Rehabilitation Programs

for example, that have ORs above 1.5, implying that participation in the program increases the odds of success (e.g. reductions in crime or recidivism) by 50%.

But the figure also illustrates that there are average effect sizes that are close to 1 (meaning a null effect), or below 1 (suggesting that interventions may even cause harm). This points again to the importance of recognizing that not all programs have been found to be effective. It is critical to subject crime prevention and rehabilitation programs to rigorous evaluation. Not every logic model or theory will produce positive outcomes in practice and some will cause harm. We must carefully evaluate programs and practices before they become widely established in crime prevention systems. But nonetheless, across all the domains we reviewed crime prevention and rehabilitation programs produce overall encouraging findings of effectiveness.

Additional Lessons Learned

Throughout the chapters, our authors provide insights into specific questions and issues in the seven domains we review. Three broad themes regarding additional lessons learned run across all the reviews, and we think that they are important to emphasize in our conclusions. The first is that existing reviews generally do not provide very specific guidance to practitioners and policymakers. We simply have not gotten enough into the weeds of crime prevention in these areas. The second—related to the first—is that we do not have enough primary studies, and few of the primary studies employ randomized experimental designs (or even the strongest quasi-experimental methods). Finally, we need to become more aware of the limits of evaluation studies as practice in crime and justice becomes more innovative. What are we comparing our practices to?

In each of these reviews, authors refer to the lack of specific guidance and the failure of existing studies to cover a broad array of programs. Gill notes, for example, that research on community interventions is surprisingly limited, especially given the broad array of such programs in practice. Bowers and Johnson (Chap. 4) examine just seven systematic reviews covering specific situational crime prevention practices. Situational crime prevention has become one of the most widely practiced crime prevention approaches. Yet, we have only limited information about it. Telep and Weisburd (Chap. 5) note that most standard police practices (see Weisburd & Eck, 2004) have not been examined, and the reviews that exist provide police with little guidance regarding what specifically they should do. Reading the chapter by Perry (Chap. 6), one is struck by the extent to which studies seem serendipitous, a sort of random sample of possible treatments. In a vast array of sentencing options, only a very few are covered.

It is not just that certain areas are not covered. There is a broader problem that one can observe in these reviews. Even when we show that certain areas of treatment or intervention are effective, the systematic reviews generally do not provide adequate guidance to practitioners or policymakers who need to make very specific decisions about what works. As David B. Wilson remarks in his chapter, "more research is needed to shed light on the effective change mechanisms" in correctional treatment (p. 215). Even in the case of hot spots policing, which is generally regarded as providing the strongest evidence base in policing (Telep & Weisburd, 2012), we have just a small number of studies covering specific types of interventions. If criminology is to provide guidance for evidence-based practice, it must begin to provide evidence that tells practitioners what specifically they must do.

The reviews in this book tell a very positive story about crime prevention, but they are, in some sense, what might be called "first-generation" studies. They provide enough evidence to overturn the narrative of nothing works and suggest that in each of the seven areas we have examined there is potential for successful crime prevention and rehabilitation programs. However, they generally do not provide information that is key to what can be called "second-generation" studies (see Weisburd & Telep, 2014). Second-generation studies would provide specific guidance regarding what types of programs are effective, for which types of offenders, and which types of settings.

Of course, some of the limitations in what we can learn from these systematic reviews derive simply from the lack of a sufficient number of primary studies. This is not a new problem and has been raised numerous times by scholars (Lipsey, 2003; Lösel & Schmucker, 2005). But a book that lays out what we have learned from systematic reviews starkly emphasizes this point. Given the importance of crime prevention and rehabilitation in society, we have a paucity of primary studies. Telep and Weisburd (Chap. 5) identify 285 independent studies in their policing review. One could argue here that this is very positive news, especially when just a few decades ago there were few rigorous studies in policing. But even here, one has to ask whether 285 studies could possibly cover even a fraction of the entire range of policing practices. Therefore, we are left with admiration for what criminology has achieved in this area and others. But it is time to use the positive evidence of existing studies to advocate for a major increase in evaluations across crime and justice.

More generally, our book emphasizes just how important it is to conduct systematic reviews. Again, the number of systematic reviews identified in this volume is encouraging, especially when one considers that just a decade ago there were only a handful of systematic reviews on crime prevention and rehabilitation. The Campbell Collaboration, which began in 2000, deserves considerable credit for this growth in systematic reviews in crime prevention and rehabilitation. Specific funders, such as the UK National Policing Improvement Agency, US National Institute of Justice, and UK Home Office, also have at various times encouraged the development of systematic reviews in criminology. But there is still a vast array of areas that have not been reviewed. And without systematic review it is difficult to identify just how many studies we have in a particular area. We cannot really take stock of the state of primary studies more generally in criminological interventions until we have a broader array of systematic review studies.

Of course, it is not simply the number of studies, but their quality that is important for developing a convincing evidence base for interventions. In all of these chapters the authors note the limitations in drawing inferences from weaker studies. Bowers and Johnson (Chap. 4) note that very few of the studies included in the systematic reviews they examined used randomized experimental methods. Telep and Weisburd (Chap. 5) find a larger number of randomized field trials relative to many of the areas covered, but still fewer than a quarter of the evaluations use random assignment. Although our conclusion here is not different from that of others (Lum, Koper, & Telep, 2011; Weisburd, Petrosino, & Mason, 1993), we think that it is important to continue to emphasize the need for strong evaluation methods. We have come a long way in many areas in terms of implementing strong quasi-experimental and experimental studies, but this remains a concern in systematic reviews in crime and justice.

A final concern is raised by David Wilson in his assessment of correctional interventions:

> Most of the evaluation studies contributing to these reviews rely on comparison conditions that involved some level of rehabilitative effort. This is simplified to the phrase "treatment as usual" in the meta-analyses and primary studies and may reflect anything from a purely sanctions-based treatment (e.g., incarceration) to involvement in other programs designed to help the offender. This greatly complicates the interpretation of findings from these studies as the results generally do not reflect the pure effect of the program of interest but rather the added value of the program relative to the background noise of existing practices and services. (p. 213)

This problem appears throughout the systematic reviews in our book. In general, we do not compare treatment to a placebo condition, but rather to an established or conventional treatment. In part, this is because we simply cannot remove treatment from offenders or places in crime and justice, or at least can only do that in very rare situations. A hot spot of crime cannot be relegated to a status of receiving no police attention. At the very least such places receive whatever is the standard treatment, usually emergency response to calls for service. And in this regard, we are not very different from medicine. Where there is a proven treatment, the innovation is ordinarily compared to that treatment; it is uncommon for an effective treatment to be withdrawn from people who suffer from serious illness, a practice that is regarded as highly unethical in medical research (Rothman & Michels, 1994; Miller, 2000). Of course, the standard practices in crime and justice are often unproven. But nonetheless, political realities mean that it is unlikely that an innovative intervention can be compared with a placebo condition.

Over the course of decades of improvement in criminal justice, this problem of the comparison condition has worsened. For example, police agencies throughout the USA and the UK are using innovative technologies and strategies. It is becoming more difficult to identify jurisdictions that use only the standard model of policing that was common five decades ago. In part, due to a growing evidence base, the comparison conditions we face will have more and more treatment options included. This strikes us as a reality to be faced across criminal justice systems in the next generation of studies. It is certainly something that we need to consider. What is the meaning of a null finding in the context where the control condition is receiving effective treatment as well? How can we adjust effect sizes to take into account unknown control group effects without any treatment? Finally, can we or should we begin to develop ethical standards that at least place nonproven strategies on par with medical nonproven strategies? In other words, can we justify placebo control groups where there are standard practices but those practices have no evidence base?

Extending Meta-Analytic Methods

Three chapters in our book examine how we can expand systematic review and meta-analytic methods so that they have broader relevance and dig more deeply into the mechanisms underlying what works. Chapter 9, by Mimi Ajzenstadt, explores how qualitative studies can be integrated into systematic reviews. In Chap. 10 Michael Caudy and colleagues examine how we can improve methods for summarizing systematic reviews. Finally, in Chap. 11 Jacqueline Mallender and Rory Tierney bring us back to Martinson's call for greater involvement of economic methods in systematic review in crime prevention and rehabilitation through a discussion of cost-benefit analysis and related approaches.

We included a chapter on qualitative methods in systematic review because we recognized at the outset the importance of such methods for providing depth to our understanding of what works. Many times we are confronted with a black box of findings in which we know there was an impact, but it is unclear which mechanisms produced that impact. In part, better quantitative data on treatments and outcomes can add important information to the question of how or why a treatment worked or did not work, but qualitative data are particularly well-suited for such questions. Moreover, qualitative data are particularly important for process evaluations, and can help us to better distinguish between theory failures and program failures. This is an issue we will discuss more in detail below when we refer to Caudy et al. (Chap. 10), but it is critically important in summarizing findings to know whether, for example, implementation problems caused a failure to show effects or whether the program model was problematic. In her chapter, Ajzenstadt lays out the potential benefits of systematic reviews of qualitative data:

> Data generated from studies utilizing qualitative methods can contribute to the improvement of knowledge in new areas… Indeed, researchers use systematic reviews based on qualitative methods to assess the nature and extent of knowledge—especially in areas that are understudied. This type of systematic review can also contribute to a broader understanding of the process and dynamics of the phenomenon under investigation, further contributing to theory-building … Findings from studies utilizing qualitative research design can generate a comprehensive understanding of a phenomenon, adding depth and breadth to systematic reviews of effectiveness by focusing on participants' views on the intervention … Finally, qualitative research sheds light on the complexity of the examined phenomenon and facilitates the generation of new evidence relevant for practice and policy (p. 240).

The importance of this review of systematic reviews is illustrated in part by the relatively small group of studies identified. Only 15 articles were found that summarized qualitative studies from an exhaustive search of thousands of documents. Systematic reviews of qualitative studies in crime prevention and rehabilitation are rare. This is not surprising, but again the review method allows us to see starkly what we have assumed.

Systematic reviews of qualitative data face more complex problems in summarizing information than traditional quantitative data reviews. However, Ajzenstadt describes that she found a number of techniques developing in this area, such as meta-summary, meta-synthesis, meta-interpretation, and meta-ethnography. Qualitative reviews face additional complications in sampling and evaluating data quality. There is simply not as much agreement for qualitative methods in reviews as has become the case for quantitative reviews. This suggests that traditional systematic review groups such as the Cochrane and Campbell Collaborations could play an important role in helping to develop methods of qualitative synthesis.

The rewards seem significant to us. For example, one review examining programs to reduce stress among police officers (Patterson, Chung, Swan, 2012) reported that the lack of significant improvement in reducing excessive alcohol consumption, smoking, and stress symptoms among police officers who participated in the studied intervention was due to the lack of trust held by police officers toward the law enforcement organization's involvement in health issues. Ajzenstadt goes on to note that:

[P]articipants felt that alcohol consumption was a private matter and that the use of alcohol was an accepted coping mechanism in the context of police work and a central part of the police culture for bonding among officers (p. 25). Similarly, the qualitative data showed that officers did not feel that experiencing stress symptoms made officers less prepared for police work. At the same time, officers' "significant others" reported observing positive changes in their spouses following participation in the stress management interventions. (p. 252)

Caudy, Taxman, Tang, and Watson (Chap. 10) describe a method for systematizing reviews of systematic reviews. This is not an easy problem since reviews overlap, and it is not clear which methods will yield the broadest understanding of studies. They provide some initial results from their efforts to develop the Evidence Mapping to Advance Justice Practice project. They report on their experiences in developing 18 reviews of health-related correctional interventions in crime and justice. These reviews summarize 300 systematic reviews.

Their findings are intriguing. Among studies that specified a control or comparison condition, it was most common for the efficacy of interventions to be tested against a comparison group not receiving treatment (65.4%). This is important given our previous discussion, and suggests that in health-related studies, it is simply more likely for the treatment to be compared to a placebo condition. But this systematic review of reviews also raises another problem that was common in reviews of the seven broad areas of crime and justice practice examined in our book. There was a lack of consistency in how authors report the findings of systematic reviews and meta-analyses. This problem is often defined as descriptive validity (Farrington, 2003; Lösel & Koferl, 1989) and has been noted in many discussions of meta-analyses (e.g., see Gill, 2011; Perry, Weisburd, & Hewitt, 2010). But Caudy et al. (Chap. 10) suggest that this problem becomes even more significant in the compilation of systematic review studies.

More generally, Caudy et al. provide encouraging confirmatory evidence of our general findings in this book. Looking at health-related correctional interventions in crime prevention and rehabilitation they conclude that: "the findings from these syntheses were generally positive suggesting that correctional treatment programs can effectively reduce recidivism and promote other positive outcomes (e.g., reduced substance use, improved vocational/educational skills)" (Chap. 10, p. 13).

The final chapter in our book examines cost-benefit analysis in systematic reviews in crime prevention and rehabilitation. Mallender and Tierney begin Chap. 11 by arguing that cost-benefit analysis is key to understanding whether programs are worthwhile to implement. The economic costs associated with a program must be contrasted with the benefits achieved. Such assessments of costs are now becoming more common in criminal justice settings. Nonetheless, Mallender and Tierney note that:

Given the four decades of established research in the costs of crime, policymakers who want to know whether investment in particular types of criminal justice interventions provide value for money might expect to find a bank of research from which they can draw conclusions, but sadly this is not the case. Good quality economic studies available for review are still comparatively rare (Byford, Barrett, Dubourg, Francis, & Sisk, 2010; Farrington, Petrosino, & Welsh, 2001; Marsh, 2010; McDougall, Cohen, Swaray, & Perry, 2008; Swaray, Bowles & Pradiptyo, 2005; Welsh & Farrington, 2000). (pp. 293–294)

Mallender and Tierney were able to identify just four systematic reviews where economic cost-benefit data are available. These include systematic reviews of situational prevention, developmental prevention, correctional interventions, and community interventions. However, benefits exceeded costs in a number of these interventions—a promising start for cost-benefit analysis in crime prevention and rehabilitation programs.

Clearly, this is an area of systematic review that must be focused on more directly in the future. Again, we think that this is a first-generation/second-generation problem. When criminologists were trying to show that interventions could be effective, the relative cost and benefits were not as critical. But having shown that interventions can reduce crime and recidivism, it is time to focus more attention on the relative economic benefits or liabilities of specific types of programs. A program may be beneficial but simply too costly to be implemented on a large scale. In turn, a program may have small benefits, but little cost, suggesting that it should be widely applied.

Mallender and Tierney provide a suggestion for what we can do to include cost-benefit analysis in reviews, even before the data are widely available. They argue:

> Given the limited ability of researchers and policymakers to rely on reviews to provide evidence of the economic costs and benefits of crime and justice interventions, some policymakers have focused instead on the use of economic models or "decision models". For example, the NICE public health methods guidance (National Institute for Health and Care Excellence, 2012) recommends that, in addition to systematic reviews of economic evaluations, a "cost-effectiveness analysis could be modelled [either] on a single well-conducted randomised controlled trial (RCT), or using decision-analytic techniques to analyse probability, cost and health-outcome data from a variety of published sources". NICE began producing public health guidance after setting up the 'Centre for Public Health Excellence' in 2005 (National Institute for Health and Care Excellence, 2009). As of analysis conducted in 2012, nearly 50% of the NICE public health guidelines use either a static or dynamic decision model for economic analysis (Mallender et al., 2012). (p. 298)

Whatever the approach taken, our inclusion of this chapter speaks to our strong view that it is time for crime prevention and rehabilitation researchers and policymakers to put cost-benefit analysis on the agenda of primary studies and systematic reviews. The paucity of such evidence limits the impact we can have on the real world of crime and justice.

Conclusions

It is difficult to imagine that just four decades ago, criminologists had accepted the narrative that nothing works in crime and justice interventions. We can see this today in the continued dominance of 'root causes' research in criminological studies. We certainly agree that looking into the broad sociological variables that influence crime is a valuable effort in criminology. But Martinson's (1974, 1976) critique just 40 years ago concluding that we should abandon the search for programmatic responses to crime and criminality is simply wrong. This book provides perhaps the most comprehensive evidence to date of that fact. At least for the last decade, there has developed a growing body of evidence that many programs and practices can reduce recidivism, drug use, and crime (Cullen, 2005; Lipsey & Cullen, 2007; Lipsey, Chapman, & Landenberger, 2001; Sherman, Farrington, Welsh, & MacKenzie, 2002; Visher & Weisburd, 1998; Weisburd & Eck, 2004). But our book provides the broadest review of such evidence to date, and is based on over 100 reviews that assess over 3,000 primary evaluation studies.

In the areas of developmental and social prevention, community interventions, situational prevention, policing, sentencing, correctional interventions, and drug treatment interventions, we find consistent evidence of programs and practices that work. Importantly, our conclusion is not that everything works. We think that as naïve as the nothing works narrative of the past century. Rather, we find that there is much evidence of practices that are effective. There is also evidence of less effective practices, and importantly practices that may in fact cause harm. This makes the development of primary studies, systematic reviews, and reviews of systematic reviews that much more critical in the evidence-based policy movement. We need to be able to identify the programs that work, that seem to have little impact, and that are harmful. The knowledge generated in this book takes an important step in this effort to advance evidence-based policy in the areas of crime prevention and rehabilitation.

References

Baumer, E. P., & Wolff, K. T. (2014). Evaluating contemporary crime drop(s) in America, New York City, and many other places. *Justice Quarterly, 31*(1), 5–38.

Bennett T., Holloway K., & Farrington, D. (2008). The effectiveness of neighborhood watch. *Campbell Systematic Reviews, 4*(18).

Byford, S., Barrett, B., Dubourg, R., Francis, J., & Sisk, J. (2010). The role of economic evidence in formulation of public policy and practice. In: I. Shemilt, M. Mugford, L. Vale, K. Marsh, & C. Donaldson (Eds.). *Evidence-based decisions and economics: Health care, social welfare, education and criminal justice.* Oxford: Wiley-Blackwell.

Clarke, R. V. (1995). Situational crime prevention. In M. Tonry & D. P. Farrington (Eds.) *Building a safer society: Strategic approaches to crime prevention. (Crime and justice: A review of research, Vol. 19).* Chicago: University of Chicago Press.

Coben, J. H., & Larkin, G. L. (1999). Effectiveness of ignition interlock devices in reducing drunk driving recidivism. *American Journal of Preventive Medicine, 16*(1 Suppl), 81–87.

Cornish, D. B., & Clarke. R.V. (2003). Opportunities, precipitators and criminal decisions: A reply to Wortley's critique of situational crime prevention. In M. J. Smith & D. B. Cornish (Eds.), *Theory for practice in situational crime prevention. (Crime Prevention Studies, Vol. 16).* Monsey: Criminal Justice Press.

Cullen, F. T. (2005). The twelve people who saved rehabilitation: How the science of criminology made a difference. *Criminology, 43*(1), 1–42.

Di Tella, R., & Schargrodsky, E. (2004). Do police reduce crime? Estimates using the allocation of police forces after a terrorist attack. *American Economic Review, 94*(1), 115–133.

Ditter, S. M., Elder, R.W., Shults, R. A., Sleet, D. A., Compton, R. & Nichols, J. L. (2005). Effectiveness of designated driver programs for reducing alcohol-impaired driving: A systematic review. *American Journal of Preventative Medicine, 28,* 280–287.

Farrington, D. P. (2003). Methodological quality standards for evaluation research. *The Annals of the American Academy of Political and Social Science, 587*(1), 49–68.

Farrington, D.P., Petrosino, A., & Welsh, B.C. (2001). Systematic reviews and cost-benefit analyses of correctional interventions. *The Prison Journal, 81,* 339–359.

Feder, L., & Wilson, D. B. (2005). A meta-analytic review of court-mandated batterer intervention programs: Can courts affect abusers' behavior? *Journal of Experimental Criminology, 1*(2), 239–262.

Gill, C. E. (2011). Missing links: How descriptive validity impacts the policy relevance of randomized controlled trials in criminology. *Journal of Experimental Criminology, 7*(3), 201–224.

Grove L. E., Farrell, G., Farrington, D. P. & Johnson, S. D. (2012) *Preventing repeat victimization: A systematic review*. Report prepared for the Swedish National Council for Crime Prevention. Stockholm: The Swedish National Council for Crime Prevention.

Gunaratna, R. (2008). The Islamabad Marriott in flames: The attack on the world's most protected hotel. *Journal of Policing, Intelligence and Counter Terrorism, 3*(2), 99–116.

Lipsey, M. W. (2003). Those confounded moderators in meta-analysis: Good, bad, and ugly. *The Annals of the American Academy of Political and Social Science, 587*(1), 69–81.

Lipsey, M. W., & Cullen, F. T. (2007). The effectiveness of correctional rehabilitation: A review of systematic reviews. *Annual Review of Law and Social Science, 3,* 297–320.

Lipsey, M. W., Chapman, G. L., & Landenberger, N. A. (2001). Cognitive-behavioral programs for offenders. *The Annals of the American Academy of Political and Social Science, 578*(1), 144–157.

Lipton, D., Martinson, R., & Wilks, J. (1975). *The effectiveness of correctional treatment: A survey of treatment evaluation studies*. New York: Praeger.

Lösel, F., & Köferl, P. (1989). Evaluation research on correctional treatment in West Germany: A meta-analysis. In H. Wegener, F. Lösel, & J. Haisch (Eds.), *Criminal behavior and the justice system* (pp. 334–355). Berlin: Springer Berlin Heidelberg.

Lösel, F., & Schmucker, M. (2005). The effectiveness of treatment for sexual offenders: A comprehensive meta-analysis. *Journal of Experimental Criminology, 1*(1), 117–146.

Lum, C., Kennedy, L. W. & Sherley, A (2006) The effectiveness of counter-terrorism strategies. *Campbell Systematic Reviews, 2*(2).

Lum, C., Koper, C. S., & Telep, C. W. (2011). The evidence-based policing matrix. *Journal of Experimental Criminology, 7*(1), 3–26.

Mallender, J. (2012). Economic modelling in Public Health. Presentation to European Conference on Health Economics, July 20th, 2012.

Marsh, K. (2010). Economic evaluation of criminal justice interventions: A methodological review of the recent literature. In: J. K. Roman, T. Dunworth, & K. Marsh, *Cost-benefit analysis and crime control*. Washington: The Urban Institute Press.

Martinson, R. (1974). What works?—Questions and answers about prison reform. *The Public Interest, 35,* 22–54.

Martinson, R. (1976). California research at the crossroads. *Crime and Delinquency, 22,* 180–191.

McCord, J. (2003). Cures that harm: Unanticipated outcomes of crime prevention programs. *Annals of the American Academy of Political and Social Sciences, 587,* 16–30.

McDougall, C., Cohen, M., Swaray, R., & Perry, A. (2008). Benefit-cost analyses of sentencing. *Campbell Systematic Reviews, 4*(10).

Miller, F. G. (2000). Placebo-controlled trials in psychiatric research: An ethical perspective. *Biological Psychiatry, 47*(8), 707–716.

Mitchell, O., Wilson, D. B., Eggers, A., & MacKenzie, D. L. (2012). Drug courts' effects on criminal offending for juveniles and adults. *Campbell Systematic Reviews, 8*(4).

NICE (2009). National Institute for Health and Clinical Excellence: 10 years of excellence. Retrieved from http://www.nice.org.uk/mediacentre/factsheets/NICEMilestones.jsp.

Olds, D., Henderson, C. R., Jr., Cole, R., Eckenrode, J., Kitzman, H., Luckey, D., et al (1998). Long-term effects of nurse home visitation on children's criminal and antisocial behavior: 15-year follow-up of a randomized controlled trial. *Journal of the American Medical Association, 280*(14), 1238–1244.

Patterson G. T, Chung I. W, & Swan, P. G. (2012), The effects of stress management interventions among police officers and recruits. *Campbell Systematic Reviews, 8*(7).

Perry, A. E., Weisburd, D., & Hewitt, C. (2010). Are criminologists describing randomized controlled trials in ways that allow us to assess them? Findings from a sample of crime and justice trials. *Journal of Experimental Criminology, 6*(3), 245–262.

Petrosino, A., Turpin-Petrosino, C., Hollis-Peel, M. E., & Lavenberg, J. G. (2013). Scared Straight and other juvenile awareness programs for preventing juvenile delinquency: A systematic review. *Campbell Systematic Reviews, 2013*(5).

Rothman, K. J. & Michels, K. B. (1994). The continuing unethical use of placebo controls. *New England Journal of Medicine, 331,* 394–398.

Sarteschi, C. M., Vaughn, M. G., & Kim, K. (2011). Assessing the effectiveness of mental health courts: A quantitative review. *Journal of Criminal Justice, 39*(1), 12–20.

Sherman, L. W., Farrington, D. P., Welsh, B. C., & MacKenzie, D. L. (2002). *Evidence-based crime prevention.* London: Routledge.

Swaray, R.B., Bowles, R., & Pradiptyo, R. (2005). The application of economic analysis to criminal justice interventions: A review of the literature. *Criminal Justice Policy Review, 16,* 141–163.

Telep, C. W., & Weisburd, D. (2012). What is known about the effectiveness of police practices in reducing crime and disorder? *Police Quarterly, 15*(4), 331–357.

Visher, C. A., & Weisburd, D. (1998). Identifying what works: Recent trends in crime prevention strategies. *Crime, Law and Social Change, 28*(3–4), 223–242.

Weisburd, D., & Braga, A. A. (Eds.). (2006). *Police innovation: Contrasting perspectives.* New York: Cambridge University Press.

Weisburd, D., & Eck, J. E. (2004). What can police do to reduce crime, disorder, and fear? *The Annals of the American Academy of Political and Social Science, 593*(1), 42–65.

Weisburd, D. & Telep, C. (2014). Hot spots policing: What we know and what we need to know. *Journal of Contemporary Criminal Justice, 30*(2), 200–220.

Weisburd, D., Petrosino, A., & Mason, G. (1993). Design sensitivity in criminal justice experiments. *Crime and Justice, 17,* 337–379.

Welsh, B.C. & Farrington, D.P. (2000). Monetary costs and benefits of crime prevention programs. *Crime and Justice, 27,* 305–361.

Welsh B. C., & Farrington D. P. (2008a). Effects of improved street lighting on crime. *Campbell Systematic Reviews, 4*(13).

Welsh B. C., & Farrington, D. P. (2008b). Effects of closed circuit television surveillance on crime. *Campbell Systematic Reviews, 4*(17).

Welsh, B., Peel, M., Farrington, D., Elffers, H. & Braga, A. (2011). Research design influence on study outcomes in crime and justice: a partial replication with public area surveillance. *Journal of Experimental Criminology, 7*(2), 183–198.

Wilson, D. B., MacKenzie, D. L., & Mitchell, F. N. (2005). Effects of correctional boot camps on offending. *Campbell Systematic Reviews, 1*(6).

Index

A
Abuse, substance, 95, 187, 205, 213
Academic achievement, 55
Access control, 112
Adjustment, 56, 162, 213
Adolescents, 15, 57, 62, 312
Adults, 17, 95, 101, 179, 197, 203, 211
After-school programs, 78, 80
Aggression, 17, 59, 61, 67
Alcohol, 59, 112, 157, 204
Alley-gating, 113
Analysis, 11, 67, 78, 94, 101, 121, 122, 124, 131–133, 162, 206, 208, 210, 212, 215, 222, 248, 280, 291–294, 297, 298, 305–307, 312, 322, 323
Antisocial behavior, 15, 17, 54, 56, 57
Arrest, 17, 55, 57
Awareness space, 112

B
Behavior change, 10, 100, 203
Behavioral management, 95, 99, 104
Bias, 6, 7, 17, 66, 253, 280, 281
Bibliographic database, 7, 17, 66, 113
Boot camps, 173, 181, 187
Brief interventions, 234
Bullying, 16, 17, 54, 59–61
Bullying cyber, 60
Buprenorphine, 206, 221, 228, 232, 234
Bureau of Justice Assistance, 293

C
Calls for police service, 4, 129, 157, 320
Campbell Collaboration, 8, 9, 54, 66, 82, 83, 96, 105, 113, 114, 132, 137–139, 171, 275, 276, 296
Campbell Crime and Justice Group, 3, 82
Campbell Social Welfare Group, 82
Child development, 15, 16
Child maltreatment, 57
Child training programs, 17, 55, 63
Children, 9, 15, 17, 54, 55, 57, 59, 60, 312
Civic engagement, 9, 77
Closed-circuit television, 114, 313
Cochrane Collaboration, 8, 82, 139, 153, 170, 262, 265, 272
Cochrane Library, 8, 17, 221
Cognitive skills, 16, 207
Cohen's d, 151, 161, 162
Collective efficacy, 79, 100, 102, 105
Community, 2, 79, 80, 83, 94, 101, 103, 104, 119, 169, 205–207, 213, 228, 232–234, 302
Compstat, 160
Conduct disorder (CD), 9, 17, 56, 59
Confidence intervals (CI), 17, 55, 57, 60, 61, 181, 198, 206, 228
Consolidated Standards of Reporting Trials (CONSORT), 265–268
Constructs, 250, 254
Context, 10, 78, 124, 130, 132, 133, 170, 197, 203, 207, 238, 239, 251, 263
Contingency management (CM), 233, 274
Corporate crime prevention, 9
Corrections, 1, 10, 54, 77, 102, 183, 185, 194, 197, 198, 206, 214, 273, 279, 280, 294, 295, 311, 313, 319, 322
Correlation, 131, 198, 202, 204
Costs, 111, 292, 293, 295, 297–299
Counseling, 16, 205, 207, 213, 273, 315
Counter-terrorism, 114, 122
Court-mandated interventions, 181, 185
Courts, 173, 180, 181, 183, 184, 187, 188, 314
Crime, 2, 8, 9, 153, 155
Crime control, 1, 105, 151, 154, 156, 164
Crime pattern theory, 112

Crime Prevention Through Environmental Design (CPTED), 113, 120
Criminal thinking, 215
Critical Appraisal Skills Program (CASP), 248
Custodial sentence, 80

D

Death penalty, 187, 189, 314
Delinquency, 5, 9, 17, 55, 56, 59, 80, 102
Demonstration project, 66, 67, 210
Design quality, 66
Designated driver initiatives, 114, 123
Deterrence, 15, 78, 79, 81, 95, 99, 100, 169, 171, 185, 186, 314
Detoxification, 220
Deviant peer contagion, 102
Diffusion, 132, 153, 154
Diplomatic protection, 122
Directed, 121, 152, 156, 159, 314
Disorder, 77–79, 151–153, 156, 157, 159
Displacement, 114, 122, 132, 153, 154, 159
Diversion, 80, 94, 98, 99, 184
DNA testing, 152
Dosage, 16
Driving while intoxicated (DWI), 153, 183, 186, 187
Drug Abuse Resistance Education (D.A.R.E.), 139, 154, 314
Drug enforcement, 152, 157
Drug market, 152
Drug substitution programs, 206
Drug testing, 99, 220, 232

E

Early-childhood, 9, 16
Economics, 295, 297, 306
Education, 8, 61, 101, 122, 124, 193, 194, 198, 238
Educational programs, 202, 206, 315
Effect size, 2, 7, 8, 16, 17, 57, 62, 67, 99, 121, 129, 194, 222, 263
Electronic monitoring, 81, 96, 100, 171
Elementary school, 61
Eligibility criteria, 7, 234
Employment, 57, 95, 101, 215
Environment, 81, 128, 251, 252
Evaluation, 5–7, 54, 56, 59, 61, 67, 96, 113, 118, 126, 130, 210, 233, 321
Evidence mapping, 282
Evidence Mapping to Advance Justice Practice (EMTAP), 11, 261, 263, 264, 282, 322
Executions, 186

Externalizing behavior, 16, 59

F

False confessions, 154, 158, 314
Families, 9, 15, 16, 77, 312
Family programs, 56
Firearms, 152
Focused deterrence, 95, 98–100, 151, 164, 314
Follow-up measurement, 66
Forensic Assertiveness Community Treatment (FACT), 184
Forest plot, 96, 155, 228

G

Gang, 83, 94, 102
Generalizability, 185, 188, 275
Government, 9, 161, 183, 291, 293, 306
Grey literature, 183, 295–297
Guardianship, 78–80, 112, 119
Gun, 6, 83, 95, 97–99, 152, 156, 159, 314

H

Harm reduction, 235
Health, 8, 54, 56, 169, 184, 189, 212, 213, 219, 246, 251, 253, 264, 265, 274, 280, 282, 306
Hedge's g, 61
Heroin, 206, 220, 232
Heterogeneity, 8, 57, 152, 155, 156, 162, 170, 232
High school, 59, 198
Hijacking, 122
Home Office (United Kingdom), 293, 306, 319
Home visitation, 9
Hormonal medication, 211, 213, 315
Hot spots, 2, 100, 151, 154, 156, 159, 160, 162, 163, 165, 314
Housing, 80, 119, 212

I

Ignition interlock devices, 186
Implementation, 10, 16, 61, 65, 67, 113, 121, 122, 129, 131, 234, 238, 264, 268, 277, 279–282
Incapacitation, 15
Informal social control, 79, 80, 98–100, 119, 203
Information gathering, 139, 159
Intensity, 16, 60, 64, 129, 131, 190
Intensive probation, 81, 95, 99, 100
Interpersonal problem solving, 16, 215
Inter-rater reliability, 276

Index

Interrogation, 154, 157, 314
Interventions, 1, 2, 4, 6, 7, 10, 11, 16, 17, 55, 59, 65–67, 77, 78, 80, 81, 96, 100, 104, 111–113, 118, 119, 125, 126, 128, 130, 132, 138, 151, 155, 171, 187, 228, 233, 237, 238, 246, 252, 254, 261, 264, 270, 273, 274, 276, 293, 295, 298, 306, 312, 315, 316, 318, 322

J
Jail, 10, 184, 197, 252
Justice, 1, 2, 9, 11, 56, 80, 96, 98, 99, 105, 137, 154, 158, 163, 171, 189, 207, 232, 246, 255, 274, 280, 291, 293, 299, 302, 305, 314
Juvenile delinquency, 80, 94
Juveniles, 9, 77, 94, 99, 185, 193

K
Knowledge translation, 261, 265, 268, 278, 279, 282

L
Law enforcement, 152, 159, 164, 185, 189, 238, 246, 321
Legitimacy, 102, 105, 138, 153, 154, 158, 313, 314
Life-course, 9
Lighting, 113, 118, 295

M
MacArthur Foundation, 305
Management, 67, 95, 99, 104, 155, 157, 237, 246, 322
Martinson, 1–4, 311, 315
Maryland Scientific Methods Scale, 296
Mechanisms of effectiveness, 77, 98, 101, 313
Mediators, 61, 96, 124
Mental health, 56, 169, 181, 184, 187, 213, 274, 314
Mental illness, 173, 179, 184, 189, 194, 213
Mentoring, 9, 10, 94, 98
Meta-analysis, 7, 11, 16, 82, 83, 95, 99, 102, 114, 119, 120, 122, 152, 155, 161, 162, 180, 183, 194, 202, 203, 206, 208, 210, 213, 221, 263, 270, 316
Meta-ethnography, 250, 321
Meta-interpretation, 250, 321
Metal detectors, 114, 122
Meta-summary, 250, 321
Meta-synthesis, 250, 253, 321
Methadone, 206, 220

Methodological quality, 7, 54, 66, 94, 101, 120, 153, 214, 275, 281
Middle school, 139, 158
Model, 298, 299, 305–307, 320, 323
Moderator variable, 55, 61, 129, 133
Motivation, 65, 263
Motivational interviewing, 233
Multi-agency interventions, 152, 164
Multi-modal interventions, 16, 64

N
Naloxone, 235
Naltrexone, 228, 230, 232, 234
Narcotics maintenance programs, 206
National Institute for Health and Care Excellence (NICE), 292, 298, 323
National Institute of Justice, 319
National Policing Improvement Agency (NPIA), 137
Neighborhood watch, 77, 83, 98, 100, 121, 125, 313
Non-custodial sentence, 10, 94, 104, 171, 314
Nothing works, 1–3, 5, 10, 311, 316, 318
Nuisance abatement, 113
Nurse-Family Partnership, 17

O
Odds ratio (OR), 17, 59, 96, 97, 114, 118, 161, 173, 198, 202, 205, 206, 208, 316, 317
Offending, 9, 17, 54, 121, 185, 210, 212, 214, 274, 275
Office of Community Oriented Policing Services (COPS), 137
Operation Ceasefire, 83, 151
Opportunities, 10, 79, 80, 94, 102, 112, 124, 214, 313
Oppositional Defiant Disorder (ODD), 56
Organizational climate, 65
Outcome measurement, 66

P
Parent training, 56, 60
Parole, 96, 187, 189, 232
Patrol, 4, 152, 156, 159, 160, 314
Peer review, 6
Penitentiary, 193, 203, 215
Pew Charitable Trusts, 305
Place-based intervention, 79, 100
Poisson distribution, 124
Police, 2, 4, 77, 98, 105, 137–139, 152–155, 157, 160, 161, 163, 164, 238, 252, 299, 314, 316, 319, 321, 322

Policing, 4, 10, 83, 98, 102, 105, 131, 137–139, 151, 153, 156, 158–161, 163, 165, 171, 313, 314, 318, 320
Policy, 5, 67, 122, 170, 189, 238, 255, 262, 279, 291, 299, 306, 307, 311
Population turnover, 79
Post-booking schemes, 187
Post-diversion schemes, 184
Poverty, 79, 252
Preferred Reporting Items for Systematic Reviews and Meta-Analyses (PRISMA), 173, 268, 282
Pregnancy, 16, 57
Preschool, 57
Prevention, 1, 2, 4, 5, 8–10, 15, 16, 54, 58, 61, 64, 65, 77–81, 83, 94, 97, 100, 104, 111, 119, 208, 210, 233, 273, 294, 295, 313
Primary school, 61
Prison, 1, 2, 4, 10, 94, 197, 203, 205, 206, 302, 305
Probation, 77, 80, 95, 99, 184, 252
Procedural justice, 154, 158, 314
Program fidelity, 98
Program integrity, 66
Property marking, 131
Protective factors, 15, 65
Protocol, 9, 249, 267, 277, 296
Public health, 15, 237, 238, 298, 323
Publication bias, 6, 66, 253, 280, 281
Pulling levers strategies, 83
Punishment, 170, 186, 313
p-value, 60

Q
Quality-adjusted life-years (QALYs), 292
Quasi-experiments, 95, 99, 138, 153, 159, 162, 295

R
Random assignment, 183, 205, 209, 319
Random preventive, 152, 160
Randomized controlled trials (RCTs), 57, 59, 61, 66, 95, 100, 101, 185, 210, 275
Reasoning and Rehabilitation, 81, 208, 210
Recidivism, 1, 3, 78, 94–96, 180, 183, 184, 188, 197, 205, 212, 261, 323
Reentry, 10, 77, 102, 103, 105
Reflexivity, 248
Regression to the mean (RTM), 130
Rehabilitation, 1–3, 5, 194, 198, 215
Rehabilitative ideal, 193, 215
Reintegration, 228, 233

Reintegration and recovery programs, 228, 233, 234, 315
Release, 4, 95, 99, 198, 203, 206, 220
Religion, 203, 204
Religious programs, 194, 204
Repeat victimization (RV), 114, 121, 122, 313
Replication, 6, 16, 276
Research, 10, 11, 164, 187, 237–241, 249, 253, 254, 262, 263, 265, 272
Residential security, 295
Respondent validation, 248
Restitution, 96, 101
Restorative justice, 80, 96, 98
Results First Initiative, 305
Return on investment, 292, 299
Review, 2, 6, 8–11, 16, 54, 63, 77, 96, 102, 114, 121, 137, 139, 156, 173, 185, 197, 203, 219, 237, 238, 241, 246, 251, 254, 256, 262–264, 266, 272, 274, 277, 280, 282, 297, 314–316, 320, 322
Risk, 9, 15, 17, 61, 62, 65, 78, 81, 98, 100, 112, 120, 124, 173, 183, 194, 280
Risk-Need-Responsivity (RNR), 194

S
Sample size, 55, 66, 185
Sampling, 240, 248, 249
Sanctions, 80, 98, 101, 170
Scanning, analysis, response, assessment (SARA) model, 151
Scared Straight, 181, 186, 302, 314
School dropout, 59
Schools, 17, 61, 62, 77, 81
Second responder program, 155, 314
Secondary school, 61
Security guards, 120
Self-control, 59, 215
Self-esteem, 56, 194
Self-evaluation, 66
Sentence, 10, 80, 94, 101, 171, 186
Sentencing, 10, 169–171, 173, 185, 187, 189, 314
Setting, 78, 101, 104, 185, 189, 202, 205, 247, 281, 298
Sex offenders, 194, 211–213, 251, 315
Situational crime prevention (SCP), 112
Sobriety checkpoints, 153
Social, 2, 8, 9, 16, 59, 78–81, 98, 101, 102, 104, 105, 186, 207, 234, 239, 313, 315, 324
Social information processing, 61, 62
Social interventions, 100, 316

Social programs, 9, 316
Social work, 237, 238
Socio-emotional, 55
Spending, 292
Staff factors, 65
Staff-client relationship, 65
Stake in conformity, 79, 80
Standardization, 294
Statistical significance, 234, 263
Stress management, 155, 237, 238, 246
Studies, 318
Subutex, 232
Supervision, 1, 60, 65, 78, 94, 100–102, 185, 232, 234, 315
Surgical castration, 211
Surveillance, 78, 81, 95, 99, 104, 113, 114, 119–121, 133, 302
Sustainability, 264, 281
Synthetic opioid medication, 232

T
Target hardening, 113, 131
Temporary home leave, 95, 99
Theory, 5, 16, 80, 111, 112, 250
Therapeutic community, 95, 99, 205
Therapy, 55, 57, 62, 81, 185, 207, 211, 233, 273
Thick, 248, 253
Time series, 82, 114, 139, 159
Traffic accidents, 139, 153
Training, 16, 155, 233
Transparency, 263, 265, 266, 268
Transportability, 262, 265, 268, 276, 278, 279
Treatment, 10, 102, 103, 131, 189, 204, 206, 212, 230, 232, 233
Treatment Foster Care (TFC), 58
Treatment matching, 279
Triangulation, 248, 254

U
U.S. Department of Justice, 293
Unemployment, 79
United Kingdom, 137, 158
United States, 10, 102, 103, 193, 203, 204, 261, 314
Urinalysis, 232

V
Validity, 10, 58, 130, 158, 161, 248, 277, 279, 295, 312, 322
Vera Institute of Justice, 293
Victim-offender mediation, 80, 96
Victims of crime, 169, 299
Violence, 61, 122, 155, 185, 187
Vocational programs, 198, 202, 213, 315
Vote counting, 273

W
Washington State Institute for Public Policy, 291, 299, 300, 306
Wilderness challenge programs, 56
Women, 180, 184, 185, 187, 246, 247, 249, 251–253
Work release, 95, 99
Work-related programs, 198
Wraparound programs, 56

Y
Youth, 9, 16, 54–56, 67, 77, 98, 102, 181, 313

CPSIA information can be obtained
at www.ICGtesting.com
Printed in the USA
LVOW02*1804150916
504783LV00002B/2/P